Contagion in Prussia, 1831

Contagion in Prussia, 1831

The Cholera Epidemic and the Threat of the Polish Uprising

Richard S. Ross III

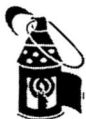

McFarland & Company, Inc., Publishers
Jefferson, North Carolina

LIBRARY OF CONGRESS CATALOGUING-IN-PUBLICATION DATA

Ross, Richard S., 1948–
Contagion in Prussia, 1831 : the cholera epidemic
and the threat of the Polish uprising / Richard S. Ross III.
    p.   cm.
Includes bibliographical references and index.

ISBN 978-0-7864-9772-0 (softcover : acid free paper) ∞
ISBN 978-1-4766-2010-7 (ebook)

1. Cholera—Germany—Prussia—History—19th century.
2. Cholera—Poland—History—19th century. 3. Cholera—
Political aspects—History—19th century. 4. Medical policy—Germany—
Prussia—History—19th century. 5. Medical policy—Poland—History—
19th century. 6. Public health—Germany—Prussia—History—19th century.
7. Borderlands—Germany—Prussia—History—19th century. 8. Soldiers—
Poland—History—19th century. 9. Refugee camps—Germany—Prussia—
History—19th century. 10. Social conflict—Germany—Prussia—
History—19th century. I. Title.
RC133.G4P787 2015   614.5'14094318—dc23   2015030989

BRITISH LIBRARY CATALOGUING DATA ARE AVAILABLE

© 2015 Richard S. Ross III. All rights reserved

*No part of this book may be reproduced or transmitted in any form
or by any means, electronic or mechanical, including photocopying
or recording, or by any information storage and retrieval system,
without permission in writing from the publisher.*

Front cover: (top) Human skull engraving by William Miller, 1818;
(bottom) illustration of Castle Square in Warsaw, 1831

Printed in the United States of America

*McFarland & Company, Inc., Publishers
Box 611, Jefferson, North Carolina 28640
www.mcfarlandpub.com*

To my son Rich, my daughter Nikki,
and especially my wife Christine,
without whose love and encouragement this
book could never have been completed

Acknowledgments

I would like to thank the following for their invaluable contribution to this work:

Library of Congress, Washington, D.C.
National Archives, Records of Great Britain. Foreign Office.
National Library of Medicine, Washington, D.C.
Geheimes Staatsarchiv Preussischer Kulturbesitz, GStA PK, Berlin
Staatsbibliothek zu Berlin, Berlin
Trinity College Library, Hartford, Connecticut
Wellcome Library, London

I want to acknowledge those who helped me years ago at the German Central Archive in Merseburg, East Germany, and who provided me with the microfilm documents I have used to continue my investigation. After German re-unification in 1993–1994, the Prussian Secret Archives were relocated to Berlin and I have referenced them by their now official location, Geheimes Staatsarchiv Preussischer Kulturbesitz, GStA PK.

I must also thank the librarians I have known over the years, especially the interlibrary loan librarians at a number of the academic institutions at which I was employed, who were tireless in acquiring for me official documents, books, articles and newspapers, both domestically and from abroad. However, I am especially indebted to the interlibrary loan librarians at Trinity College—Mary Curry, Alice Angelo and Yuksel Serindag—who have been instrumental in acquiring the materials that allowed me to complete this book. I would also like to thank Nancy Smith and Lisa Corson in the Trinity College Library Imaging Unit for their assistance in preparing the images for this book.

I would like to acknowledge my son Richard and daughter Nicole, who both grew up with this project, and my wife Christine whose editorial assistance, patience and understanding allowed it to finally come to completion.

Contents

Acknowledgments vi
Preface 1
Introduction 3

1—Cholera Approaches 9
2—Public Health Administration in Prussia Before 1831 23
3—Cholera in Poland 38
4—First Response to Cholera: Misery in Danzig 59
5—Prussian Cholera Policy and the Russian War Effort 73
6—Cholera Policy on the Prussian Border 85
7—Cholera in East Prussia and the City of Königsberg 110
8—The Cholera Tumult in Königsberg 135
9—Cholera Enters Berlin 154
10—Berlin Organizes to Combat Cholera 183
11—The Medical Legacy of the Cholera Epidemic of 1831 196
12—Prussia, Cholera and the Polish Refugee Crisis 221

Conclusion 244
Chapter Notes 255
Bibliography 281
Index 289

Preface

This book grew out of my interest in both Germany and epidemic disease. It was originally inspired by a graduate seminar on cholera and history at Northeastern University in the late 1970s under the direction of Professor John Post. Investigating the cholera epidemic in Germany, I quickly became aware that little work had been done at that time in either Germany or the United States on this topic.

I went on to Boston College to obtain my PhD and decided I would investigate this topic for my thesis. My advisor, Professor John Heinemann, allowed me to pursue this topic with one caveat—I had to travel to the Prussian State Archives in Merseburg, East Germany, and discover what documentation was available. I quickly became convinced that there was sufficient material and focused on the Prussian administrative response to the first cholera epidemic to invade Europe. I did this for two reasons. My youth had been epidemiologically quiet. As a child, I had heard of polio but with the discovery of the Salk vaccine the fear that crippling epidemic disease had held for my parents and neighbors was diminished. It seemed that public health measures adopted in the United States had triumphed and our new enemies were the chronic diseases of old age, cancer and heart disease.

Then in the early eighties, a new disease arrived that our doctors and government did not understand: the AIDS epidemic had begun. This was a new and misunderstood illness. It seemed to strike down people in the prime of their life. Initially, no one knew how it spread, only that it was deadly and there was no cure. This reinforced my interest in this topic. The basic question for me from a historical and public health perspective was how do governments cope with new deadly diseases? What affect do their policies have on the public? How does the public react when no one seems to know how a disease is spread and how to combat the disease? What are the short- and long-term consequences of various government public health policies? Finally, what can be learned about past societies that have confronted diseases for which they had no previous experience?

Prussia in 1831 was an excellent example of a country that saw itself as a bulwark against the new disease, cholera. The historical literature on this first epidemic is in agreement that Prussia's initial response was to institute a strict military quarantine, but then Prussia abruptly changed course in the middle of the epidemic. Why this happened was one of the basic questions I was looking to answer. I also discovered that there was a direct link between Prussia's domestic cholera policy and foreign policy during the Polish uprising in 1831. The totality of the problem had not been thoroughly examined probably for two reasons. First, public health issues like cholera were quickly forgotten and just noted in passing in the historical writing about this event. The resulting quarantine policy on the border most agree was established to prevent western assistance to Poland during the revolt. There seemed to be no need for further investigation. Second, historians had not until recently investigated Prussia's overall domestic response to cholera during this first epidemic. After all and especially in Germany disease and public health was traditionally the purview of medical historians. As I discovered, there was overwhelming documentation that the intent of Prussian cholera policy was primarily to preserve its people from the expected ravages of cholera. The evidence is found in the strict laws and detailed documentation regarding cholera policy in private and government publications and is easily available to researchers who choose to look for it.

Following my original thesis in 1992 there have been subsequent studies on cholera published in Germany but no adequate study in English on the first epidemic in Prussia and especially not on the relationship between Prussian cholera policy and the Polish revolt. This book provides new information on the results of the Prussian government's strict health policy and its consequences, including social unrest, and resulting reforms. It also investigates cholera and public health policy in Poland in 1831 in light of the needs of the revolutionary government. For the first time in English, it describes and shows why Prussia established cholera camps in July 1831 to quarantine Polish soldiers who crossed into Prussia as refugees during the Polish uprising.

Recently I had found my original work being noted in scholarly literature in the United States, Germany and Poland, and I believed a proper book length study containing corrections, new information and an expanded argument was required. I hope I have been successful in this endeavor.

Introduction

Epidemic disease has played a critical part in modern European history.[1] Cholera, a disease of the nineteenth century, has been investigated from different perspectives, including its psychological and social impact. Cholera also played a part in the political turmoil of the nineteenth century, acting as an agent to promote a sanitary revolution in the countries affected.[2] The response of the affected European nations provides us an opportunity to study their differing state structures to investigate how they adapted to the challenges posed by this disease.[3]

Cholera was a new disease to nineteenth century Europeans and little understood by the medical community. It was a destabilizing force in newly emerging urban environments that were witnessing unprecedented population growth and accompanying unsanitary conditions. The disease presented a serious challenge to the medical community and the political structures in these countries as they attempted to understand the epidemic and determine the most effective measures to protect their populations.[4]

Until recently, research on the first cholera epidemic in Germany and specifically in Prussia has been limited. While research on cholera's impact in other European countries has been underway for many years, this has not been the case in Germany. Earlier German studies examined traditional medical history themes including prevention of disease and the treatment of the sick.[5] However, recently German historians have struck out in a new direction to focus on the social history of the cholera in Prussia.[6] In England, Richard Evans has made a significant contribution to the study of cholera in the latter part of the nineteenth century in Hamburg, Germany. In the United States, there is my own earlier study on the Prussian administration, the first cholera epidemic and its impact on domestic and foreign policy decisions, as well as future public health policy in Prussia. Recently, Robert Baldwin published his comparative study on various European government responses to contagion, including their reactions to the first cholera epidemic in Europe.[7]

For example, the French focus on social, gender and age inequalities with regard to cholera. The English concentrate on cholera's effect on the development of public health. In other areas of Europe there is a greater attention on *mentalities* or group attitudes on the problem of sickness."[8]

This book addresses the political, administrative and diplomatic response of the bureaucratic absolutist Prussian state in responding to the 1831 cholera epidemic. The country was threatened by the recent revolutionary government change in France and a large, restless Polish population in its recently acquired eastern provinces on the Polish border. Its Polish neighbor, inspired by the successful revolution in France in 1830, revolted against its imperialist master, Russia, on November 29, 1830. By February 1831, the Russian army was on the march to quell the uprising in Poland. Russia continued to expect cooperation in its war effort from its ally, Prussia but Prussia declared neutrality.

This book is intended to provide new information on Prussia's response to the first cholera epidemic and to put this response into a context that goes beyond the public health and medical debate. It will shed new light on Prussia's domestic policies and Prussia's actions regarding Polish military and civilian refugees on the border during and after the Polish uprising.

Non-German readers have gotten most of their knowledge of the cholera epidemic in Germany from Richard Evans' book *Death in Hamburg*, which examines the city of Hamburg as a model of the nineteenth century liberal tradition of "laissez-faire." He noted the cholera epidemic of 1892 finally initiated a transformation of the "victory of Prussianism over liberalism and the triumph of state intervention over laissez-faire." Evans admits that his selection of Hamburg represented a conscious effort on his part "to counteract the narrow Prusso-centrism of much writing on German history at this time."[9]

This book takes a more measured view of Prussian "bureaucratic interventionism" and places the Prussian response to cholera in 1831 in the context of a domestic medical policy. This policy is best summarized as "disease prevention." It was not based on a response to Prussia's international concerns with regard to Russia's invasion of Poland. Also, as a result of the Prussian experience with the cholera in 1831, for the first time a statewide contagious diseases law was enacted in 1835. The new law attempted to bridge the needs of the "liberal" aspirations of Prussian economic bureaucratic interests and a bourgeoisie sympathetic to "free trade." At the same time, the law was written with the understanding, advocated by the official medical bureaucracy, that there was still a need to retain quarantine and isolation measures to prevent the spread of contagious diseases like the plague into Prussia.

The Cholera Problem in 1831

From the beginning, Asiatic cholera was not properly understood by the governments and the medical communities of the early nineteenth century. At the beginning of 1831, Dr. Ernst Horn, a Prussian privy councilor and state physician, wrote a history of the disease and its course. He described it as a "new and terrible form of sickness" that first occurred in the city of Jessore, in the lower Bengal region of India, in August 1817.[10] The local Medical Board in Bengal reported in September 1817, in contrast to what usually prevails, "it has proved far more fatal than at any former time within recollection."[11]

English doctors in India reported that this "new cholera could scarcely be equated with other earlier choleras." The new disease seized the victim more rapidly, its symptoms were unique, and it had a fearful death rate. The disease was also highly infectious. These symptoms and the rapid spread of the disease gave rise to the idea that it originated from an "atmospheric influence."[12]

Prussian doctors were familiar with the reports of English physicians in India on the "Asiatic cholera" and informed of cholera's origins and its progress. Horn reported to the Prussian medical community how the disease spread to Calcutta and, later in the autumn of 1818, to Madras, Bombay, all of India and then to Sumatra. He wrote that cholera spread by troop movements from India to Ceylon and then southwest, extending 3,000 miles to the island of Mauritania—demonstrating its ability to cross the sea—and then by trading ships from Hindustan to the Persian Gulf. From here it was and carried by caravans and troop movements to Astrakhan, Russia, in 1823. The Prussian physician concluded that it had spread along trade routes, or "in one word by human traffic."[13]

In 1824, the sickness spread into Hindustan, Persia and Arabia, then to China, Java and to upper Asia, and in late summer 1829 by caravan to Orenburg in Russia. It also traveled via Astrakhan and Persia into southern Russia where it was carried into the Russian interior along trade routes. It reached Moscow in 1830. Cholera "gripped the southwestern provinces of Russia" and in spite of "protective quarantines" the disease quickly spread to Poland, Prussia, Austria and Hungary.[14]

During the nineteenth century, the pandemic form of cholera spread five times from its home in Bengal, India, reaching out to ravage most of the known world. Cholera's last and most devastating outbreak in Germany occurred in 1892 in the port city of Hamburg.[15]

Cholera is a classic disease of the nineteenth century, primarily because population growth and unsanitary conditions prevailed in the major cities of the world. It was aided by increasingly rapid trade around the world. A lack of the knowledge of the germ theory and transmission of disease created an environment that the cholera *vibrio* easily exploited.[16]

The etiology of the cholera was unknown until 1883, when Dr. Robert Koch isolated the cholera *vibrio* and demonstrated the origin and transmission of the disease.[17] Prior to this discovery the inability to understand how cholera spread had led to one of the most heated controversies in medical history: Was cholera a contagious or a non-contagious disease?[18] It was not "until the theory of inanimate contagion was replaced by a theory of living germs" and the recognition of the critical role of water and animal carriers over long distances that cholera was finally recognized as a contagious disease.[19]

This contagion controversy had medical implications as well as economic and political associations. This resulted from the basic role quarantine was to play for the supporters of the theory of contagion in the government in opposition to the liberal beliefs of many private physicians and supporters of the doctrine of free trade.

The contagion debate was particularly heated in Prussia but occurred in nearly all European countries. Medical opinion was divided between anti-contagionists, who believed in "atmospheric" or "miasmic" influences—poisons arising from decaying animal or vegetable matter, "filth"[20]—and other physicians who upheld the older, more accepted theory of contagion, with roots in the plague epidemics of prior centuries. At this time, adherents of the "miasmic" or infection theory were considered proponents of "advanced ideas in medicine."[21] Dr. Becker, a Prussian physician, described the distinction between the two views at the time of the epidemic as follows:

> Some English as well as French authors have laid down a distinction between contagious and infectious diseases, restricting the word contagion to those cases in which communication of a disease takes place, evidently and exclusively, by actual contact, while they employ the other term to express that propagation of disease which is caused by human effluvia, without actual contact, and by means of an impure atmosphere.[22]

There were various supporters of different degrees of contagion or anti-contagion, but generally they could be divided along the lines of those who saw the direct transmission of the disease from one infected person to another or those who looked to a general miasma. The fundamental problem that the Prussian government faced was deciding which medical opinion should serve as the basis for the government's cholera policy. The consequences were important because, as Dr. Becker wrote when the disease appeared in Europe, attention was diverted from the medical question. Physicians and the public were more absorbed by "discussions as to the propriety of certain preventive measures, which most European governments have adopted in order to arrest the march of the disease; and the animosity with which these discussions are carried on has materially prevented the progress of calm scientific inquiry."[23]

Each position was taken seriously. It was reported that one doctor was threatened with the words "Kill him, he is a contagionist."[24] Ackerknecht later wrote that contagionism had found its "material expression in the quarantines and the bureaucracy." The discussion was never one of contagion alone, but always of "contagion and quarantines."[25] Contagionism, because it was linked with the old bureaucratic powers, would always be suspect to liberals, "trying to reduce state interference to a minimum."[26]

The basic problem was that the "conflict symbolized the antagonism between two systems of thought, one liberal and progressive and the other conservative and regressive." Those who argued in favor of quarantine were bureaucrats with their eyes fixed firmly on the past. "Bureaucratic behavior was "allegedly dictated by routine and self-interest." Those who supported non-contagion argued that the "liberalization of trade was crucial to new industries.... Freedom of travel and freedom of trade went hand in hand; both were important to business interests."[27]

Because cholera was a new disease and its etiology could not be satisfactorily explained, it initially inspired fear, disorder and a sense of helplessness among governments, the medical community, and the general population. No government in Europe was convinced of the proper way to combat cholera, nor was the medical community prepared to adequately explain its origin, cause or cure. Europe appeared to be on the eve of confronting a crisis which it had not experienced since the last plague threat in 1720.[28]

In studying the cholera epidemic in Prussia and gauging its reactions to this threat it is critical to understand recent historical developments within the Prussian government and the Prussian population. This was the same generation that had recently overcome the Napoleonic occupation of Germany, the Russian campaign, and the war of liberation.[29]

After 1816, Germany underwent massive migrations (both external and internal) and experienced mass poverty as a result of an agricultural slump in the 1820s and early 1830s.[30] This gave rise to what would be called the "social question" in Germany: essentially, what was to be done about the poor? In fact, this issue finally came to a head in 1844, with the Silesian Weaver's Revolt.[31]

Politically, Prussia had embraced the Carlsbad decrees in 1819 and turned away from the political liberalism of the West and allied with reactionary Austria and Russia. However, the cholera epidemic threatened to de-stabilize Prussia just as the government was coping with revolutionary fears created in 1830 in Paris, and by France's overt interest in the Belgian throne. Prussia viewed the Polish insurrection in November 1830 with alarm.[32]

Overpopulation, poverty, revolutionary activity in Europe, and liberal elements demanding reform in the other German states as well as in Prussia created a politically explosive situation. The Prussian government was aware of the gravity of the situation and when cholera struck found itself facing the dilemma of having to choose how to defend itself based on whether the cholera was contagious. Medical officials had to decide how they were going to obtain more information on this new disease, which state agency would make decisions as to the public health measures to be implemented and whether the public health infrastructure in place was adequate to cope with this new disease.

Initially troops were stationed at the Polish border not to present a *cordon sanitaire,* but to control border crossings during the Polish insurrection. Nevertheless, this policy led to suspicion and mistrust of the government, declining employment and a scarcity of food. Later, when combined with quarantines, travel restrictions, border closings and fear of cholera, the ingredients were in place to fuel violence and inspire hatred. Even doctors were viewed as government agents out to poison the poor.[33]

As early as November 1830, the Prussian government was aware of the danger cholera posed to the country. It cautiously watched the Russia response to cholera. At this early stage it was suggested that a Doctor's Commission be sent to Russia to determine how Prussia should respond to this disease. Prussia did not arrive at a strict cholera policy based on the theory of contagion until May 1831, following the reports of the Commission's doctors. The official policy of contagion began in May 1831, when Frederick William III issued a cabinet order mobilizing a preliminary defense commission previously appointed on January 5, 1831. On May 3, 1831, he appointed adjutant Major General Ludwig von Thile to head an *Immediat-Kommission zur Abwehrung der Cholera* (Immediate Commission to Prevent Cholera). This Commission derived its authority directly from the king, "it acted independently of the different boards (each of which, however, has its representatives in the Commission)" and issued "its orders to the provisional, civil, and military authorities, all of whom are, for this particular object, placed under the direction of the Commission."[34]

The Commission was composed of members of the administration, several military men and civil medical officers. The Immediate Commission was mobilized because following the Battle of Iganie on April 10, 1831, between Russian and Polish forces, cholera spread to the Polish army and soon broke out in Warsaw. From Warsaw it spread to a number of Polish provinces where Russian prisoners of war had been sent. The Prussian king ordered preparations to defend his kingdom and these preparations included the mobilization of the Immediate Commission.[35] The medical policy initiated by the Commission was formulated by Dr. Johann N. Rust, head of the medical administration in Prussia. He was a strict contagionist whose policy toward cholera was modeled on the "principles adopted on the Austrian frontiers against ... plague."[36]

With the formation of this Commission, Prussia embarked on a public a sanitary policy that provoked heated controversy and domestic unrest. The Commission's inflexibility in the face of the public's reaction eventually led to a more conciliatory response on the part of the king and the administrative structure. The decision of the king and his officials to modify the policies of the Commission was critical in determining the short- and long-term effects of cholera on Prussian society and the people's continued trust in the state. The Prussian experience with the cholera in 1831 led to the first Contagious Diseases Act in Prussia in 1835. To understand the administrative infrastructure that was in place and that carried these developments forward is the subject of the following chapters.

1

Cholera Approaches

Asiatic cholera was not well known by European doctors outside of India before the second pandemic of 1826–1837. The little that was known was reported by English physicians in India who had a greater experience with the disease. The disease had its origin in the Ganges delta in India and was endemic to this area. English physicians subsequently published their reports on cholera and these found their way to the various capitals of Europe. These reports provided Prussian doctors with their first introduction to the symptoms and experimental treatments for a new and especially virulent foreign disease.[1]

A modern description of the symptoms of cholera indicates that the disease is marked by the onset of "diarrhea, acute spasmodic vomiting and painful cramps." Dehydration leads to the telltale blue color in the face, and cold limbs. The skin becomes clammy, cold and puckered.[2] Toxins released by the cholera *vibrio* "alter the exchange of sodium and chloride ions" in the small intestine disrupting the natural exchange of fluids in the body, leading to watery stools, severe dehydration and finally death. Today the treatment for cholera is "fluid and electrolyte therapy along with feedings of rice or grains."[3] The etiology of cholera was not known at the time of the first cholera epidemic in Prussia although, as we will see, this did not prevent Prussian physicians from attempting experimental cures, as well as expressing their opinions as to the cause and infectiousness of cholera.

A description of the disease by a Prussian physician in 1831 confirmed the same outward symptoms. Besides the vomiting and diarrhea:

> The facial expression of the sick shows great pain. The whole face is pinched; the eyes dulled and sunk in deeply.... The neck throat and tongue, the chest ... especially the fingers and toes, rarely the entire surface area showed itself a blue, livid opalescent color, as at the beginning of decomposition.... The blue of the nails, somewhat less constant ... the fingers and toes as well as the palms of the hands and the soles of the feet, and a wrinkling of the skin like a washer woman's.[4]

However, this knowledge, and fear that cholera would create among the people, came later. Before the entry of the disease into Prussian territory, the symptoms and virulence of cholera were unknown to the public, and most physicians and government officials in Prussia. In fact, the great fear in Prussia in the summer of 1830 was not cholera but "revolution." The revolutionary spirit had lain dormant for a number of years but was awakened in Europe following the July revolution in France and the ascension of Louis Philippe to the French throne on August 9, 1830. This "revolutionary spirit" was compared to an "infectious sick-

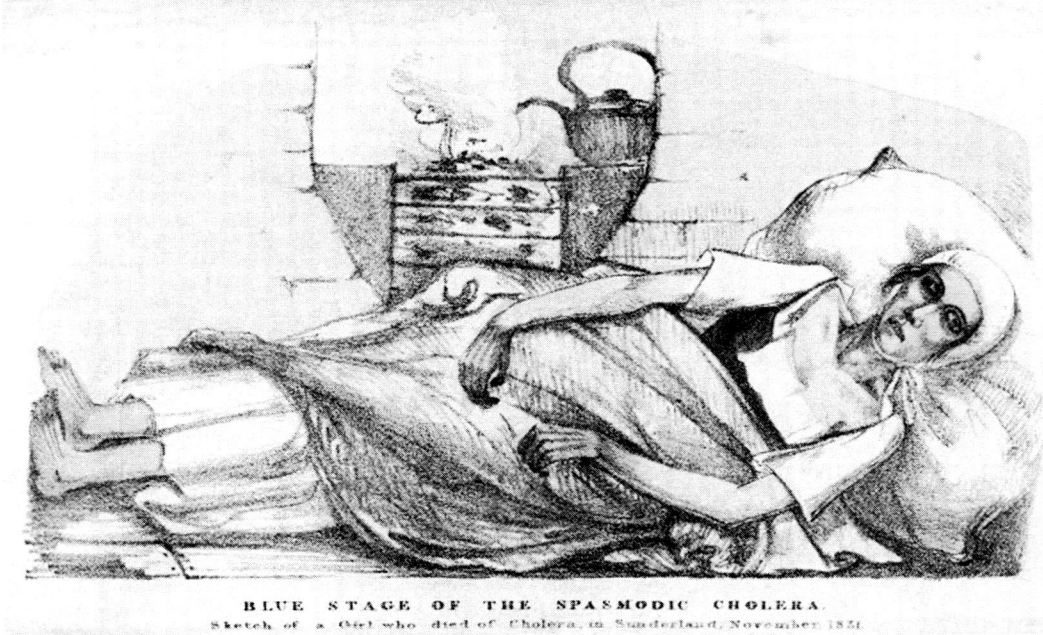

"Blue stage of spasmodic cholera." Sketch of a young woman who died of cholera at Sunderland, England, November, 1831. By Thomas Wakley. First published in the *Lancet*. 1832, volume 1 (courtesy the Wellcome Library, London).

ness," and spread to Belgium, parts of Germany and finally to Poland.[5] It was quickly supplanted by the frightening reality of a real plague. During the last half of 1830, cholera came to "occupy Berlin exclusively to the extent that politics was hardly thought about."[6]

It is no wonder that high-level government officials were occupied with cholera. The key function of any government is security and in the face of a potential epidemic, "policy makers must make timely decisions even with incomplete information" that include "value judgments of the acceptability of risk and the reasonableness of the costs."[7] These issues confronted Prussian policy makers as they assessed the potential impact of cholera. Their concerns began to play out almost immediately. European governments at the beginning of the epidemic expressed contagionist views and developed measures based on previous experience with plague prevention.[8] One of the more successful models invoked immediately was the plague prevention quarantine system along the Austro-Turkish border.[9] However, Freiherr vom Stein zum Altenstein, the Minister of Religion, Education and Medical Affairs was doubtful this could be effectively duplicated and informed the king "the Prussian situation with its Russian and Polish borders was an entirely different matter than the well-executed quarantine that Austria maintained on its border with Turkey."[10]

In November 1830, the Prussian government began taking a cautious attitude. Medical officials were determined to discover the nature of the disease and to decide whether or not it was contagious before acting.[11] They were especially aware of the financial burden that their own government would incur by imposing a land and water quarantine. Officials had to be assured that the disease was contagious and that quarantine would work. For this they looked to Russia for guidance. From the beginning some medical officials suspected cholera was contagious and wanted to impose a blockade immediately. The chief officials in the medical division were also inclined to suspect contagion. The Cholera Commission investigated the issues surrounding cholera and presented a plan to the king in December 1830. In early May, the plan was initiated by the newly established Immediate Commission. This led to the cabinet order of June 6, 1831, which imposed strict controls on the Russian-Prussian border. By the end of May, because of the outbreak of cholera in Poland, the Prussian border from the Nieman River to Upper Silesia was cordoned off by the military. Next came the Act of June 15, 1831, which "determined that those persons who violated the provisions adopted for the prevention of cholera, should be severely punished." All persons who violated the quarantine or crossed the border illegally could be shot immediately; those who violated the other provisions were threatened with prison sentences of up to ten years.[12]

Almost immediately there was a conflict between those who wanted the protection of these measures, and commercial and business interests who complained about strict measures impeding trade locally and on the border.[13]

The question of quarantine and the contagious nature of cholera was a critical question for the liberal middle classes, who saw quarantines as an impediment to one of their most cherished beliefs: "free trade." This key question was first raised by the German medical historian E.H. Ackerknecht,[14] who wrote regarding the nineteenth century quarantine controversy:

> Contagionism had found its material expression in quarantines and their bureaucracy, and the whole discussion was thus never a discussion of contagion alone, but always on contagion and quarantines. Quarantines meant, to the rapidly growing class of merchants and industrialists, a source of losses, a limitation to expansion, a weapon of bureaucratic control that it was no longer willing to tolerate.[15]

Indeed those who believed quarantines were unnecessary were not looked upon as scientists but as "reformers, fighting for the freedom of the individual and commerce against the shackles of despotism and reaction."[16] It was this ideological controversy that served as the background over which the government's approach to the cholera epidemic in Prussia was fought.

The first cholera pandemic broke out in India in the spring of 1817, and lasted until 1823. It spread eastward through Asia, Oceania and touched on Africa, Arabia and Persia. The disease subsided over the winter of 1821, but returned in the spring. It reached the Persian city of Tabriz in August 1822.[17]

The ravages wreaked by cholera in Persia and the imminent threat to the Russian empire stirred the Prussian Ministry of Foreign Affairs following the receipt of a report from Dr. Mazarowitsch, the Czar's *chargé d'affaires*, at the court of the crown prince of Persia in Tabriz. The report described the outbreak of cholera in 1822, with a "detailed description of the disease, specification of its symptoms, many things about its treatment ... [but] ... on ... its alleged causes few and uncertain words." He concluded that the rapidity of its action "resembles arsenic poisoning."

The outbreak in Tabriz was important because it is the first eyewitness report given to the Prussian government of the medical description of the disease as well as its effects on an unprepared and unsuspecting population. It was also the first suggestion the progression of the disease was so rapid that it was similar to arsenic poisoning. This would later feed rumors that doctors were poisoning victims on behalf of the rich in the European capitals.

This report along with news from the Russian city of Astrakhan, in southern European Russia, was sent to Altenstein, Head of the Ministry of Religion, Education and Medical Affairs. When cholera subsided and returned to the Indian borders medical and government interest in the disease declined in Prussia and Europe.[18]

The second pandemic began in 1828, and by the end of 1830 cholera had spread into European Russia. At that time the "danger of its penetration into the Prussian State ... seemed unlikely, it still seemed so far away," wrote a doctor in 1832.[19]

The Prussian Government Prepares

The communications that were being received in the Medical Division of the Ministry of Religion, Education and Medical Affairs, "seemed contradictory in part, and the doctors could not make a sound judgment about the nature of the disease." When they compared the official and extra-official reports, there were too many conflicting messages. When they took into account the unfavorable reports concerning the imperial Russian quarantine stations, the Ministry had doubts about the true nature of the contagion.

The Minister of Foreign Affairs requested news from the Prussian legation in St. Petersburg about cholera. The Prussian ambassador in St. Petersburg reported that the physicians of the city had reversed their previously held opinions (based on that of the English doctors) and now declared cholera was contagious but "not as contagious as plague."[20]

Meanwhile, the Austrian government notified the Prussian Ministry of Foreign Affairs that it had already begun to take measures against cholera; "Metternich had ordered the formation of a commission" of high ranking Austrian officials including members from the "Vienna medical faculty" to determine the most "expeditious means" to deal with the epidemic.[21] On November 6, 1830, the Prussian Foreign Ministry asked the Prussian Ministry of the Interior if "precautions against the spread of cholera" should be taken in the event that the "Russian measures were insufficient."[22] On November 9, 1830, the Minister of the Interior and Police, Gustav von Brenn, wrote to Altenstein concerning reports he had been receiving about cholera. He inquired about the customs officials stationed near the infected Russian province and wanted to know if they should be taking precautions similar to those being discussed by the Austrian government on its Russian border. Because the precautions under discussion were adopted by Austria on November 21, 1831, he asked if it would be advisable for Prussia "to maintain quarantine stations to prevent the spread of the sickness."

Altenstein replied that the evidence for whether the disease was miasmic or contagious was contradictory and only after this was resolved would they be able to specify the measures needed to limit the spread of the disease. This was necessary because "going through a too hasty establishment of quarantine stations would disturb trade with neighboring states and give rise to exceedingly costly facilities."[23] With regard to the Austrian measures recently implemented, he thought it impractical for Prussia. Austria, unlike Prussia, was "thoroughly prepared to initiate a sanitary cordon, if Prussia did this it would only make trade difficult, there would be enormous charges against the state treasury," and it would cause "unnecessary anguish."[24]

The background to his response has to be seen in the division of the medical administration between the Ministry of Religion, Education and Medical Affairs and the Ministry of the Interior that occurred in 1825. The division was not amicable and led to many conflicts over areas of responsibility as well as competencies. Altenstein later used the suggestion by von Brenn for the immediate implementation of quarantine measures as an example of this conflict. Essentially, von Brenn wanted the sanitary police to impose plague like measures without any investigation. He wished to do this because of the evidence he received from Russian reports and the recent Austrian decision to quarantine its border. However, according to Altenstein, Interior Minister von Brenn also thought "decisions concerning the defensive measures should be made by his department alone."[25]

Nevertheless von Brenn had posed questions that needed to be answered over the nature of the cholera. He addressed his questions to Altenstein's medical division in order to determine what measures would have to be taken by the sanitary police. Could its spread be limited? Was it epidemic in nature? Could the infection be spread by the healthy as well as the sick? What type of commerce should be limited? What goods might carry the disease?[26]

Von Brenn's questions could not be answered immediately by medical officials in Altenstein's ministry. Yet, Altenstein did not want rely on the plague measures that would have been implemented by the sanitary police in the event that the cholera was not contagious. The members of the medical division realized a complete quarantine would be costly to the kingdom and an impediment to trade. They did not want to commit themselves to an expensive plan until they were satisfied cholera was an immediate threat to Prussia or before they had ascertained its degree of contagiousness. The Ministry of Religion, Education, and Medical Affairs required a more informed opinion before it would recommend policy. It also needed to develop a plan.[27]

Three days later Altenstein replied to von Brenn, suggesting that physicians with medical policing experience be sent to areas where cholera existed to observe and report back whether the disease was "purely miasmic or of a contagious nature." Von Brenn replied on November 15, 1830, he was in agreement with the request and understood that an investigation was necessary. Sending experienced physicians to Russia to report back to the Prussian government was appropriate and he went on to suggest the name of a physician to head this mission.[28]

Meanwhile, Altenstein had recently received two disturbing reports. The first from the Prussian east province of Posen that cholera had broken out in Lithuania. The second from the Prussian general consul in Warsaw, stating that no cholera security measures had been initiated in Poland and that the epidemic in Russia had "intensified" and had not spared the upper classes.[29] Altenstein concluded that the Russian measures were "inadequate" to prevent the spread of cholera and that it would be necessary to take precautionary measures. On November 14, 1830, the cholera matter was transferred to the *Geheimen Ober-Medizinalrat* (Privy Medical Councilor) and Professor at the University of Berlin, Dr. Johann Nepomuk Rust, Head of the Medical Division in the Ministry of Religion, Education and Medical Affairs, and Chief of the Scientific Deputation for Medicine.[30] Dr. Rust was given responsibility for coordinating all cholera administrative matters.[31]

The Scientific Deputation for Medicine met the same day and formed a Cholera Commission. It included members of the Medical Department in the Ministry of Religion, Education and Medical Affairs, the Ministry of the Interior and Police, a representative of the General Staff, representing the military, a representative of the Finance Ministry and the Ministry of Foreign Affairs. Additional members included a city physician and the chief of the military medical administration. The objective was to coordinate the response to the impending epidemic among the ministries. Secondly, the Deputation elected four of its members to a technical commission to investigate the medical issues associated with the cholera. The technical commission was ordered to report its findings to the newly formed Cholera Commission and make its recommendations in response to von Brenn's inquiries.[32]

On November 24—the day designated for the meeting of the Scientific Deputation for Medicine to consider what was to be done about the disease—Rust sent a hastily written note to von Brenn arguing that strict measures should be taken against the cholera, probably including the assignment of the military on the borders of countries where the cholera existed. Rust also informed von Brenn that the Scientific Deputation would try to establish the true nature of the disease and determine policies to prevent its spread into Prussia.[33]

The first order of business for the technical commission was to reply to the series of questions from the Ministry of the Interior and Police posed on November 9, 1830. Did the cholera develop a contagium? How did the sickness spread? Was cholera epidemic in nature? Did cholera infect goods? Was it spread through human contact? What kind of quarantine measures (if any) should be applied?[34]

The members of the technical commission realized that a decision concerning the contagiousness of cholera could not be determined because of the overwhelming number of contradictory reports. It reported that a definite "finding" could not be "pronounced" at that time.[35] Nevertheless, the Deputation met under Rust's leadership on November 24, 1830. Documents, letters, reports, and communications were gathered. The matter was "extensively ... debated." The attendees settled on the following advice to the Ministry of the Interior and Police: that cholera can "probably [be] assumed" to be contagious and "measures should be taken to prevent the possible introduction of the cholera."[36]

That was not the end of the matter: the degree of contagiousness needed to be decided. The answer would inform how stringent the precautionary sanitary measures would be. Preventive measures were discussed within the technical commission under the direction of Privy Councilor Dr. Ernst Horn and Dr. Charles Ferdinand Von Graefe of the General Staff. Part of their task was to determine the level of the "contagiousness" of the cholera and use this to minimize the quarantine measures recommended. The categories included human-to-human and animal-to-human infection, personal property and wares, such as money, letters, clothing, and imported goods. Other areas of concern included what measures to impose for travelers on land and water as well as how to instruct customs officials dealing with travelers on main roads. Other issues included correcting "false dietary instructions to evade the cholera," and communicating to local governments the "signs and hazards" of the disease so that proper arrangements could be made to prevent it from spreading.[37]

The two physicians also discussed the level of response necessary as it related to the nature of the contagion. Was the contagion "fixed or volatile?" Did it depend on an individual's "predisposition for the poisonous substance?" Was the disease more like typhus or like plague or the more virulent "bubonic plague?" For example, a disease like typhus would require measures that were "milder, modest and less cumbersome" than the more infectious diseases like bubonic plague. If the cholera was like bubonic plague and its contagium, then it had to be dealt with in the same way that the "Austrian government deals with its Turkish border with fortunate results."[38]

Prussian officials and physicians in these discussions were informed by the Austrian example. The last great plague epidemic had occurred in Prussia in the early part of the eighteenth century. Prussian doctors had no experience with a disease that looked to be as infectious as plague. On November 21, 1830, in the midst of the Commission's deliberations Austria established a "strict blockade along the Russian border, individuals suspected of plague "second grade" were quarantined before crossing from a cholera infected area.[39] The cordon in Austria was based on a military border that originated in the early 1600s and eventually extended from the "Adriatic to the mountains of Transylvania" or over one thousand miles. Originally established to protect the Austrian lands from Turkish incursions it eventually became a sanitary institution protecting Austria and some would argue Western Europe from plague that had been endemic in Turkey for hundreds of years.[40]

Initially in Austria, frontier posts were established as well as patrols. Orders were given to shoot at all crossing points, small stations and larger quarantine stations. The Austrian quarantine stations performed fumigations and purification of goods. They served as "check points and crossing points for travelers." All this was based on three "alert stages" with corresponding quarantine times ranging from twenty-one to forty-eight days.[41] By 1785 new regulations reduced the quarantine time so during "normal times" quarantine was eliminated and during plague, quarantine was "reduced to twenty-eight days." The Austrian *Pest Kontumaz Patent*, although modified in 1827, was essentially unchanged from the *Patent* of 1770.[42] There is little doubt that the Austrian system was highly regarded. Even the French, who controlled the "four western most regiments of the military border" from 1809 to 1813, maintained the integrity of the Austrian system. Napoleon himself was convinced that the system should be "preserved in its entirety." When Austria once again regained control in 1813, plague broke out in the following year. Although "thousands died in adjoining districts of Serbia and Bosnia, the plague was contained and did not spread into Austrian territory.[43]

The physicians responsible for determining Prussia's response to the cholera referred to the Austrian system a number of times in their discussions and were determined that if cholera was as contagious as plague they would follow the Austrian model. Dr. Horn and Dr. Graefe in a reply to the level of quarantine needed if the cholera proved to be as contagious as plague wrote, "If on the other hand the sickness should be analogous to plague this matter would be handled like the Austrian-Turkish border with a strict quarantine and the usual purification procedures should be undertaken."[44] After the cholera outbreak in Prussia, Rust wrote the eminent Prussian scientist, Alexander von Humboldt, that he was convinced that if the "cholera had come by way of Turkey across Transylvania, Austria by its proven sanitary institutions" would have prevented cholera just as it had previously prevented plague.[45]

The members of the Cholera Commission reported that the dreaded disease appeared in many different climates and was therefore not "caused by a miasma but was contagious." Evidence for this was demonstrated by the fact cholera moved from the Ganges delta in India to Astrakhan in Russia to the harbors of the Mediterranean Sea, traveling by "men and goods along the caravan routes." Cholera Commission members referred to the reports of the English doctors Steuart and Phillips who in their 1819 report to the government of Bombay noted that the disease was contagious. In addition, Russian doctors in Astrakhan also reported cholera was contagious.[46]

The final report from the Cholera Commission authored by Horn and Graefe was contagionist, but did not immediately recommend a sanitary quarantine.[47] The report was more nuanced. Both were mindful of the "cost and inconvenience" to trade without additional proof of how cholera spread. They needed additional evidence to justify stringent measures. Because "scientific and political considerations were so important," the Cholera Commission looked at the possibility of bringing into balance the competing doctrines of miasma vs. contagion by noting that cholera originated in Bengal India (miasmic) and later as it spread it became contagious.[48] This theory did not appear in any official subsequent reports.

Besides, the government was not finished investigating cholera. It was preparing a Doctor's Commission to go to Russia to gather more information to develop a more informed policy.[49] On December 4, 1830, Altenstein aware of the situation in Russia and conflict among Russian doctors on the efficacy of quarantines reported because of the lack of "clarity" on cholera's contagion he could not recommend quarantine stations on the border.[50] On December 10, 1830, the king authorized Altenstein and von Brenn "without delay to take appropriate measures" to prevent cholera "from reaching the Prussian States."[51] Altenstein was awaiting direction from the Cholera Commission to determine what had to be done next. Undoubtedly, pressure from the cabinet order influenced the Commission's internal discussions to try to come to terms with the two competing doctrines mentioned previously (especially in regard to the interference with trade).

On December 13, 1830, the Cholera Commission made less stringent recommendations to Altenstein and von Brenn. Copies were sent to the Ministry of Foreign Affairs and the Ministry of Finance. The Commission recommended the introduction of a health pass, the erection of a sanitary advisory line, and the designation of a provisional health cordon. These measures drafted in December but were not published until April 5, 1831.[52] Undoubtedly, the provisional recommendations combined with the king's order prompted Altenstein to order Rust and another member of the Commission, *Ober-Medizinalrat* Behrnauer "to draft more expansive preventive and helpful measures for the population."[53] To assure ministry unity across the government and the military, the king ordered the establishment of a defense commission on January 5, 1831. This commission would not meet until May 5, 1831, as the Immediate Commission to Prevent Cholera.[54]

The Cholera Commission concluded cholera was plague-like and was transmitted from person to person.[55] According to Rust, the Austrian sanitary policy when applied to contagious diseases like plague was proven effective and he was convinced that quarantine measures if handled correctly would prove effective against this new disease as well.[56] Rust was Austrian and trained as a physician there. He gained experience "with sanitary policy during the war in 1805." In addition, in 1809, during an epidemic sickness in Cracow, he was recognized for his leadership and support in the local hospital there.[57]

Even the doctors on the Cholera Commission were not completely convinced of the severity of contagion but recognized they had better be prepared. After all, they were responsible for many lives and "the men of this time had learned not to put much hope in the art of medicine during plague ... to prevent or even assist in healing, but to depend on military discipline." However, the situation had not yet reached the "military stage" and there were still intermediary steps that could be recommended to "first responders," customs officials, town, village and other local government and medical officials as well as the local militia. For example, in early December, Theodor von Schön, provincial president of East and West Prussia demanded stations be established on the Russian border for disinfecting, purifying and washing wares. If cholera became a threat, Schön said he would establish a "military cordon" by calling up a "contingent of local militia."[58]

However, there was still more investigating to be done. Cholera had not yet appeared at the Prussian boundary so a cautious approach was a reasonable recommendation by the Cholera Commission at the time.[59]

The Commission realized that strict plague quarantine and its consequent interruption of commerce and the movement of people and goods would impose too high a cost on the public. The Cholera Commission proceeded with deliberate caution and expected that it would later receive more reliable reports from the Doctor's Commission sent to Russia.[60] Commission members agreed some early precautions had to be taken. However, there is no evidence of a quick bureaucratic "reflex action" to impose strict quarantine restrictions immediately. At this early stage, Rust did not get a full commitment to contagion nor did he obtain his military cordons.

In January 1831, instructions were drafted by the medical technical unit for customs officials. The instructions concerned the approaching cholera as well the outbreak of the cholera. They were developed for quarantine officials on the border. They outlined disinfection practices for travelers and for goods and animals originating from areas where cholera was present. Other regulations concerned the introduction of health passes for travelers coming from infected areas. These preliminary measures were necessary as a precaution in the event the government did not have time to impose stricter sanitary measures on its border. Other measures were added to assist officials in cholera awareness and treatment. Finally there were instructions for the preservation of health and for the "greater public." However, it was believed that these instructions should be precautionary and it was too premature to implement them. If made public, they would only "create fear before its time and in this way more damage ... than would be useful."[61] The Cholera Commission wanted to wait until the Doctor's Commission had the opportunity to observe the epidemic in Russia and report back to the Cholera Commission before releasing the instructions.[62]

The Doctor's Commission to Russia

Although not usually given credit by historians, Prussia was one of the earliest countries to send an official commission to study cholera in Russia, to acquire more scientific knowledge and learn the most practical therapies.[63]

The idea to send this delegation was proposed in November by Altenstein in a letter to von Brenn. Dr. Johann Christoph Albers, a physician from the *Regierungsbezirk* of Gumbinnen in East Prussia and "a close friend" of Rust, was appointed to head the Commission. Other members included two professors of medicine, Dr. Edmund Dann from Danzig (who we will find later working in a cholera lazaret in Danzig), and Dr. Quincke (of whom there is little biographical information). The fourth appointee was Dr. Barchewitz, a *Stadtphysikus* from Silesia.[64]

On December 12, 1830, Rust outlined the scope of the mission. The doctors were instructed to go to infected areas in Russia "to observe and investigate" the nature of the disease and determine what public health measures and therapies were most effective. As discussed by the Cholera Commission, Dr. Albers was to determine if the contagion was similar to "plague, smallpox or typhus."[65] Similar letters were sent to Quincke, Dann and Barchewitz.[66]

Rust wrote to Foreign Minister Bernstorff that the king had authorized the delegation's trip to "investigate and observe the spread of the cholera" in Russia. The doctors were requested to depart immediately. He added that it would please the king if "all impediments could be set aside."[67] Bernstorff expedited the Commission's travel to Russia. Provincial President Schön, of East and West Prussia, was informed that the doctors would meet in Königsberg, receive instructions, and report to him and the Ministry of Religion, Education and Medical Affairs.[68]

The four doctors met in Königsberg on January 15, 1831. Barchewitz and Dann were ordered to Moscow, Albers and Quincke to St. Petersburg. Barchewitz and Dann were sent to investigate sanitary policy, Albers and Quincke to investigate causation and potential therapies.[69]

Dann and Barchewitz traveled to Vilna in Russian Lithuania where it was rumored there were cholera cases. They reported from Vilna they observed no cholera. They were told cholera had broken out in Kiev. However, outbreaks were not easily communicated to the doctors and hard to confirm due to unrest in Poland and the on-going Russian preparations for war. They decided to travel on to Moscow where they expected to observe cholera cases.[70] The team of doctors was delayed reaching Moscow as a result of the cordons they had to pass through to reach Moscow. The two doctors arrived in Moscow on February 2, 1831, and were met by two Russian medical state officials, Dr. Loder and Dr. Marcus as well as the Governor-General of Moscow, Count Galitzen. Along with other doctors in Moscow, they discussed the history of the epidemic in Moscow, the effectiveness of various therapeutic methods and visited a number of cholera hospitals.[71] They saw their first cholera case on February 4, 1831. Dann later reported visiting a lazaret in Moscow that contained the "most violent cases" in which nearly all ended in death. The impression of the effects of cholera symptoms on the patients he reported was extraordinary.[72]

By the time Dann and Barchewitz arrived in Moscow the cholera epidemic was beginning to wane. Dann reported that on average approximately five out of seven infected people died. After February 14, 1831, deaths decreased further and for many days there were no reported deaths. The last new sick case occurred on March 22, 1831. By March 29, 1831, the epidemic ended in Moscow. The last cordon was lifted on April 6, 1831, and "communication with all of Russia was restored."[73]

However, the debate over the contagious nature of the cholera continued to rage in Russia. In Moscow, it was reported that of the twenty-four members of the Moscow Medical Council three were weak supporters of contagion, two were strong supporters and nineteen confirmed anti-contagionists.

Albers and Quincke had departed on January 25, 1831, for Riga and then St. Petersburg.[74] During the early stages of their trip neither team made any recommendations concerning the cholera or the usefulness of quarantine. In St. Petersburg Dr. Albers and Dr. Quincke found the situation reversed from that in Moscow. Dr. Mudroff, the Head of a five member Central Cholera Commission, and a "moderate contagionist" was in charge of the government's defense against the cholera. In conjunction with the Russian Minister Sakrewski and the Central Cholera Commission, he insisted on strict quarantine and sanitary police regulations.[75] St. Petersburg would not have a cholera outbreak until June 26, 1831. Therefore the Prussian doctors had no eyewitness accounts to report to Berlin. They used information gathered from official government and independent reports of physicians who had treated cholera victims in other parts of Russia. They also reported on the methods the central government in Russia used in attempting to prevent the spread of the disease.[76]

The Result of the Doctor's Commission

The Doctor's Commission provided more eyewitness reports from Russia concerning the epidemic in Moscow. Dr. Barchewitz and Dr. Dann observed a number of cholera cases in Moscow. Dr. Dann found Dr. R. Lichtenstadt's, contagionist book, *Die Asiatische Cholera in Russland* that appeared on February 1, 1831, "convincing" and could not understand how such a work was possible in such a "time of general calamity."[77] Official opinion in Russia, which included the Medical Council of the Russian Ministry of the Interior, held that the cholera was "contagious." In April, the Moscow Cholera Council argued that the cholera was "contagious" but, "less so than bubonic plague."[78]

Official opinion in Russia, as well as respected physicians like Dr. Lichtenstadt, advocated the contagionist doctrine. Berlin required an urgent answer from the Commission. In late March, Dr. Albers, reported to Berlin that he was convinced that cholera could be spread from person to person but that he had "met with no instance which could render it at all probable that cholera is disseminated by inanimate objects."[79]

This was undoubtedly the information that Dr. Rust needed. As one physician wrote, his position was "strengthened by the report of a doctor that had been sent to Russia ... [Albers] ... and perhaps through the weight of such fearful responsibility." Altenstein concluded, "together with his colleague ... [Rust] ... cholera should be stopped utilizing official plague prevention policy."[80] Officially it was reported that at the end of April, the Doctors Commission reported to the Ministry of Religion, Education and Medical Affairs the "sickness belonged to the kind that was infectious ... [contagious] ... and only prevented through quarantine regulations, which makes impossible the communication and spread of the contagious matter."[81] Three of the doctors, Albers, Quincke and Dann, agreed cholera was contagious. Only Dr. Barchewitz because of his direct experience with cholera in Russia was convinced it was not contagious. He became an outspoken advocate of this opinion. However, Rust remained convinced cholera was contagious. His opinion became official Prussian government policy and he became the chief architect of the government's response.[82]

Cholera had already appeared on the Polish-Russian border when the revolution in Poland broke out in Warsaw in November 1830. But it was not until late March and early April, after the battle of Iganie near the Prussian-Polish border on April 10, 1831, that cholera began spreading through the Polish army and subsequently reached Warsaw and its vicinity.[83]

The proximity and magnitude of the disease forced the Prussian King, Frederick William III, to take action. The previously established defense commission appointed in January 1831 was now established as the Immediate Commission to Prevent Cholera. The Immediate Commission was charged with carrying out policies in line with the recommendations of the Doctor's Commission. Dr. Rust was appointed head of the medical section of the Immediate Commission.[84]

Dann and Barchewitz finished their work in Moscow and traveled to Kiev in what was then southwest Russia to investigate the only area in Russia where cholera was active. The two doctors met with Quincke and Albers in the Russian city of Saratov on the Volga River in early May. The Commission was recalled because of the cholera outbreak in Warsaw and the establishment of the Immediate Commission. Due to the unrest in Lithuania in early May, the only way back to Prussia was by way of St. Petersburg. Meanwhile Czar Nicholas ordered a Commission to meet in St. Petersburg to settle the question of whether the cholera was contagious or not. The Prussian doctors traveled to St. Petersburg to attend the conference prior to their return to Prussia. They arrived in St. Petersburg on June 5, 1831.[85]

The doctors arrived while the meeting was underway. Dr. Marcus, the temporary secretary of the Moscow Medical Council represented the anti-contagionist viewpoint and Dr. Mudroff represented the Central Commission in St. Petersburg with the opposing view. Dann reported, there were approximately forty government doctors from St. Petersburg, as well as doctors representing the governments of Austria, Prussia and England. The third and final meeting was held on June 17, 1831. Dann later reported the subject of the last meeting was a contentious debate on an article published in a German journal. In addition a poll was taken as to whether cholera was or was not contagious. Dr. Marcus continued to use the example of the description provided by the doctors in Astrakhan as evidence of the non-contagious nature of the cholera. Still a few doctors believed the question could not be resolved. The majority of doctors "voted for contagion."[86]

Why had the majority of doctors in St. Petersburg voted for contagion? Dann explained when he and the other Prussian doctors left Moscow to travel into southwest Russia things had "suddenly changed." While they were away for a "few weeks" to undertake further studies, cholera "showed itself" and "spread from southwest Russia up to Archangel." It was now raging in Riga. The people of St. Petersburg were "frightened." The city was currently surrounded by three cordons and the quarantine was increased from twenty to sixty days, a plague level quarantine. The people of St. Petersburg had been spared the previous autumn and thought that they would be spared a second time, but by the end of the month cholera was epidemic.[87]

Dr. Dann wrote upon his arrival in St. Petersburg he had received reports cholera had broken out in Danzig. He was determined to "hasten as quickly as possible to his home city of Danzig." Getting there required passing through new quarantine measures established by the Prussian government. Returning by way of Riga would require a three week stay in a quarantine station on the Prussian border. Instead all four doctors traveled by ship, Barchewitz and Albers to Memel, Quincke and Dann to Kronstadt and then to Danzig. After an eight day journey with inclement weather, they dropped anchor near Danzig and spent time in quarantine from July 3, to the morning of July 6. Dann was permitted to go on to Danzig.[88]

There is little further information on Dr. Quincke. Dr. Dann remained in Danzig from July 6, 1831, and did not return to Berlin until October 16, 1831. He continued his investigations, reported them to Berlin and later published his experiences in a leading medical journal. He lived and worked in a cholera hospital during the epidemic in Danzig.[89] Dr. Albers later became one of the editors of the contagionist *Cholera Archiv* and an advocate of Rust's policies.[90]

Carl Lorinser, who later became a prominent physician and an important voice in the cholera debate, referred to Albers as Rust's "trusted servant," and claimed Rust later rewarded Albers for his unwavering support with an appointment as Head of the Veterinary School in Berlin in 1832.[91]

Of the four doctors, Dr. Barchewitz had the greatest influence, not as a supporter of official government policy but as an anti-contagionist outside the confines of government circles. After May 7, 1831, official policy supported the contagionist position. There had been earlier debates in Prussia but it was primarily among officials within the medical community and within the government.[92]

Dr. Barchewitz later wrote that after his observations in Russia he had been "wholly freed of the official theory of infection, and came after a month to be a decided opponent." He found "scarcely any sanitary policy in Moscow." Curiously, his support of anti-contagionism over contagionism was not expressed by his partner Dr. Dann. Dr. Barchewitz remained on good enough terms with the government and continued as a member of the Commission until its dissolution after its return from St. Petersburg.[93] Nevertheless, Barchewitz later made an enemy of Rust who wrote bitterly, that "non-contagionists" were his enemies.[94]

Dr. Barchewitz was influential because he had been selected to go to Russia as a representative of the Prussian government. His views carried weight outside of official medical circles in Berlin. His greatest influence came when he returned to East Prussia in July as an opponent of the official theory. His writings were used by the doctors of Königsberg as the basis for opposing the official doctrine of contagion as well as by Schön who came to accept the anti-contagionist view.[95] His writings were also used to oppose police and military "preventive measures" later imposed in the various districts of East Prussia.[96]

Doctors and officials like Schön in East Prussia were not yet wholly convinced of the reliability of Barchewitz's observations. Provincial President Schön sent two doctors in late May to investigate the cholera in Poland and Lithuania. Dr. Jacobi was sent to the Augustowoschen region in Poland and Dr. Burdach (the younger) was sent to Lithuania. Both doctors returned in June to report to Schön. They confirmed Dr. Barchewitz's opinion. This information compelled Schön to ask the Immediate Commission in Berlin to reverse its regulations or to at least modify the severity of the measures.[97] Berlin refused and Schön continued to advocate for anticontagionism as the basis for modifying the strict measures imposed by the Immediate Commission in Berlin. His advocacy would eventually lead to his calling on Berlin on July 25, 1831, to modify the strict cholera regulations.[98] During the time leading up to his decision Schön continued to refer to Barchewitz in his disagreement over the strict cholera regulations with the Chief of the Immediate Commission, General Thile.[99]

Barchewitz's views were not limited to Prussia. When cholera appeared in St. Petersburg, the Swedish ambassador, Baron Palmstierna, requested Barchewitz provide him with written reports of his experiences with the disease. His influence was extended throughout Germany when his views were hurriedly published in the *Swedische Staatszeitung* and subsequently picked up in smaller German state newspapers.[100]

The inability of the medical community to resolve the contagion debate lay at the heart of the government's decision to continue its strict sanitary policy. The Doctors Commission accomplished its mission, to investigate and recommend measures to prevent and treat cholera. It supported the contagionist doctrine and subsequent policies which the government adopted. At the same time, it exposed Dr. Barchewitz to the anti-contagionists in Moscow and provided him with the opportunity to bring the anti-contagionist message to Prussia. As the champion of these views he had both a domestic impact in Prussia and an international influence. Dr. Barchewitz was not alone in his anti-contagionist views and the debate raged on in Prussia during the epidemic and in subsequent years.

2

Public Health Administration in Prussia Before 1831

Prior to 1806 the Prussian medical administration was a highly centralized organization, purposely established under the auspices of *cameralism* in the eighteenth century to increase the population. At that time, population was seen as a critical resource for increasing wealth and for the defense of the state. This centralized medical administration continued even under the Napoleonic conquest.[1]

Following the defeat of Napoleon there was a conscious effort on the part of the "reform administration" in Prussia to decentralize all aspects of the Prussian government. This included decentralizing public health and medical administration. The health system was changed from a highly centralized system to a "communal and decentralized" system. A second change, after 1817, was a health infrastructure of shared responsibility between two fractious Ministries. In 1825 this led to a strident public medical debate concerning bureaucratic paralysis. The overlapping areas of responsibility, unclear divisions among offices and the lack of proper qualifications among office holders were the major issues of dispute. The debate was public and included physicians, officials, lay people and other professionals.[2]

Finally, many of the agencies and most of the medical bodies responsible during the cholera epidemic had been established during the "reform era" and did not exist prior to 1806.[3]

"Prussianism" and Medical Reform

Prussia was heir to a State organized medical administrative infrastructure with ideological roots originating in the seventeenth century. These roots are generally analyzed in terms of the development of the "power State." This idea of the "power State" was described by historians in the development of the Prussian public health administration and medical community throughout the nineteenth century.[4]

However, the reform administration in Prussia that began in 1806 as a response to the defeat of Prussia by Napoleon transformed the general governmental organizations in Prussia. This included reforms in the public health and the medical sectors. This effected a fundamental change in the way that the Prussian government organized itself to lead the response to the cholera in 1831. The reform administration in Prussia and its impact on the social, economic and political organization has been well studied. What has been little analyzed is the impact on the public health system and its consequences.[5]

What was the impact of the medical reforms on the Prussian sanitary system in relation to the first cholera epidemic in 1831? How did general philosophy of the reformers affect the sanitary and medical administration from the local level and how did this affect the dismantling of the centralized Sanitary Board at the beginning of the reform period?[6]

Prussian medical reforms also had implications in the greater context of the development of public health policies in Europe in the nineteenth century. For example, the observation put forward by Ackerknecht about the conflict over quarantine that arose during the first cholera epidemic that "contagion and quarantine corresponded to authoritarian political instincts ... miasmatism and sanitationism to liberal."[7] Historians of the cholera epidemic in Prussia are in general agreement with this thesis.[8]

A brief review of the Prussian public health system and infrastructure is warranted to explain why Prussia when faced with the threat of cholera took an interventionist approach. There are three significant reasons that had important consequences for Prussia's choice and these cannot simply be attributed to an authoritarian regime out to "disrupt the everyday lives of its subject peoples."[9]

The regulative State or *Polizeistaat* evolved in the seventeenth century. Prussia is acknowledged as the leading example of this type of State. Today the term carries a pejorative connotation but the word *Polizei* originally referred to the idea of administration in its widest sense. The *Polizeistaat* which was created in the seventeenth century should be more closely identified with the term *Wohlfahrstaat*.[10]

The idea of the *Polizeiordnung* and *Landesordnung* developed out of the paternalistic ideas of medieval society and was later nourished by individual towns. The ideas were developed further by the larger States which in turn provided the rationale for State intervention in all areas of community life, including medical affairs. By the middle of the seventeenth century the concept of "general welfare" had given way to the authoritarian and absolutist State, concepts which developed out of the state's need to foster population growth.[11]

A direct result of a policy to increase population as fundamental to the increase in national wealth led cameralist writers in Prussia to emphasize public health intervention.[12] Charles Rosen a critic of the medical policies of the cameralist states in the seventeenth and eighteenth centuries noted that their policies were "rooted in a particular economic, political and social system."[13] Public administration emphasized the problems of health and welfare because they were direct concerns of the state. Others have also seen a link from the early modern Prussian State to the later "enlightenment" period in the eighteenth century. This approach was identified by the hospitalization of the poor, additional social disciplinary action in medicine and the medical administration, and educating the population in a healthy lifestyle.[14] For example, Johann Heinrich Gottlob von Justi, advocated "measures to advance health and medical provisions" and defined them as a critical "part of police science." Further positive population growth was necessary for "agriculture, industry and trade as well as other service areas, and was central to the wealth of the state." These "three sectors were the key to the state achieving its primary but abstract aim of "happiness." In order to attain this "coercive means might be necessary," including social and medical relief.[15]

By the end of the eighteenth century, Prussia had undertaken "administrative and regulatory activities. These regulations dealt with communicable disease control, organization, and supervision of medical personnel, environmental sanitation and the provision of health care for the indigent."[16] These activities were not undertaken for social or charitable reasons but to serve the needs of the newly emergent power State. Originally state intervention in such areas was based on the idea of the common good. By the middle of the eighteenth century this idea had been transformed and the "cultural and welfare purpose receded before the power purpose."[17]

With the emphasis on power, the needs of the absolutist State now precluded a broader social approach to medicine. By the early nineteenth century health problems associated with the new industrial order required an approach to public health that should have been "calculated to increase the welfare of the people rather than augment the power of the state."[18] The State's approach based on the use of medical police was "outmoded and reactionary."[19]

Unfortunately, there was no break with the older view of the "medical police." This did not occur until legislation deregulated medical practice in Prussia in 1869. However, there were antecedents for change, for example, the debates to reform the medical system in Prussia in the 1820s. One important suggested reform put forward was the "idea of remedying the social question" by calling for a more locally controlled public health structure.[20] The Prussian administration (especially the Ministry of Interior where the medical police resided) was not prepared to change direction and expected individuals to obey orders and continue to follow tradition.[21]

The primary purpose of "health policy in the eighteenth century exhibited a clear priority" to increase the state's population. Prussian bureaucrats were trained to support this policy well into the early nineteenth century. However, due to the pauperism debate and obvious overpopulation in Prussia in the early nineteenth century this outmoded policy no longer agreed "with the demographic observation." Some officials "acknowledged" this as a problem. It was not until the 1840s that the conflict over the role of the medical police as providers of welfare took on a more scientific and humanistic orientation that reformers demanded. The anachronistic ideas from the enlightenment remained in place throughout the 1820s and 1830s.[22]

Even with philosophical ideals introduced in the early part of the nineteenth century that promoted humanistic values and self-cultivation, the Prussian bureaucratic apparatus was not able to supplant or replace the idea that the individual was a "cog in a machine." These lofty goals were also never widely adopted in the administrative realm during the 1820s and 1830s.

More effective in bringing real change to the medical administration were the decentralizing actions of the Reform period. The appointment of provincial officials, of local medical organizations and the strengthening of the authority of local medical officials led to increasing confrontations by these authorities "with the realities of urbanization and industrialization in the form of the social question." While the "bureaucratic apparatus was still enmeshed in the model of the last century" the reformers initially prospered at the local level with the appointments of provincial officials who brought practical experience and planning, attributes that were brought into discussions concerning the health system.[23]

Nevertheless, it could be argued that the strength of the decentralized system was at its weakest when confronting a disease like cholera. In Prussia one aspect of the old "medical police" system was the ability of the medical police to cope with communicable diseases.[24] However, it was precisely at this time that the Prussian medical administration was at its most decentralized therefore least capable of coping effectively with this medical crisis and thus it fell back on the plague regulations of 1709.[25]

The medical profession in Prussia held an official monopoly on health care as a result of the requirement of State certification for all medical personnel. The general population did not always recognize their professional expertise for a variety of reasons or could afford them. People turned to unlicensed individuals, clergy and even quacks. At this time, a physician's status was not necessarily based as much on medical knowledge as social origins, relationships and general education. The physician also had to share responsibility for educational qualifications and appointments to practice with the bureaucratic State.[26]

Early Medical Organization in Prussia

In 1685 the Elector Frederick William initiated State control of medicine in Prussia, by establishing a *Collegium Medicum* (Board of Medicine) in Brandenburg, Prussia.[27] In 1692 Frederick appointed a privy councilor as president of the Board of Medicine. The Board's function was to license medical personnel and to raise the standard of medical practice in Prussia.[28]

On September 27, 1725, he issued a decree that created a *Provinzial-Collegia Medica* (Provincial Medical Board) in each of the twelve provinces. On December 17, 1725, the Chief Board of Medicine in Berlin now functioned as a central medical board.[29] The provincial medical boards reported to the Chief Board of Medicine in Berlin. Besides regulating the qualifications and fees of provincial and city doctors, the edict regulated medicines and outlined a physician's responsibilities in the event of plague.[30]

Following the Edict of December 17, 1725, there were additional modifications regarding the practice of medicine in rural areas. After 1727, "medical ordinances seemed to meet with considerable success in improving standards of professional qualifications and conduct."[31] State regulations forbade the unauthorized practice of medicine by traditional healers and clergy.[32] Up to the early part of the nineteenth century the relative insecurity of income "motivated many physicians to acquire ... a city or State office" along with their private practice.[33]

The *Collegium Sanitatis* (Board of Sanitation) was established in 1719 and originated from the Plague Board (*Pest Collegium*) established in Berlin during the plague threat of 1709.[34] The Board of Sanitation was responsible for "preserving and protecting the provinces and country from pestilence and other infectious diseases ..." as well as overseeing trade, food quality, and ensuring clean water.[35]

By 1762 provincial sanitary boards existed in each province in Prussia, subordinate to the Sanitary Board in Berlin. The provincial sanitary boards were responsible for local responses to disease human and animal. Physicians reported instances of infectious diseases to Berlin. The sanitary Board instructed local sanitary officials when to begin quarantine measures in the event of an epidemic.[36]

In 1786 Frederick William II issued a royal order placing the Chief Medical Board in Berlin under the authority of the General Directory.[37] The oversight of medical and sanitary boards was moved to the General Directory which was now also responsible for all decisions and appointments concerning the number of doctors, surgeons, apothecaries and midwives.[38] The non-medical control of this function lasted until 1797 when a new *Obermedizinal Department* (Chief Medical Department) headed by a Chief Medical Officer, was appointed to the General Directory.

In 1799 the responsibilities of the Chief Sanitary Board were merged with the Chief Medical Board in Berlin. The new Chief Medical and Sanitary Board was responsible for issuing plague regulations "to the cities, market towns and villages," providing general health information; protective measures for animals; and when necessary establishing quarantine measures with the now merged provincial medical and sanitary boards.[39] The merged boards were responsible for the prevention of epidemic diseases, empowered to issue regulations concerning impure foods and vapors from tanneries and cemeteries, and ensure the quick internment of the dead. On April 21, 1800, the state issued additional edicts concerning the responsibilities of the provincial medical and sanitary boards.[40]

For the first time the medical administration was not only centralized but raised to the status of the other departments in the General Directory. The Chief Medical Officer had immediate access to the king. Dr. Johann N. Rust wrote, this change in the status of the medical administration was like a "shining star on the medical horizon."[41] This new status was short lived as a result of Napoleon's defeat of Prussia in 1806 and the implementation of "reforms" in Prussia.

The Reform Era 1806–1815

The catastrophe of 1806 and the collapse of old Prussia initiated the need to rebuild the Prussian State that was "so thoroughly defeated" by Napoleon. Prussia was a State composed of multiple feudal interests and, above all, the competing interests of the "monarchy, nobility and bureaucracy." The Prussian bureaucracy saw as its "overarching goal" the need to assert its dominance in Prussia, to modernize and rationalize the state and to make it once again an important player in European politics. It also saw itself as "the real soul of the state, the champion of reasonable opinion, of law and of the common good, of progress and modernity."[42]

Prussia had not been a unified state but a country of "states, provinces and territories." The king was advised by his ministers, advisors, and councilors from whom he would draw guidance and make decisions. Called "anarchic and irrational" by his senior bureaucrats, the reform of the Prussian administration was considered essential to the future success of the Prussian State. The reforms were begun with the aim "from above to below" and from "within to the outside" to establish the advancement of a state civil society.[43] The reformers looked to modernize the Prussian State by adopting "new ideas of a civil society, grounded on civil liberties and equality under the law." They adopted the liberal economic philosophy of Adam Smith. They demanded the modernization of government and administration by decentralizing authority "to permit State Power to penetrate into the countryside." They enacted a Municipal Ordinance to allow "citizen participation in public affairs" and cleared away old privileges and traditions of the feudal society. In 1807, the peasants were freed, individuals could freely dispose of their land and occupations were open to everyone.[44]

Intellectually, Prussian reformers were influenced by William von Humboldt and neo-humanism with its emphasis on education, individualism and self-cultivation. Critical here, and of importance to later developments in the founding of universities and medical education in Prussia, were his ideas concerning *Wissenschaft* or "scholarly knowledge." This was differentiated from the passing on of knowledge by tradition or by the trades. *Wissenschaft* was defined as the search for knowledge for its own sake and to the reformers this was more useful and important to society.[45]

In the "reform era" and later the reaction, the Prussian medical and public heath sector underwent a series of changes that drastically changed its earlier organization and structure. During the "reform era" it was decentralized, the result was a period of overlapping areas of responsibility and organizational paralysis in the medical and public health sectors that lasted beyond the cholera epidemic. This forced the Prussian government to respond to its greatest public health threat by falling back on traditional measures that were in conflict with the new ideas of liberalism and free trade.[46]

The Prussian Health Administration from 1806–1817

The rationale for the reformers coming to power in Prussia was the loss of territory, the military and administrative weakness as well as the financial burden placed on the state. The first minister, Baron Heinrich Frederic Karl vom Stein was in power from 1807–1808. By 1807, the Prussian ministry was reorganized along departmental lines. There was now a "twin leadership of bureaucracy and monarchy." The king had to work alongside his ministers turning what had been an "autocratic authoritarian state into a bureaucratic state."[47]

Stein advocated increased provincial administrative responsibility and demonstrated his willingness to place more responsibility in the hands of local authorities. With the Municipal Ordinance of November 1808, local governance control was transferred to the cities including their own public health measures.[48] Also, in keeping with his reformist views, more responsibility was delegated to the provincial level. On December 26, 1808, medical and health matters were assigned to local *Regierungen-Präsidenten* (administrative executives). The new medical responsibilities included oversight of the medicinal trade, certification of medical persons, responsibility for dealing with infectious diseases, bad food and the protection of the public from unqualified medical persons. Other responsibilities included the administration of hospitals, insane asylums and other public institutions.[49]

Initially the provincial officials seemed to have a new level of authority as a result of the Stein edicts. However a clearer line of authority was necessary and was reflected in the strengthening of the authority of the recently established *Oberpräsidenten* (Provincial Presidents) of the Provinces.[50]

In December 1809, under the Dohna-Altenstein Ministry, Alexander von Humboldt was appointed Head of a newly established Medical Department located in the Ministry of the Interior. In order to decentralize authority in Berlin and to provide greater responsibility to local officials the Chief Medical and Sanitary Board in Berlin as well as the provincial medical boards were dissolved.[51] As long as the Board existed in Berlin local governments looked to the Board for guidance rather than assuming local responsibility.[52]

Following the Dohna-Altenstein Ministry 1809–1810, Carl August Freiherr von Hardenberg was appointed Chancellor in 1810 and remained chancellor until his death in 1822. While Stein favored "decentralization and collegial government" Hardenberg advocated a "strong state and a tightly organized and centralized administration" on the French model.[53] Both approaches had a lingering effect on the organization and structure of the Prussian medical system as well the later retrenchment of reformist values that followed the reaction that set in after Hardenberg's death in 1822.

The former responsibilities of the Chief Medical and Sanitary Board were now divided into administrative and advisory bodies in the Ministry of the Interior. The administrative sector did not have a "research agenda" as part of its portfolio. Humboldt protested.[54] He resolved this by moving this section to the Medical Department in April, 1810. This led to a ten year conflict between the role of police administration, oversight of medical personnel and the role of medicine and social welfare.[55]

The advisory duties of the Chief Medical and Sanitary Board were transferred to a new sub-medical section in the Ministry of the Interior. Within this department the better qualified members of the old Chief Medical and Sanitary Board were assigned to the *Wissenschaftliche Deputation für Medizinalwesen* (Scientific Deputation for Medicine). This replaced this function on the Chief Medical and Sanitary Board. It was strictly advisory.[56] Nevertheless, the Scientific Deputation emerged as one of the more important medical bodies. It was founded as a clearing house for medical research and new therapies. It also functioned as an advisory body to the Ministry of the Interior. On January 23, 1817, the Scientific Deputation's duties were expanded to include advising the state on criminal cases, the revision of medical legislation, medical statutes and on sanitary conditions in the cities and larger districts.[57]

The Medical Department located in the Ministry of the Interior was responsible for all medical practice, policy, institutions, and health legislation. It reviewed physician qualifications, other medical personnel, hospital heads, medical police regulations, and measures for the care and treatment of the poor. The latter measures were expected to be negotiated between the Police department and Medical department within the Ministry of the Interior.[58]

The dissolution of the Chief Medical and Sanitary Board along with the local medical sanitary boards had been in keeping with the goals of the reforms of 1806 by strengthening the authority of the city physicians. The cholera epidemic in 1831 would challenge this new orientation.[59]

Chancellor Hardenberg was more interested in medical reform on a state wide level. He later appointed Freiherr Karl vom Altenstein who had previous medical administrative experience at the provincial level and who became the architect behind later medical reforms in Prussia.[60] Altenstein entered service in his home province of Ansbach-Bayreuth in southern Prussian under the leadership of the future Chancellor of Prussia, Hardenberg, administrator of Ansbach-Bayreuth. In 1803, Altenstein had been responsible for the medical administration of the province as well as that of Silesia and established a general hospital system in the province after the Vienna model.[61]

In exile in Riga with Hardenberg in 1807, Altenstein collaborated with Hardenberg on the *Riga Memorandum* in September 1807. The memorandum reflected his view and "concept of the science of administration." It incorporated a neo-humanist emphasis on science, scientific research, and self-cultivation. Although "abstract" in nature regarding medical reforms, a number of his ideas served as a model for the establishment in 1817 of the *Ministerium für Geistlichen, Unterrichts—und Medizinal Angelegenheiten* (Ministry of Religion, Education and Medical Affairs). The Ministry was headed by Altenstein from 1817 until 1837.[62]

In 1807 Altenstein proposed that in the administration of health care scientific research and education should be independent and separate from the police within the Interior Ministry. These areas should be under the "general management of the medical department."[63] Altenstein's views were in contrast to the way that physicians and other medical personnel were traditionally trained. Medicine was viewed as a trade rather than a profession and based on little or no formal scientific research. For example, on medical issues Altenstein initially supported the *Gewerbefreiheit 1810* (freedom to pursue trade) that abolished the guild system, including the surgeons guild. He maintained that the basic function of the state was to "clear away obstacles by abolishing the guilds, to [support] ... freedom of the press, academic freedom and the individual's freedom to learn." And further, by the "respect for and the appreciation of science" and hiring competent individuals and their supporters.[64]

Altenstein's evaluation of the health care system in 1807–1810 was focused on improving the formal education of doctors as the basis for a forward thinking medical care system. He believed in the inherent "progress of science" and that the two needed to be "directed by legislation and within the organization of medical care."[65] Essentially there were three principles applicable to the role of State health care: promoting citizen health in the sense of clearing away harmful things that the individual could not correct or avoid; respect for a healthy lifestyle through the promotion of good health; and concern for the welfare of the poor sick."[66]

Altenstein was a strong supporter of bureaucratic absolutism; he identified with the Prussian State and "advocated absolute loyalty to the Prussian monarchy." He supported Prime Minister Hardenberg who advocated the central control of all ministries and that government should be run on rational scientific management principles.[67]

Humboldt had originally envisioned a Medical Department composed of licensed physicians with representation from the Police department and the Education department. He wanted university educated physicians trained in scientific theory and practice. With the establishment of the Medical section in the Ministry of the Interior in 1810 and the transfer of the administrative body to his department, this led to a conflict over traditional coercive "medical police" functions versus the role of social welfare and its place in the medical administration.[68]

These issues would have been difficult to resolve but were not pursued, because of the intervention of an unrelated political crisis. Humboldt resigned his position in protest. Humboldt's resignation was unfortunate because he was attempting to unify the many State medical responsibilities. The pursuit of medical unification later emerged as a point of controversy with the founding of the Ministry of Religious, Educational and Medical Affairs in 1817.[69] Humboldt's main contributions were the humanist ideals and educational perspective that he brought to this task as well as the concrete shape that he gave the Medical Department.[70]

The inability of the Prussian government to avoid overlapping authority and clear lines of responsibility even in the administration of health services can be attributed to the conflict between to divergent philosophies of organization. Those like Humboldt, who advocated collegial organization and others like Hardenberg who insisted on a more hierarchical organization. This difference existed even at the non-ministry level in the organizations responsible for governing at the provincial and local levels. It reached to the highest levels and existed between the newly established Ministry of Religious, Educational and Medical Affairs and the Ministry of the Interior. But first some background on the various government organizations and positions with health care responsibilities.

The office of the *Oberpräsident* (Provincial President) was established in 1808 to unite the various provincial branches in the provinces and to serve in an advisory capacity.[71] It was designed to exist at the highest level of provincial administration in Prussia and its role in medical administration in the state was derived from its peculiar role as the direct representative of the king in the provinces. It supported the "statist" desires of those in the government who wanted to ensure greater uniformity at all levels. The Provincial President "ruled but did not administer."[72] His force was moral rather than formal empowerment and he reported directly to the king.[73]

With the establishment of the new Medical department in 1809, in the Ministry of the Interior, medicine and medical research was transferred to the Scientific Deputation for Medicine. As noted earlier, local medical and sanitary responsibilities were placed in the hands of the chief executives of the government districts. The reform was seen as ineffective because the responsibilities of the medical councilors in the various administrative districts were not clearly defined *vis à vis* the recently established office of the provincial president. In 1815, new provincial medical boards and sanitary commissions were established and subordinated to the local governments but were still not answerable to a central medical authority, instead, they now answered to the provincial president.[74]

The role of the provincial president was reviewed in 1825. One major area at issue was under what circumstances could the provincial president act independently without necessarily waiting for orders from Berlin. The issue was later highlighted during the cholera epidemic in 1831.[75] Nevertheless, the provincial president's position had been strengthened somewhat in December 1825 within the provinces. They were given greater responsibility for the welfare of the province. They coordinated the activities of the provincial government and the general security of the province. This included the economy of the province, educational, religious and medical affairs (including authority over the new provincial medical boards).

As a quasi-independent entity within the Prussian government and chief member of the provincial medical board, a provincial president, like Theodor von Schön of East and West Prussia, had a legitimate base to later challenge the health policies of the government.

Provincial medical boards were established in 1815. Each was located at the seat of a provincial president.[76] The instructions for the medical boards were issued in October 1817. They were collegial advisory bodies for the local governments and the law courts. They had no administrative authority but had responsibilities in the following areas; the education and certification of medical personnel, the formulation of general medical regulations, and they had decision making powers concerning medical-legal matters within the provinces. The medical boards advised the local governments through the state medical councilor.[77]

The provincial medical boards were the chief sanitary advisory agencies for their provinces. They were composed of at least five members that included physicians, surgeons, and veterinarians, a State medical councilor and the provincial president. The provincial president headed the board. If he could not be present the state medical councilor took his place.[78] In 1815, Chancellor Hardenberg established within each administrative district (that lacked a provincial medical board) a *SanitätsKommission* (sanitary commission) to advise local authorities. The local sanitary commission was composed of local physicians, surgeons and apothecaries. In general, it was at the district and local government that medical measures were now formulated and reports communicated to the state government or central authorities on the progress of epidemic diseases in humans and animals.[79]

At the lowest official level a *Landräte* (district administrator) functioned as both the *Kreis-Polizei-Behörde* (county police) and the *Kreis-Medizinal-Behörde* (county medical official). He received assistance from the county physician and the county surgeon. The district administrator was instructed take an official interest in all health and sanitary matters within his jurisdiction. The county physician and county surgeon served in an advisory capacity for "epidemic sickness, smallpox vaccinations, and animal sicknesses" and received their orders from the district administrator.[80] The district administrator was responsible for the administration, health and the sanitary conditions of local institutions for the poor, prisons and hospitals.[81]

Due to a series of conflicts in the Prussian Ministry between "statists" versus collegial administrative supporters it was difficult to reform the administration and establish clear lines of authority. Nevertheless, there were some attempts. For medical affairs the problem was partially resolved using the provincial presidents who were authorized to preside over the provincial medical boards in a "direct attempt to target the decentralized provincial functionality" and who could report directly to the Ministry of the Interior on health matters where the medical section was housed. It was not an effective solution because the medical boards served in a purely advisory capacity to the provincial presidents. The medical police reported separately to the Ministry of the Interior. Also, the medical boards had little influence in "shaping health care" as the "real duties were handled by the local government medical councilor."[82]

The Ministry of Religion, Education and Medical Affairs

In November 1817, Hardenberg appointed Altenstein to head a new Ministry of Religion, Education and Medical Affairs. This Ministry was not part of the Ministry of the Interior. From the outset there were questions of the overlapping administrative roles of the provincial medical boards and also the responsibilities of the two ministries. Count Friedrich von Schuckman (Interior Minister from 1819–1834) raised the question of differentiating the medical administration from poor relief. He wrote to Altenstein, "The separation of the Charité [hospital] from the administration of poor relief was certainly desired by different parties with different motives, but was not realistic."[83] Also built into the new Ministry were overlapping areas of responsibility and a lack of a strong financial footing as compared to the Ministry of the Interior. The commissioner who negotiated the separation of responsibilities between the two Ministries, Wilhelm Anton von Klewitz, assured Schuckmann that the Ministry of Religion, Education and Medical Affairs "would not acquire the entire medical administration." Schuckmann and Altenstein initially agreed on a "partly shared arrangement on common issues" but that they would "separately manage" their ministries. In short, the "top management of medical matters outside of the military was not concentrated in one Ministry" but shared by three, the Ministry of Religion, Education and Medical Affairs, the Ministry of the Interior and at times the Ministry of War.[84]

The overlapping responsibilities and confused lines of authority were partly due to the inability of officials to consider the "necessity of a health service with social and political responsibilities." Conflict over this issue would come to a head in 1825 and would eventually be resolved in 1848.[85]

The medical responsibilities that remained with the Ministry of the Interior and Police following the creation of the Ministry Religion, Education and Medical Affairs in 1817 included supervision of the local medical police and carrying out the edicts and executive measures issued by the Ministry of the Interior to whom local officials reported. Its duties included administration of the medical police, supervision of hospitals, poor relief, food quality, disease prevention and forced inoculations.

The Ministry of Religion, Education and Medical Affairs was assigned supervisory responsibility for the medical system, advised on medical matters, appointed physicians and supervised sanatoriums and nursing homes. It had oversight of medicines, disease prevention and was responsible for a voluntary vaccination system. The provincial medical boards reported to the Ministry of Religion, Education and Medical Affairs and were responsible for the "supervision and administration of disease etiology."[86] The Scientific Deputation for Medicine was transferred from the Ministry of the Interior to the Ministry of Religion, Education and Medical Affairs but continued to advise the Ministry of the Interior.[87]

In 1819 Altenstein issued an important memorandum defining the purpose of the Ministry of Religion, Education and Medical Affairs to the rest of the state administration. He wrote that the aim of the Medical Department in the Ministry was to "organize ... public health assistance that individuals should be able to secure from the state."[88] He advocated better education for medical personnel and stricter laws against unlicensed persons practicing as physicians.[89]

He also asked for an increase in the number of surgeons. Ironically, Altenstein blamed the shortage of surgeons on the recently enacted "freedom to trade" law (that he had originally supported) that allowed the free movement of the population. He also recommended that a school of surgery be established in Prussia, because of the abolition of the surgeon guilds the manpower required to meet the increasing need was not available.[90]

Altenstein urged the state stop treating physicians like common tradesmen. He recommended it stop taxing physicians, increase the salaries of State physicians and place more doctors where they were badly needed, along the Russian border. He also recommended a revision of current medical legislation, the implementation of a standard medical ordinance concerning vaccination, and better administration of insane asylums, hospitals and doctors charged with the care of the poor.[91]

Altenstein suggested a uniform and comprehensive public health system for Prussia envisioning the effective role that educated medical personnel could play in gaining support for the state from their patients. He wrote:

> The earnestness, the moral conscientiousness and prudent activity of the physician affects the public profitably. A rough, impudent, vulgar, charlatan practicing is a visibly detrimental influence. The ethical and moral responsibility of the physician appears to be a more important object rather than the work of the doctor itself.[92]

Altenstein urged that the Prussian government do more to minister to the unfortunate in the interests of humanity.[93] This could be accomplished by appealing to the "highest sense in the people and by awakening the communal spirit."[94] The State had to play an active role at the local level but the chief part of reform had to be stimulated by the state. The commune, county, and province were responsible for intervening when necessary. The development of relations between these political organs on medical affairs should fall to the state.

Altenstein also complained about a lack of financial support for the Ministry. The various Savings Commissions and the on-going struggle with the Finance Minister to fund his department "handicapped its efficiency." He argued the 50,000 talers he received annually was not enough to alleviate the medical needs of Prussia. This was an insufficient amount to meet the spiritual and physical needs of ten million inhabitants.[95] He concluded that "Idealism, a free hand, individual engagement, and commitment to a secure existence through adequate payment" were the real "drivers of health conscious political actions for the administration."[96]

Altenstein made little progress administratively because he was not able to increase the financial support for the Ministry. He was not able to clarify areas of responsibility with the Ministry of the Interior. The fact that the two ministries worked together at all for a few years was attributed to Hardenberg who "up to his death had served as a mediating presence between the two Ministries."[97] This fractious relationship between the two Ministries brought continued criticism of the ministries that finally culminated in the medical reform debate of 1825.[98]

After Hardenberg's death in 1822, Altenstein made no further attempts to reform the Ministry of Religion, Education and Medical Affairs because he said he was waiting for an expected "new reorganization of the State Ministry in 1824." He was also aware that there was a "hardening of the fronts" (reactionaries were assuming power in the government) and he thought he could make better progress "though individual efforts on his part."[99]

The Medical Order of January 29, 1825

The joint medical administration between the Ministry of Religion, Education and Medical Affairs and the Ministry of the Interior came to an end in 1825. An Immediate Commission charged with investigating the financial affairs of the state was ordered to reduce the state budget by cost savings and personnel cuts. At the higher administrative levels two provincial presidents and two districts governments were eliminated. The middle layer of the administrative civil service was reduced by one-sixth. As one historian wrote "the Immediate Commission's recommendation was "a rare historical example in history" in which "government expenditures and personnel cuts were actually carried out."[100] However, because the elimination of personnel and the criteria was worked out for both ministries separately, there was no relief from overlapping areas of responsibility.[101]

As a result of the Medical Order of January 29, 1825, the scientific and technical medical and police functions which had been unified within the Ministry of Religion, Education and Medical Affairs were separated. Those with police functions were transferred to the Ministry of the Interior and the strictly medical stayed with the Ministry of Religion, Education and Medical Affairs. The Ministry of the Interior supervised public health concerns. These included medical police functions, food quality, infectious diseases in man and animals and oversight of institutions for the poor. Altenstein's medical department was responsible for general medical policy and therapeutic treatments. For example, it was responsible for the administration of "mad houses," supervised smallpox vaccinations, administered the *Charité* in Berlin, coordinated medical training and approved the administration of different therapeutic treatments in the larger hospitals of Prussia.[102]

The result of this division continued to leave the lines of authority between the two Ministries blurred. On March 25, 1825, the two Ministries agreed to share written information and decided which Ministry should first be informed "in the event of a dangerous disease."[103] Such confusion was not unique to the medical administration, but was symptomatic of most of the state administrative bodies including the local governments the provincial presidents and other Ministries.[104] The order of January 29, 1825, was seen by the chief medical officer in the Ministry, Dr. Rust, as a severe blow to medical administration and medical education. Officials with only theoretical knowledge and no practical experience lacked the perspective to write effective health legislation. Rust wrote that the resolution to this problem lay in the unification of all medical services and personnel in one of the two Ministries.[105] The solution was finally achieved in 1911 when a Medical Department was formed in the Ministry of the Interior.[106]

The solutions that eventually arose out of the medical reform debate in 1825 are beyond the time period we are considering. The debate was a consequence of the one hundredth anniversary of the Medical Edict of 1725 in Prussia. The basic issue was over the classification of health personnel, especially the new two part surgeon classification. This was an attempt to increase the number of surgeons in Prussia. It was also a broad based debate that included doctors, State officials, lay people, and other professionals over the complex and unclear authority within the Prussian medical administration, complaints concerning individual office holders and their lack of medical qualifications.[107]

After 1825, these issues along with the place of social welfare in medicine and public health became popular themes in literature and were often connected with the emerging "social question."[108]

In 1825 the medical police and other health personnel were divided between the Ministry of the Interior and Police and the Ministry of Religion, Education and Medical Affairs. As a result of this cost cutting measure, theoretical medical matters were separated from practical and policing of public health and medicine.[109] The re-organization and movement of medical departments and personnel between ministries over the years from 1806 on made it difficult to establish a stable chain of command and a clear pattern of administrative order. This was reflected in the overlapping lines of authority in which ministries and departments attempted to define responsibility. It was also demonstrated for example, in the local medical boards that found themselves simultaneously responsible to the local governments and to the king through the office of the provincial presidents, and the Ministry of Religion, Education and Medical Affairs. This problem was not resolved especially after medical police functions were transferred to the Ministry of the Interior in 1825.

Criticism of the first reaction to the cholera epidemic in 1831 in Prussia is predicated on a view of the Prussian administration that suggested a unified medical administration centralized and prepared to make decisions from the top down. With the arrival of the cholera in 1831, there was no single agency with the complete authority to orchestrate a unified response. The two ministries responsible for organizing against the epidemic—the Ministry of Religion, Education and Medical Affairs and the Ministry of the Interior—continued their fractious relationship under the leadership of Altenstein in the former and von Brenn in the latter. Neither could agree as to which ministry should have responsibility for this emergency. This would change with the appointment by the king of the "Immediate Commission to Prevent Cholera" in May 1831. Responsibility for fighting the epidemic was moved to this Commission under the leadership of a military man, General Ludwig Gustav von Thile, adjutant to the king.

That Prussia did not consolidate and unify its medical infrastructure or reform the medical system toward a more humane health and social welfare system before 1830 resulted initially in the inability of Prussia to gain the support of the public in confronting the epidemic. The administration was left to confront a newly emergent disease that required both a centralized public health program based on strict quarantine regulations and the support of the people as well as government officials. The strict regulations required the trust and confidence of the population in the actions of the authorities and doctors. Not surprisingly, there was a definite lack of trust in physicians and officials during the epidemic.

The Immediate Commission was formed to deal with the crisis from a centralized perspective. It relied on all State agencies, the military, as well as local administrative and medical bodies established during the reform era as part of the existing infrastructure to execute policy and ensure local adherence to regulations. Ironically, it was the local medical organizations and provincial bodies established during the reform era that served as a place to oppose the central authorities in Berlin. It was at the local and provincial level where the most vigorous and sometimes violent opposition was found to reverse the strict quarantine policy. This opposition was found not only among the public, but among those provincial officials in areas of Prussia that experienced cholera and the strict measures they came to see as economically ruinous and ineffective in combatting cholera.

3

Cholera in Poland

While Prussian officials were engaged in determining whether the cholera was contagious, events in Poland and Russia created a crisis that affected Prussia's border policy and emerged as a serious concern for Prussia's international relations. Even before the issue of cholera presented itself in Prussia, the government was confronted with what it saw as the moral disease of "revolution."[1] In July, revolution broke out in France and brought the bourgeois king, Louis Philippe to the throne. This immediately put a strain on the conservative powers of Europe, the Holy Alliance of Prussia, Russia and Austria. For the "Holy Alliance" Louis Philippe's ascension to the French throne undermined the "principle of legitimacy." Nowhere was pressure more evident than in Prussia. Czar Nicholas of Russia was Frederick William's son-in-law. He was determined to take action against France and expected his father-in-law's support.

Prussia's Foreign Minister, Christian Bernstorff, recognized Prussia was in no position to initiate a war against France even with Russian support. He was negotiating with the French ambassador to secure a peaceful recognition of France by Prussia. In England there was public support for peace. Louis was recognized as king by England on August 27, 1830.[2]

Metternich in Austria was not pleased. Nevertheless, Austria recognized Louis Philippe as king on September 8, 1830. In Prussia, the recognition of Louis was delayed because the king was not convinced by Bernstorff's arguments to recognize Louis. He finally relented and on September 9, 1830, recognized Louis as the French king.[3]

Russia refused to recognize Louis. Nicholas was convinced that the "revolution in France was a danger to his kingdom and his house."[4] The first dispatch from Prussia to the czar after the fall of the legitimate king, Charles X, in France, was that Prussia could not "mix in French internal affairs" but would "repel any attack ... [initiated by the French] ... with the greatest force."[5] Nicholas sent his emissary, Field Marshal Diebitsch, to Berlin with a letter outlining his concerns about the legitimacy of Louis Philippe. He included instructions that in the event of a war with France, Nicholas would aid Prussia and that the king should put its troops on a war footing.[6]

Diebitsch reached Berlin on the night of September 8, 1830. He was received by the King's Adjutant General, Job von Witzleben. This was a delicate time in Prussia's relations with France. His arrival was an embarrassment. Louis had just been recognized by Great Britain. Prussia was about to recognize him as well. Even so, Diebitsch instructions concerned military measures to be taken against France. He forwarded the czar's concerns to the Prussian Chief of the General Staff, General von Krauseneck. By this time, Prussia did not fear a "surprise attack" by the French. The king had received a letter from Louis stating that he wished "to maintain the peace of Europe."[7]

Diebitsch continued his "warlike" rhetoric and appeared before the members of the Prussian Cabinet stating that a general war between the legitimate powers and the "hydra of revolution" could not be avoided and would soon break out. Diebitsch wanted Prussia's cooperation with Russia to prepare for war.[8] The Prussian General Staff was not as confident as Diebitsch in its ability to fight an offensive war. Carl von Clausewitz had argued in 1819 that Prussia was better suited to "fight a defensive war" since its army, the *Landwehr* (militia) was more of a territorial armed force. Witzleben remarked when he heard of the July revolution in France that Prussia should not intervene "since the militia could not be called up for such a campaign."[9]

On August 25, 1830, revolution broke out in Brussels. When Frederick William was informed of this he stated that he was "committed to maintaining peace in Europe." He told his Chief of the General Staff, General von Krauseneck, that he "would resist a French attack, but would not interfere in the affairs of other states.[10] On October 11, 1830, following further revolutionary activities in Brussels and the Netherlands, Nicholas sent a note to Prussia and Austria requesting the establishment of a "barrier against revolution."[11] Nicholas was asked by the king of the Netherlands for assistance and replied that "the king of the Netherlands should not for a moment be in doubt, that Russia would hesitate in his request for assistance."[12] Prussia refused to act without the cooperation of England. On October 20, 1830, the English called for a conference to be held in London. It was agreed that Holland and Belgium be separated as decreed by King William of the Netherlands. The Prince of Orange was to be named General Governor of Belgium.[13] Nicholas was enraged by these decisions and from the beginning "viewed the Belgian revolution as part of a subversive threat to all of Europe."[14]

Diebitsch under orders from Nicholas continued his warlike talk in Prussia and advocated a "joint Russian-Prussian operation in Flanders." The king was even more uncomfortable with the Diebitsch mission. Bernstorff and Witzleben did their best to "neutralize the Russian field marshal's bellicose proposals."[15] Nicholas said he was "prepared to march 150,000 men into Western Europe."[16] It was unlikely that Nicholas could mobilize that many soldiers quickly. Secondly, there was little support by the other powers. Nicholas finally "agreed to support efforts to settle the Belgian question by the mediation of the great powers."[17]

In Russia preparations were underway for the "great campaign," a war against "revolutionary" France. This was a prospect that "No major leader, with the possible exception of Nicholas, contemplated ... with any enthusiasm."[18]

Diebitsch continued to plead with the king that he be permitted to return to Russia. The king was greatly concerned with his "appetite for war" Frederick knew that the Lithuanian corps, as well as two Reserve Corps were mobilized. Warsaw was already on a war footing. Diebitsch, the hero of the Russo-Turkish War in 1828–29, was to be appointed chief commander of the Russian troops. Diebitsch had been notified that troops would be ready for him to lead on January 1, 1831. The plan was to unite Russian troops with the Polish troops and march from the Prussian cities of Tilsit and Königsberg on the 'great road" to Berlin. Prussian troops were expected to join the Russian and Polish troops.[19]

In Berlin, it was feared that Russia's actions would not only "cause unrest in France and Belgium but England as well." Without a doubt the "execution of the Russian plan would inevitably lead to a general war."[20]

For Prussia, two events occurred one political, the Polish Insurrection and the other natural in origin, cholera. Both combined to prevent the Emperor's plan from going forward and dragging Prussia into a war that it seemed no one but Nicholas wanted.

On December 3, 1830, Diebitsch was informed by Count Bernstorff that on November 29, 1830, a revolution had broken out in Warsaw. The czar had a revolution in his kingdom, preventing him from proceeding with a war against France. Diebitsch left Berlin believing that he could count on Prussian support in suppressing the Polish insurrection.[21]

The second development that affected the czar's plans in a war against France was the outbreak of cholera. In 1830, the cholera was inexorably spreading from the east by way of the Caucuses, then along the navigable rivers through the rest of Russia, paralyzing trade and transport. When Nicholas attempted to put his troops on a war footing in November to attack France, he called up the Lithuanian third and fifth corps. The two units were stationed in the cholera infected eastern governments of Kherson (today in southern Ukraine) and Kursk. The troops were subsequently moved to the western boundaries of Russia to the governments of Podolien (today part of the Ukraine) and Wohlynien (today part of Poland) and temporarily stationed there. These troop movements "carried the cholera to these latter governments" and spread cholera to the Russian troops in the spring. These Russian troops infected the Polish troops.[22]

The international situation informed Prussia's cautious relationship with Russia and its stance toward revolutionary Poland. Poland exploited its relationship with revolutionary France, as well as garnering sympathy for the Polish cause in the East Prussian provinces. This sympathy was evident in the Polish territory recently ceded to Prussia following the Congress of Vienna in 1815. In Prussia, ethnic Poles and liberal intellectual and business groups were sympathetic to the Polish cause. Later Poland used Prussia's strict cholera quarantine policy as an opportunity to gain international sympathy for its own cause, while implementing a domestic sanitary policy designed more for political gain than for the protection of its citizens.

Polish Insurrection

The Polish Insurrection began on November 29, 1830, in Warsaw and was received with alarm by the Prussian king and his advisors. Prussian officials were concerned with the influence that the insurrection would have on the recently acquired "former Polish provinces now a part of Prussia."[23] The Prussian king responded to the threat by mobilizing four army corps under General Gneisenau and ordered them to the Grand Duchy of Posen in early December 1831.[24] The king informed the other European countries these were "precautionary measures" to secure the "Polish provinces."[25] There was no concern about cholera or its spreading to Poland during this initial call up. European opinion did not associate the spread of cholera into Poland until the Russian campaign in Poland in the spring of 1831.[26]

The Polish uprising was inspired by the July revolution in France. French radicals aware of czar's plan to begin a war against France and use the Polish army as an advance guard supported the Polish insurrection to prevent the Polish army from active involvement in the czar's plan.[27]

The plan to instigate the Polish revolt was to murder the Great Count Constantine, brother of the czar and disarm the Russian troops with the aid of the cadets at the officer's school. The plan failed.[28] On November 30, 1830, the Prussian General Consul in Warsaw, Julius Schmidt, reported that at seven o'clock in the castle of the Great Count Constantine twenty junior officers began the attack. Two people including the Police President were bayoneted to death. Fortunately, the cavalry arrived to save the Count and his wife. The entire Polish garrison was in on the plot. The arsenal was looted and the people armed. A government was established under Prince Adam Czarotoryski and Michael Radziwill. The next day the military stood aside while the mob plundered Warsaw. Finally the national militia restored order.[29] Count Constantine "offered no resistance and marched homewards with his Russian regiments."[30] Czarotoryski, a moderate was challenged by more radical elements in the government. Following failed negotiations with Nicholas, on January 25, 1831, the Polish government declared the Polish throne "forfeited" by Nicholas and "Poland separated from Russia."[31]

As early as December, Nicholas expected that it would be necessary to invade Poland and that he would have the support of Prussia and Austria. Count Alopeus, ambassador to the court in Berlin, delivered the following note on December 19, 1830, to Count Bernstorff:

> The governments of Prussia and Austria have without doubt heard of the news of the events that have taken place in Warsaw and taken the necessary measures to assure the peacefulness of their States and to impede the revolt and prevent its propagation in the former Polish provinces of the two monarchies. To this end and to neutralize at the same time the revolutionaries of Poland, it is of the utmost importance to forbid as much as possible contact between the Kingdom and the rest of Europe and intercept all communications that the rebellious Poles would be able to have with French agitators and agents acting as travelers.[32]

Nicholas wrote that he had prepared a resolution to adopt measures to "quickly isolate" the Kingdom of Poland from the other European states. He wished to know what measures Prussia intended to adopt so that Prussia's intentions "could be communicated back to the emperor's cabinet."[33]

Prussia, concerned with the former Polish province of Posen, had already issued a cabinet order on December 10, 1830, ordering its customs officials prohibit the export of "weapons, powder, lead and other war necessities."[34] Later other items were affected, like horses, food wagons and forage as these could be considered war related too. Eduard Heinrich Flottwell, provincial president of the Grand Duchy of Posen, decreed that "in trading areas ... legitimate travelers would be permitted to cross over the boundaries with horses as long as they used caution and displayed an authorized pass. Moreover, there were to be daily warnings against those who attempted to smuggle weapons, horses and munitions" as well as any other activities, "not expressly forbidden" but of a "mischievous" nature.[35]

The Prussian government had been unnerved by reports from Silesia and Posen. During the July Revolution in Paris, some inhabitants had greeted the revolution with "jubilation" and in no place was it more "festive" than in Posen. Some of the Posen noblemen had been in Paris and participated in the revolution. There was a report from Posen on November 16, 1830, about preparations for a "renewed Polish Kingdom."[36]

In December 1830, the Prussian government established a military cordon to prevent people traveling from Prussia to Poland to participate in the Polish uprising, and conversely to prevent agitators coming from Poland into Posen and Silesia. Prussia also issued orders to its customs agents along its border to prevent the smuggling of weapons and munitions.[37] On February 7, 1831, the Russian government responded to the Polish insurrection by sending a Russian army of 79,000 men under Field Marshal Diebitsch to march on Warsaw. In return the Polish Diet declared war.[38]

The Prussian ambassador to Russia, General Schöler, wrote, Diebitsch "had begun the war too early and with inadequate forces."[39] Nevertheless, Diebitsch marched on Warsaw. He defeated the main body of the Polish army on February 25, 1831, at the battle of Grochów. He did not complete his victory action and take Praga, "the bridgehead of the capital," which might have ended the war immediately. He was short on supplies and cholera had begun to appear among his troops. The Russian army retreated across a country "devoid of roads, an unexpected early thaw, and with cholera raging in its ranks."[40] On May 26, 1831, Diebitsch fought the Poles at the Battle of Ostroleka and for a second time he refused to follow-up his victory and finish off the Poles.[41]

In April, Frederick William wrote to his son-in-law, Nicholas that he had been following Diebitsch's operations and that he had complete "confidence ... that the valor of your troops and energy of their chiefs will ... obtain a decisive success."[42] Public opinion was not as supportive of the invasion as the king.[43] Alopeus had to exercise damage control in Prussia when an anti–Russian article appeared in the *Militär-Wochenblatt*. The author, a colonel on the Prussian General Staff, criticized Diebitsch and after analyzing the battle at Grochów wrote that the Poles "in the details of their tactics showed a much greater knowledge of combat."[44]

Diebitsch's inability to defeat the Poles was criticized in Prussia and Russia. Shortly before June 10, 1831, Nicholas' emissary, Count Orloff, met with Diebitsch under the pretext of discussing the provisioning of the Russian army. Orloff reported that the "Field Marshal was making preparations to carry out the czar's campaign plans."[45] On the night of June 10, 1831, Diebitsch became acutely ill. A few days previously, he had eaten his regular meal and gone to bed quietly. He awoke a few hours later "heavily discomfited." His physician was called. He diagnosed his illness as a case of cholera. Diebitsch died a few hours later. A rumor circulated immediately that he did not die from natural causes. In a letter to the czar on June 6, 1831, Diebitsch wrote of his "true devotion" to the czar. However, the czar replied in a "bitter and scoffing" letter to the Field Marshal asking why he had taken five weeks to cross the Vistula River. The letter did not reach Diebitsch before his death.[46]

Diebitsch's death was a shock to many in Europe and rumors were rampant that it had been arranged. These rumors were not quieted when Count Orloff returned to Berlin for further negotiations. He "showed little concern about Diebitsch's death, acted mysteriously and equivocated" on the matter. For the Russian army there was a smooth transition to General Ivan Paskievitch who it seemed had been waiting in the wings for this command.[47]

From the Russian viewpoint the quickness with which the Polish revolt spread across the entire Kingdom of Poland inhibited any attempt by the Russian government to prevent the spread of the cholera between these "two neighboring populations." One contemporary wrote that the "Russian government misjudged the moral sickness" of revolution as more of a threat than the "physical" sickness of cholera. This in turn led to the "unfortunate consequences" of the rapid spread of cholera into Poland by infected Russian soldiers.[48] The first cases of cholera among the Poles were identified after the Battle of Iganie on April 10, 1831, and occurred among Polish soldiers in the camps.[49]

Cholera in Poland

The first outbreak of cholera in Poland and the response to the epidemic had specific consequences for the Polish government and its relationship with Prussia. The government accepted a non-contagious policy with the support of its newly formed Central Health Committee. In turn, it criticized the Prussian quarantine policy on its border. To the western powers, the Polish government, military and medical establishment appeared to be united in their view that cholera was not contagious. The Polish government was able to take advantage of what appeared to be a united front. They vigorously complained that the Prussian *cordon sanitaire* on the Polish border was simply a ploy to prevent aid from France, England and the smaller German states from reaching Poland. Prussian policy was undermining the Polish insurrection.[50]

The sanitary policy in Poland was more nuanced than the Polish government's complaints against Prussia indicated. Internally the domestic sanitary policy was more complex and controversial. The immediate decision that "the cholera was not contagious" was based on the judgment of the doctors in Moscow. The decision was made without investigating the disease and was controversial and was opposed by two important military men—the Governor General of Warsaw and the Chief Medical officer of the Polish army—and a number of foreign doctors who advocated for contagion. It was argued at the time that Central Health Committee was influenced "by the country's internal situation" and this contributed to its decision.[51]

In late March and early April, there were a few reports of cholera in the Polish military. A number of doctors had deep suspicions. Initial medical investigations reported that there was no sign of cholera in Poland in early April. When cholera appeared, the quick acceptance that it was not contagious was seen as a means to relieve the anxiety and fear created by cholera. Others believed there were political considerations involved and the hasty decision was in "support of the insurrection."[52]

The immediate acceptance of the "Moscow doctor's judgment" also had a foreign policy advantage for Poland. Once the government made the decision to accept the opinion of the Central Health Committee and not implement quarantine policies in Poland, the latter was free, after Prussia imposed quarantine on its border, to criticize Prussia. Prussian sanitary policy was not viewed as a rational response to a non-contagious disease (as the Poles saw it) but as an impediment to travel and trade.[53]

The non-contagious pronouncement of cholera by Poland's leading health authority was desired by the Polish National Government because it would be useful to the revolutionary government of Poland in its international criticism of Prussia's strict border controls. Secondly, the government was able to garner international sympathy because of its obvious effect on the Polish war situation.[54]

The first observation of cholera in the Polish army was sent to Warsaw in early April. Two Polish doctors, Dr. Malcz (who was later appointed head of the Central Health Committee), and Dr. Woyde were sent from Warsaw to investigate the case. They returned on April 9, 1831, and reported "the rumor was unfounded."[55]

Dr. Carl Julius Remer traveled to Poland from Breslau to observe the cholera. He was critical of this report. He wrote, the government wanted "to suppress" the diagnosis of cholera as long as possible to avoid an anxious public. Remer did not doubt that the two doctors had observed a cholera patient, because the next day, April 10, 1831, he saw a case of cholera in the army in Warsaw. He wrote, there were "earlier cases of cholera," acknowledged primarily in the military, prior to the Battle of Iganie. Also, military physicians believed this sickness to be contagious. From the beginning, the question of the contagious nature of the cholera and how the medical community and the civilian authorities should respond to its origin, cause and how it spread was not settled.[56]

Dr. Leopold Leo, a doctor practicing in Warsaw, arrived at the hospital in Minsk to tend the wounded. He reported on April 10, 1831, that a Polish officer, a prisoner, at a Russian hospital in Minsk, had contracted cholera.[57] On April 16, 1831, a foreign physician, Dr. Bernstein, diagnosed cholera among Russian prisoners of war in the local hospital. He immediately informed the Polish Kingdom's General Medical Council in Warsaw.[58]

Meanwhile, on April 12, 1831, the Chief Medical Physician of the Polish army, Dr. Karol Kaczkowski, diagnosed cholera among the soldiers in Kałuszyn (near Minsk). He ordered isolation of the sick. He informed the General Medical Board in Warsaw of the cholera outbreak and the Commander in Chief of the army, General Jan Zygmunt Skrzynecki. General Skrzynecki had previously reported his cholera concerns to Warsaw. Several doctors warned the government that it should prepare to take precautions. Others argued that "not much could come from quarantine measures" and claimed "in this respect there was nothing to fear."[59]

Following the Battle of Iganie on April 10, 1831, General Skrzynecki received reports cholera had shown itself in a number of war prisoners from General Pahlen's corps. The prisoners had been removed but several had died. It seemed the disease was contagious. Another medical commission was sent to investigate. It returned to report there was no sign of the cholera. This finding was made known to the public, "and there was great joy in Warsaw." The joy did not last long. Soon after, Dr. Kaczkowski reported to the government cholera had broken out in the Polish army.[60]

Meanwhile, General Skrzynecki notified President Adam Czartoryski, that cholera was "already spreading in our army." Skrzynecki turned to the General Medical Council and asked what "precautionary" measures the government should take "to combat the ... epidemic." The General Medical Council was composed of four doctors, a pharmacist, the Minister of Health, the President of the National Militia, the Head of the military hospital, a priest and the Director General of the Commission on Internal and Police Affairs. They met on the evening of April 13, 1831. They initially based their decision that there was no need to immediately "observe precautionary measures" on the January 4, 1831, opinion of the Moscow doctors.[61]

At the same time, Dr. Kaczkowski's medical report on April 12, 1831, unsettled many of the doctors on the General Medical Council. They simply refused to believe cholera had spread to Poland. The next day the Council met to consider Kaczkowski's report. The Council ruled the description of "the symptoms for cholera were insufficient for a proper diagnosis. The doctors Malcz and Le Brun were dispatched to the headquarters of the army at Jędrzejów and the nearby village of Mienia. Doctors, Brandt, Fijalkowski and Wojdego were sent to Praga, a suburb of Warsaw, on the eastern side of the Vistula. The National Government sent the French doctors Brierre de Boismont and Le Gallois to a temporary cholera military hospital housed in a local convent in Mienia and directed by Dr. Kaczkowski.[62]

The delegation sent to Jędrzejów reported the outbreak was "sporadic cholera" and not the "epidemic Indian cholera" reported in Moscow. In a direct criticism of Dr. Kaczkowski, Dr. Malcz and Le Brun reported they did not consider the hospital in Mienia "properly equipped" nor did the patients have "adequate protection or proper care."[63] At Praga, the doctors observed that among the prisoners there were no cases of cholera but "stomach colds" as well as illnesses brought on by a lack of "clean drinking water." In both instances the delegations raised questions about the quality of care and medicines the sick were receiving.[64]

This disagreement between Dr. Kaczkowski and the members of the Council was a great embarrassment for the National Government. The French physician, Dr. Brierre de Boismont, who recently arrived in Poland with his colleague Dr. Le Gallois, observed that one of the reasons the Polish doctors could not agree on the nature of the sickness was due to the simple fact that none of the Polish doctors on the Medical Council had any direct experience with "epidemic cholera." They diagnosed the soldiers they observed with having more familiar military illnesses like typhus.[65]

But it was Dr. Brierre de Boisemont and Dr. Le Gallois who settled the matter between the Council and Dr. Kaczkowski. Neither French doctor had direct experience with "cholera morbus." Dr. Brierre de Boisemont later commented when he observed those sick from the disease that they were the same symptoms "reported in Russia."[66]

The two French physicians left on April 14, 1831, for the military hospital in Mienia to report on the cholera there and determine if the sickness was Asiatic cholera. From the beginning, Dr. Kaczkowski believed the sickness was Asiatic cholera and contagious. He "isolated cholera cases and organized the cholera hospital" in Mienia.[67]

After the two doctors arrived they met with Dr. Kaczkowski and Dr. Karol Marcinkowski. They performed autopsies on two cadavers with the cooperation of the two

Polish military doctors. After completing their examinations both returned to Warsaw convinced that the disease they had observed was Asiatic cholera.[68] They were sent to Praga afterwards, and found that among 400 patients many were suffering from cholera too.[69]

On April 16, 1831, the two doctors arrived at the government palace. In the presence of President Czartoryski, other government officials and doctors, they demanded the other physicians acknowledge their finding of Asiatic cholera.[70] They based their diagnosis on the autopsies performed at Mienia. They informed those assembled that Dr. Kaczkowski and Dr. Marcinkowski, witnessed the autopsies and agreed the disease was Asiatic cholera. The National Government was forced to accept the diagnosis of cholera and admit the disease was in Poland.[71] Dr. Boisemont later wrote that because he and Dr. Le Gallois had "warned the authorities of the country" of this disease, both were later awarded the "order of merit" by General Skrzynecki. Each was given seats on the newly established Central Health Committee.

The Government Commission for Internal and Police Affairs, concerned about the developing epidemic had recommended the creation of a Central Health Committee to protect the health of the civilian population and combat the epidemic.[72] The Polish National Government established the new Central Health Committee on April 18, 1831. It was to be subordinate to the General Medical Board. The following day on April 19, 1831, cholera erupted among the civilian population in Warsaw.[73]

The Central Health Committee was headed Dr. Wihelma Malcz, Medical Commander of the Polish National Militia in Warsaw who assumed his new office on April 21, 1831. Other members included doctors who served on the General Medical Board as well as civilian and military doctors.[74]

At this time, Dr. Remer reported that medical officials had been taking every opportunity "to declare cholera was infectious."[75] Now that cholera was officially diagnosed, the General Medical Board declared on April 19, 1831 "cholera was of a contagious nature." It recommended a *cordon sanitaire* however, "due to the war time situation it was recognized that the Russian army made such a procedure impossible."[76]

On April 23, 1831, the Central Health Committee, headed by Dr. Malcz, reversed the policy of the General Medical Board and announced cholera was not contagious. It based its opinion on Moscow doctors, who determined "cholera is not like the "plague, [it is] ... not as potent, but weaker."[77] It also published an announcement recommending dietary regulations. It advised the use of flannel abdominal belts to ward off the cholera (noting that over 30,000 belts had been distributed to the army). One contemporary physician, Dr. Hille, from Breslau, believed that many of the members of the Central Health Committee were convinced that the cholera was contagious, "but fear of cholera" was for them "worse than the disease itself." He wrote, in the beginning most doctors removed themselves from caring for the cholera sick. Initially, in a report from the Central Health Committee to the city of Warsaw on April 22, 1831, its recommendations were "contagious in nature and included limiting large assemblies of people, quick burial of the dead without services in a special cemetery, fumigation and purification of the effects of the dead with chlorine gas."[78]

These proposals were not carried out because of the recommendations later published by the Central Health Committee on April 23. Hille did not agree with the new policy. He believed these proposals had been effective in the past. But the public embraced the "new view" and basic police sanitary regulations could not be implemented. For example, at the beginning of the epidemic, houses containing the sick were to be quarantined but this "was soon done away with."[79]

Polish civilian physicians were undoubtedly influenced by the many foreign physicians arriving in Poland with the view that cholera was not contagious. This opinion was also supported by the Moscow doctors and articulated by Dr. Malcz. The opinion of the General Medical Council of the Polish Kingdom was immediately overturned and that of the Central Health Committee became the official position. One French physician later wrote, the Central Health Committee "could not see the necessity of cutting off communications" with the infected, this decision prevailed on the orders of the Polish government. He concluded, "God save us from medical radicalism born of political radicals."[80]

Nevertheless, some Polish military physicians were not convinced that this was the right course. They did not accept the Central Health Committee's decisions. Dr. Karol Kaczkowski continued to act on the belief that the cholera was contagious. Throughout the epidemic he established military hospitals, separate military camps and isolated cholera

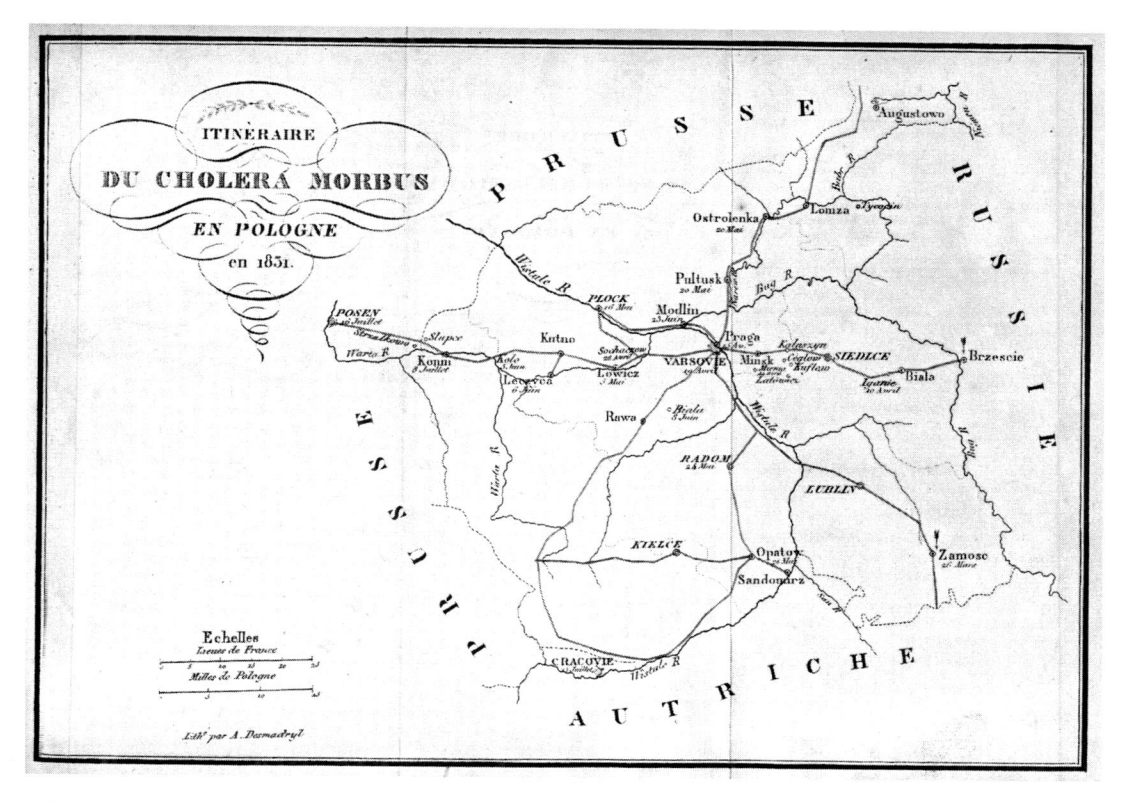

"Itinèraire du Cholera Morbus en Pologne en 1831."(Route of Cholera Morbus in Poland in 1831). Map shows the dates that cholera broke out in various cities in Poland and its progress through Poland to the Prussian city of Posen on July 16, 1831. Reproduced from Brierre de Boismont, A. *Relation Historique et Médicale du Cholera Morbus de Pologne*, Paris, 1832.

cases in these military hospitals and camps. He did this in the face of opposition from later decrees and threats by the Central Health Committee.[81]

Questioning the Sanitary Policy of the National Government and the Central Health Committee

While the Polish National Government and Central Health Committee were staunch supporters of non-contagion, this opinion was not shared by Polish officials in all quarters. At first there was confusion over the initial regulations of the Central Health Committee. They first forbade the public from gathering in cafes, taverns and tobacco shops. According to Brierre de Boisemont, the measures were not enforced because there was no demonstrated link between exposure to cholera and direct contagion. Still other directives were derived from older sanitary police guidelines. The streets were to be cleaned and no burning of refuse in the streets was permitted. Hospitals were organized to receive the sick. A central facility was established to hold stretchers. Porters were hired to transport the sick (primarily the poor and workers). The police were instructed to visit the dwellings of the poor and the Jews, because it is in these places that one sees the "ravages the cholera makes among individuals who live in these cramped and humid places." It was forbidden to sell spoiled meat, new beer and dead fish. Specific times were arranged to transport corpses. There was to be a minimum of religious fuss, special cemeteries and burial arrangements were issued for the cholera victims. Instructions for fumigating the effects of the dead were issued. Although the published regulations of the Central Health Committee concluded that cholera was not contagious, the committee recommended the sick be separated from the healthy. This led to confusion on the part of the public and the physicians.[82]

The Central Health Committee clarified its position, on May 10, 1831. Dr. Malcz announced the disease was not contagious and isolating the sick only spread the disease. More needed to be done to give "immediate medical help" to the sick.[83]

The Governor General of Warsaw

When the cholera first broke out in the Polish army, the Governor General of Warsaw, Jan Krukowiecki, ordered a quarantine of the city on April 14, 1831. He separated the military from the civilians to prevent the disease from spreading into Warsaw. He ordered any soldiers who became sick in the city to be taken to the suburb of Praga and established a camp in Powazki where sick soldiers received care.[84] Prisoners of war were to be placed in strict isolation and quarantine was imposed on the right bank of the Vistula, "three sentry lines deep."[85]

The Polish National Government reversed his orders. Krukowiecki was informed that "the capital and the army are one camp, and the military and the civilian population should be put equally at risk." Only Russian prisoners were to be put in quarantine at Praga.[86]

Krukowiecki realized that the implementation of quarantine would have been a great embarrassment to the National government. Current medical opinion had "pronounced against the strict isolation of the sick." He had no choice but to stand down. Yet, once cholera broke out in Warsaw and accounting for the unsanitary conditions in the city, he had many of the sick in Warsaw brought to the camp in Powazki. Others remained isolated in their homes.[87]

The Central Medical Committee was allocated a sum of 50,000 złoty to "organize services" to combat the epidemic. In Warsaw, General Krukowiecki actively participated in the "struggle against the cholera." He opened hospitals in the military camps at Praga and Powazki to treat those ill from cholera. He established an additional hospital in Warsaw to treat the sick. The city was divided into eight medical sections with a surgeon in charge of each as well as assistants to help in transporting the sick. Due to popular unrest in Warsaw, he asked that the Central Health Committee issue medical advice immediately to deal with the impending epidemic. The Central Health Committee distributed its new regulations as previously noted to help calm the public.[88]

The Central Health Committee regulations to assist the public were primarily of a sanitary nature. Some measures advocated quarantining the sick. They were virtually ignored or harshly criticized, but also caused confusion. Due to the uncertainty of how the cholera spread, the Central Health Committee recommended establishing a hospital for the cholera sick on the left bank of the Vistula to avoid transporting the sick into Warsaw. According to Dr. Brierre de Boisemont, the committee was harshly criticized for this measure by two foreign physicians, Dr. Leo and Dr. Foy (both later appointed to the Central Health Committee on June 17, 1831).[89]

The Central Health Committee's measures to establish hospitals and whether or not to transport the cholera sick to the hospitals led to much confusion in Warsaw. General Krukowiecki attempted to intervene and bring some order to the situation. He requested the National Government appoint Count Henry Zabiello, who had supervised a 500 bed hospital at the Powazki camp to the Central Health Committee. He requested Zabiello be given executive authority. Although Zabiello was appointed to the committee on May 2, 1831, his position was only advisory. Krukowiecki asked that Count Zabiello be given the deciding vote on the committee. On May 5, 1831, the Government decreed that the Central Health Committee had controlling authority on all matters pertaining to cholera. Krukowiecki argued against the decree and said that the committee members had made damaging claims against him and Dr. Kaczkowski (see below) and that the committee should be addressing the concerns of the hospitals. He suspected the committee did not want to share "credit for combatting the epidemic." The National Government did not change the decree. Zabiello resigned at the end of May.[90]

Krukowiecki was not able to exercise the control over the Central Health Committee that he blatantly sought through the appointment of Count Zabiello. He undoubtedly believed that by bringing more military order he could also re-introduce some of the older sanitary measures (note his ongoing support of the military physician Dr. Kaczkowski, who was in fact doing this and earning the enmity of the Central Health Committee).

Nevertheless, he increased his efforts to bring order and accountability to fighting the epidemic. He organized the large metropolitan hospitals. He personally inspected these hospitals and held the staffs accountable. He publically acknowledged the mistakes of hospital officers, domestics, doctors and apothecaries. He had doctors arrested and sentenced. His contribution to combatting the epidemic was recognized later by the Military Governor's Office in Warsaw.[91]

Dr. Kaczkowski and the Central Health Committee

Dr. Kaczkowski, Physician in Chief of the Polish Armies, found himself in conflict with the Central Health Committee. Early in April, after the Battle of Iganie and the outbreak of cholera, Kaczkowski wrote that he saw hundreds of soldiers in despair. They did not despair because they might die in battle. That would be a contribution to victory for their country, but because they might die from an ignoble disease. To maintain the spirit of the troops, the Supreme Commander, General Skrzynecki, looked to Dr. Kaczkowski to fight the epidemic. His success in this endeavor helps to explain the prominent role he played in fighting cholera and the independent role he carved out *vis a vis* the Central Health Committee. His success came from recognizing that cholera was probably of an infectious nature. This resulted in recommending hygienic measures that were in opposition to the views of the Central Health Committee.[92]

From the beginning, Kaczkowski was at odds with the Central Health Committee. On April 14, 1831, he issued a pamphlet to the military *News on the Cholera*. He discussed various chlorine preparations for disinfecting the sick and their effects. He called on doctors to perform their duties and advocated isolating the sick. On May 1, 1831, he ordered all regiments appoint a health inspector. On May 2, he ordered the "burning and destruction of all Russian camps" because the incidence of cholera increased after Polish soldiers bivouacked in the former Russian camps. However, the greater criticism from the Central Health Committee was reserved for the military doctors under his authority, who tended to the sick in the military hospitals in Warsaw, Praga and Powazki. The death rates were excessive in these hospitals. The Health Committee blamed the high mortality on "bad conditions and disorganization."[93]

Kaczkowski replied that the doctors were working under severe conditions. There were no cases of negligence. The death rate was high because there was no first aid given to the sick before they were brought to the hospitals and there were not enough doctors. Additionally, there were not enough cards with medical instructions printed for patients and the doctors. Doctors did not have the time to write out medical instructions in the field for their patients. He concluded that "he was sorry but he did not feel guilty," or forced to explain his conduct. As proof of his work he told the committee to look at the circulars, notes and letters he had issued.[94]

General Kruckowiecki came to his defense. He wrote to the National Government that the General Medical Council and Central Health Committee were not pursuing their proper tasks. Military doctors worked in hospitals while civilian doctors selected "a few hospitals in the middle of the city, with stop-watch in hand ... [he could have confused a stop-watch with a pulse watch] ... or in hospitals where they purposely did not have to spend a lot of time."[95]

The conflict with the Central Health Committee continued. On June 19, 1831, Kaczkowski traveled to Modlina to investigate an outbreak of cholera in an infantry regiment. While he was gone a delegation from the Central Health Committee, Dr. Foy and Dr. Leo inspected the hospital in Miena. They returned to Warsaw and reported "the patients in Mienia were not given proper care or support as indicated in his report and those that were cured were not suffering from cholera."[96]

Kaczkowski was highly indignant. He wrote, he would never betray the public or the Government's trust in him nor would he "blemish science with absurd lies."[97] He had "immediately recognized the infectivity of cholera and for the duration of the epidemic recommended the strictest isolation of sick soldiers." The good health of the lower ranks was due to his "positions and orders" to the troops. His management of the troops was in opposition to directives of the Central Health Committee and the non-contagion view the National Government advocated.

By May, the Central Health Committee ruled that cholera was "transported by the air." This view played into the plans of the National Government as it was preparing to launch its verbal attacks against the Prussian border quarantine policy. It stood to reason, if cholera was spread by air then quarantines and isolation policies were ineffective. However, Kaczkowski continued his "isolation" policy in the face of civilian opposition because of the support of General Skrzynecki. Kaczkowski later wrote that when he was first given responsibility for the troops to combat the cholera it seemed "the life of the entire army moved to accommodate me and my subordinates." It appears that the General's support did not waiver in his chief physician as long as he saw improved general health among his soldiers.[98]

Kaczkowski was later presented with the Polish Legion of Honor for his work during the epidemic. One historian noted that he should not only be recognized for his fight against cholera but the positive effect on the Polish military campaigns as well.[99] Kaczkowski later attributed his success against the cholera in 1831 to the fact that "God had apparently blessed the sincere and preserving steps we doctors ... took, because the epidemic weakened each day and finally ended."[100]

The epidemic in the Polish Kingdom was of interest to all the European governments. The various diplomatic missions asked the Polish National Government about its progress. The Central Health Committee issued reports on its progress every five days to the Polish Foreign Office.[101]

On April 27, 1831, the Prussian Minister of the Interior and Police made a series of inquiries to the Polish Minister of Foreign Affairs asking what information could be supplied about cholera, the establishment of hospitals and other means that the Poles were taking to combat the disease. Dr. Malcz reported on the number of cholera victims in Polish hospitals. For example, the military hospital at Mienia had 612 patients, 54 healed, 29 dead and 230 in recovery. One would expect a 50 percent mortality rate for cholera under these circumstances if all those who were sick actually had the disease. It is likely that the death rates had been minimized for political purposes in the hope the Prussian government would not erect a strict quarantine on its border.[102] Secondly, Malcz reported, with a political purpose in mind, that the "source of cholera was a miasma in the atmosphere."[103] He wrote, there had been observations cholera could be spread by "contact with dead bodies." The Central Health Committee was "not convinced that this malady was spread in this manner."[104]

On the Polish side, this early in the epidemic, opinion concerning the contagious nature of the cholera and the most effective means to combat the epidemic was not settled. However, there is no mention of this divided opinion in the document sent to the Prussian Minister of Interior and Police. The initial decision not to establish a Polish quarantine was not based on medical evidence but that the "capital city was in a revolutionary mood … it could scarcely enforce strict health regulations." Quarantine measures were simply unenforceable with the Russian army in the Polish territory.[105]

On May 10, 1831, Malcz made public the Central Health Committee's decision that the cholera was spread through a "miasma in the atmosphere," and that cholera was not contagious. One doctor wrote that this "insight" was "desired by the government," the "hope of the nation" and based on the "observations" of its medical officials.[106] This decision came shortly after the imposition of a sanitary cordon by Prussia. The Polish National Government used the strict quarantine policy to accuse Prussia in the international press of overreacting to cholera and acting in bad faith, especially in light of the Polish insurrectionary struggle.

While the Polish National Government attempted to present a united front on this question, there was not total agreement for the non-contagionist position in Poland. It was demonstrated in the views of the Governor General of Warsaw and the Chief Physician of the Polish Army. Their views were not for public consumption. It was the official voice of the Central Health Committee in conjunction with the Polish National Government that took precedence over any opposition voices to anti-contagion.

Some of the conflict among the Central Health Committee and a Polish doctor like Dr. Kaczkowski can also be attributed to the influx of over 200 foreign doctors who were invited into Poland by the National Government to help with the epidemic.[107] To be fair to the Polish government, the Kingdom of Poland only contained 335 physicians and 105 army surgeons. In Warsaw there were 76 physicians and 20 army surgeons or about "one physician to 12 thousand citizens."[108] The number of military doctors responsible for 80,000 soldiers included 4 division doctors, 22 staff doctors and 85 battalion doctors.[109]

The Government recognized that the nation was in a medical crisis and called for international assistance. General Lafayette headed up the call in Paris under the auspices of the Polish Committee, in London the Polish Legation and in Berlin the famous surgeon Karl Ferdinand von Graefe (who had been born in Poland and was sympathetic to the cause of his homeland). Graefe was both a Co-Director of the Charité hospital in Berlin and Physician to the General Staff of the Prussian Army. When foreign doctors first arrived they were greeted with "enthusiasm." The Polish War Commission "spared them no honor." Polish doctors were forced "to cede their posts in the lazarets of Warsaw to foreign physicians and they were sent to less desirable posts in the provinces." Many foreign doctors were "not up to task." Well known doctors like Graefe and the English doctor Charles Searle with his

Indian experience, continued to receive the respect of the Polish doctors but it quickly became clear that many foreign doctors lacked the appropriate credentials. In a meeting of the Council of Polish Physicians, the French physician, Dr. Foy, admitted that many of his fellow countrymen were lacking the "technical knowledge" or their "credentials were simply false."[110] This concerned the Prussian government and it later claimed that many of these doctors were simply French officers who traveled to Poland to support the Polish revolt.[111] Among those who at first received the foreign doctors with enthusiasm were the local doctors themselves. Soon many misunderstandings occurred between the two groups resulting in a decision by the Polish War Commission to prevent more French doctors from coming into Poland.[112]

The general population of Warsaw and the other cities of Poland were not as convinced as many of the civilian and foreign doctors that cholera was not contagious. By the end of May, many suspected cholera had been imported into the Prussian city of Danzig by Russian ships. The Polish public accused the Russians of "taking an unknown plague for their ally" and even the Polish government by June 1, 1831, publically accused the Emperor of Russia of obtaining an ally to assist him in the "work of exterminating the Polish people."[113]

By June, the insurrection began to go badly for the Poles. The new Russian commander, Field Marshal Ivan Paskievitch, had received reinforcements in late spring and early summer. Cholera among the Russians had begun to recede. The Polish government protested to Berlin that Prussian border authorities were using "quarantine regulations to restrict and contain the movement of Polish citizens, to interfere with the Polish war effort, and to spy on Poland." The Poles said of Prussia:

> they were using sanitary regulations to support the Russian intervention and further ... at the end of April, when the cholera appeared in our countries, the Prussian government hastened to make it a pretext for developing means still more detrimental and even hostile in regard to us, since, on the other side, those methods favored our enemies.[114]

In a "Circular" dated June 1, 1831, the Polish government attempted to gain support from the other European powers by taking a somewhat ambiguous position. The Polish government recognized that "Preventive measures, cordons sanitaire, quarantine, these will be of no use." The circular then oddly stated that "the physicians of Berlin have lately made a report upon the Cholera, which demonstrates that all precautions will be useless, and that there is nothing but a cessation of hostilities which can avert from Europe the dangers that threaten her."[115]

The Poles added that it was Count Pahlen's Russian troops that "brought the Cholera into Poland ... [and] ... the contagion, therefore, is general in the Russian army, and each contact with any body [sic] of the enemy is dangerous."[116]

The Polish government argued cholera originally in Turkey was established in Russia. The only way to prevent the danger from spreading into the rest of Europe was for Russia to cease hostilities in Poland. The Polish government wanted other European Powers to assist them in halting the hostilities to prevent the plague. They advised them cholera was "advancing towards the west" and threatened "every state." After all, according to the Polish government, Russia had used the excuse of preventing the spread of plague to go to war against Turkey in the past.[117]

In a "Note" from the Polish Ministry of Foreign Affairs to the Cabinet in Berlin, dated July 16, 1831, Prussia was accused of being too strict in its quarantine measures. The Polish government seemed willing to advocate whatever policy suited the revolutionary cause. In return it applied its own "self-serving" motives to Prussia.[118]

The Prussian Polish Border

While the Polish government did not have the complete support of its military doctors or even the public regarding how cholera spread, the Government continued to endorse the miasmic view. As a practical matter this permitted it to call for open borders and criticize Prussia for implementing a policy to protect its citizens from cholera, not as medical precaution, but to subvert the Polish revolt.

This brings us to the question of the timing of the implementation of the strict sanitary regulations on the Prussian-Polish border. Some historians have uncritically accepted the Polish position and blamed Prussia for taking advantage of the cholera threat. They argue that its policy helped to thwart the Polish insurrection by erecting a *cordon sanitaire* along the Prussian-Polish border. The Prussian government had argued that "Prussia did not attempt to be impartial toward Poland." The Prussian Foreign Minister Bernstorff, said "Prussia was an ally of Russia, not a neutral." As late as April 1831, Frederick William ordered Provincial President Schön to allow the Russian army to buy supplies in East and West Prussia and to have "access to goods in every possible way." He also ordered the "confiscation of all property belonging to any Pole residing in Posen who would cross into to Poland to fight in the rebel army." The Poles also charged that the Prussian authorities provided materials and an engineer to assist "in building a bridge across the river near Złoty."[119]

Polish opinion was that cholera "offered opportunities to neighboring powers, especially Prussia, to harass the Polish government with increasingly stringent frontier regulations." They believed the policy was political in nature and not medical.[120] The Prussian government argued that "in April-May at the outbreak of cholera, a continuous boundary cordon was put in place and traffic blockaded. "Although Poland was inconvenienced by these strict ... regulations they were necessary to "hold off the sickness ... at the border." Besides, "nothing was done on the Polish side to prevent the disease from spreading. The assumption that Prussia had not prevented the cholera but established the cordon on the boundary on a political basis is so easily exposed and visible, it must be dismissed out of hand as absurd."[121]

The regulations developed by the Cholera Commission in Prussia in January 1831 were not announced until April 5, 1831. Prior to this time, the disease was not an immediate threat. Members of the commission realized to have issued the regulations prematurely would have caused a panic. The regulations were sent to the provincial presidents of Prussia, Posen and Silesia in April.[122] They primarily targeted customs officials who were instructed to apply a limited quarantine to all people and goods exposed to the disease. Individuals had to present a health pass when traveling or face quarantine. A quarantine of Prussian harbors was imposed. Initially, these regulations were directed against Russia.[123]

3. *Cholera in Poland*   55

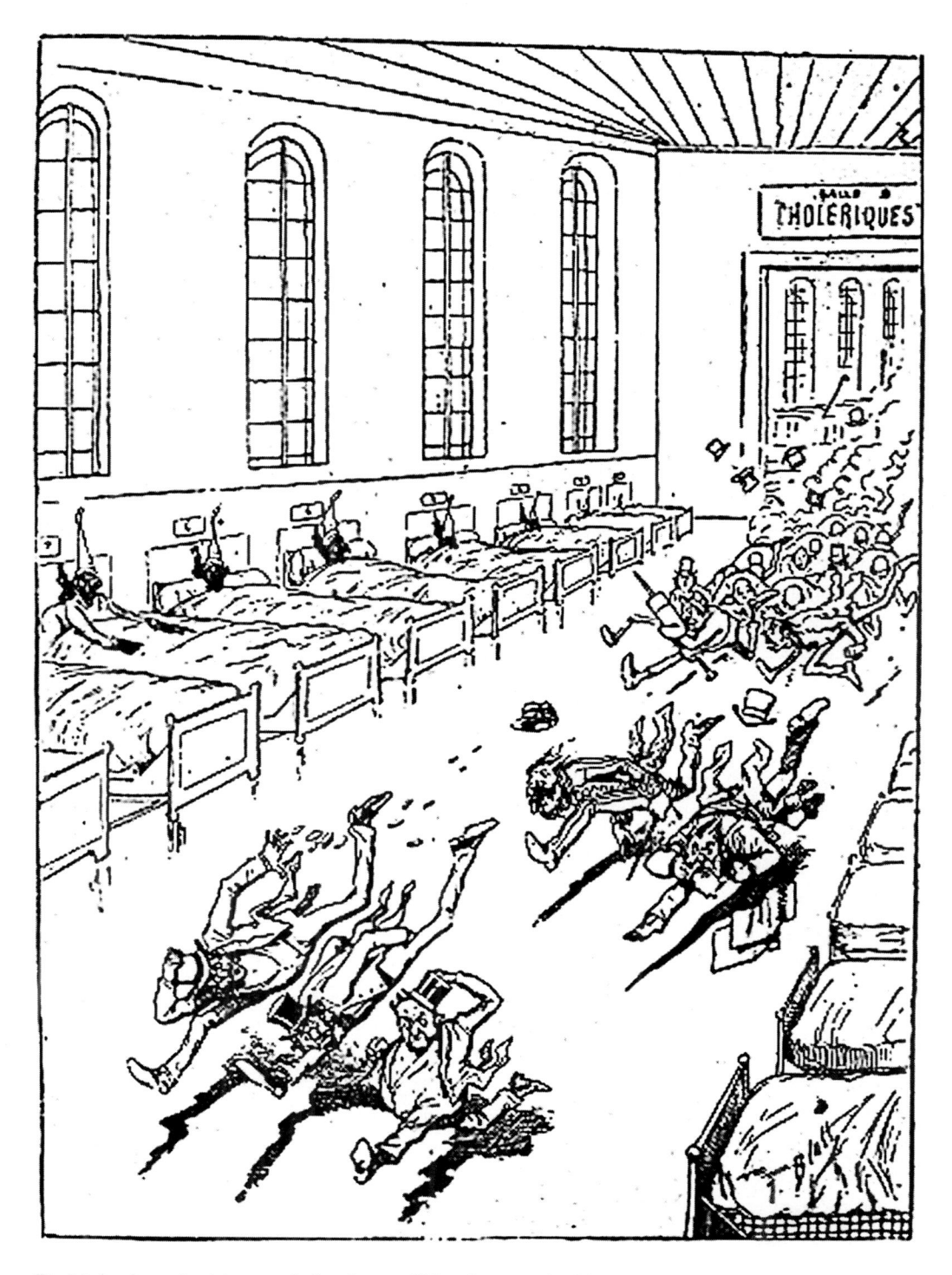

"A visit by the authorities to a cholera hospital," by Blass, 1884. Although a later caricature, the sentiment expressed about physicians and officials was not uncommon in the 1831 cholera epidemic (Courtesy of the Wellcome Library, London).

The military situation on the Prussian-Polish border at the beginning of the epidemic in Poland was still based on the original orders given to General Field Marshal Gneisenau. He was sent to the Grand Duchy of Posen and given chief command of the armies on the Polish border. On April 27, 1831, he wrote to his generals that cholera had spread to the Polish army and to Warsaw.[124] This news was reported to Berlin. He requested the Ministry of the Interior and the Ministry of Religion, Education and Medical Affairs impose quarantine between the Kingdom of Poland and The Grand Duchy of Posen.[125] Gneisenau was concerned that the disease would spread outside quarantine facilities. He was frustrated by the laxness of the civilian border guards. He privately recommended the military take over all responsibility for border patrols (during this epidemic) and in this way the cordon would "be effective." On April 29, he proposed a military cordon plan that he sent to General Witzleben. He wrote, in this way the "object of a plague cordon could be fulfilled."[126]

Gneisenau wrote to General Krafft on May 3, that cholera was spreading in Poland and President Flottwell requested they "isolate the borders against the Kingdom of Poland" and "establish quarantine facilities." Gneisenau told Krafft that even without official orders he had developed a plan for a military quarantine of the border. He only informed the War Ministry and the General Command of these measures and to please "bear this in mind."[127]

His plan was to cordon off the roads between Posen and Poland. He estimated 200 roads would need to be manned. He would need to, employ 1,200 men or three battalions for this purpose. His major concerns were scheduling and rotation. He also estimated that to do the same for Silesia and Prussia (the province) would require 1,000 and 3,000 men respectively.[128]

On May 3, 1831, Gneisenau wrote to Genera Witzleben he had learned the king had appointed a commission to prevent the spread of the cholera and that this commission was to be headed by General Thile. Gneisenau wrote, it was his duty to "anticipate orders" and hoped the commission would now "take the proper steps" that he had been recommending.[129]

The responsibility for enforcing the regulation of April 5, 1831, since the beginning of May had fallen to the "customs officials, police and men in the villages in the districts on the boundary." Yet, without military support there was little these overworked officials could do to enforce them. On May 20, 1831, the Prussian military was assigned to implement the sanitary cordon on Prussia's eastern border.[130] There were no orders issued from Berlin to erect a *cordon sanitaire* or a strict blockade of the Polish border until the first meeting of the Immediate Commission on May 5, 1831.[131]

The Prussian response rested solely on the fear of the cholera reaching Prussia. No responsible Minister, Provincial President or General had recommended a sanitary blockade of the boundaries in order to politically isolate Poland. Until the first meeting in early May of the Immediate Commission medical policy in Prussia was to some extent decentralized. The Scientific Deputation and later the Cholera Commission were responsible for the medical sections of cholera policy. The Cholera Commission coordinated actions with the Medical Department in Altenstein's Ministry. The sanitary policy was the responsibility of the Ministry of the Interior. It was up to provincial presidents and local officials to enforce sanitary policy. There was no overt military support on the border prior to the later orders of the Immediate Commission.

Gneisenau was critical of local border control and what he saw was as a lack of strict security on the Posen border. Only after receiving the recommendation of the Doctors Commission that the cholera was contagious did the Prussian government respond by calling the first meeting of the Immediate Commission to begin to officially coordinate the Prussian State ministries and the military to combat the cholera. The Immediate Commission was contagionist from the outset, an opinion vigorously advocated by the Chief medical official in Prussia, Dr. Rust.

Nevertheless, the Polish government supported the non-contagious position for strategic reasons and it obtained the endorsement of the foreign physicians mentioned above (Foy, Graefe, and Searle) as well as prominent Polish members of the Central Health Committee. This opinion played into the hands of the Polish government in its response to the Prussian sanitary policy accusing Prussian officials of "chicanery" in support of the Russian war effort.[132]

The quarantine regulations implemented by Prussia engendered "plenty of anger and hostility" by the western powers in support of Poland. Later after numerous complaints by the Polish government, that included using "cholera as a pretext for the damaging border closure of Poland" and "establishing a sanitary cordon blocking the border for residents and their goods," the Poles charged this was a violation of the Treaty of Vienna.

These complaints resulted in a public relations nightmare for Prussia. Later on September 20, 1831, privy councilor Eichhorn, in the Prussian Foreign Ministry, wrote to Provincial President Flottwell of Posen these "fiercest and most passionate attacks" on Prussia, have certainly not escaped your attention, especially in the French and English papers." These attacks "probably have their foundation in the work of the rebel leaders in Warsaw and by their representative in Paris and London."[133] Flottwell was asked to answer them because he knew the Polish language and was in "possession of ... completely trustworthy material as well as knowing the true ... facts."[134]

The Prussian position was decidedly different from the Polish view of Prussia's policy toward Poland. The strict quarantine measures enacted by Prussia were seen at the time "as a pretext to simply close the Polish boundaries" and "prevent Polish inhabitants and their cargoes from crossing the border in violation of the Treaty of Vienna."[135] The accusations that the cordon against Poland was part of a "political game to support Russia and inhibit the Polish revolt" were stated by one Polish general at the time. His view has been echoed well into the twentieth century by Polish historians and others who view the sanitary cordon on the Prussian-Polish border in 1831 as a political-military measure, rather than a sanitary measure to protect Prussia from cholera.[136]

The contagionist medical policy introduced in Prussia was based on an agreement among the medical officials of the Prussian Kingdom. It was not based on or used as a hostile act toward Poland during the insurrection. Once cholera erupted in Prussia there was a serious effort to create policies to administer the Prussian borders. Additionally, the commission developed internal policies to prevent the spread of cholera in Prussia as harsh as those on the border.

The Prussian government was excessive in its medical administrative measures. These regulations included minute and detailed instructions concerning boundary cordons, quarantine establishments, the isolation of the sick, trade restrictions, travel restrictions, and the establishment of cholera hospitals. Penalties for disobeying were harsh.

This is all consistent with an almost overwhelming amount of documentation that shows that Prussian officials were seriously concerned with the disease itself. The subject matter discussed almost exclusively concerned medical and sanitary policy with officials trying to determine the most effective means of preventing the introduction of cholera into Prussia. Once cholera was introduced officials focused on how to limit its spread among the public, how to care for those who became ill, and finally to discover cholera's cause and how it spread.

4

First Response to Cholera: Misery in Danzig

On December 3, 1830, Provincial President Schön received the news that cholera was approaching the Prussian border. The report was sent to Minister Altenstein and from there to the king. The Prussia government was placed in a difficult diplomatic position. Prussia had promised to render aid to Russia to help it suppress the Polish revolt. That support would now depend on the sanitary policy Prussia was preparing to take concerning cholera. As late as May 13, 1831, the king had ordered his government to offer assistance to the Russian army in order for it to obtain badly needed supplies.[1]

Once cholera breached the Prussian border and the Immediate Commission took charge of the situation, there was a serious effort to create strict external and internal policies to prevent its spread. The Prussian government came to be viewed by its own people as "fanatical" and "unyielding," especially after the public gained more experience with cholera. This experience gave rise to internal opposition over the strict blockades, the use of health certificates, regulations concerning burials, the forced sequestering of the sick and inflexible quarantine measures. For those sympathetic to the Polish plight, cholera was seen as a "welcome pretext for complicating all measures which King Frederick William III had arranged for the benefit of Russia." For others, Prussia's response was an excuse to prevent material help from the western powers reaching Poland.[2]

With the cabinet order of January 5, 1831, the Prussian king had established a defense commission against cholera. On May 3, 1831, Major General von Thile was appointed head of the former defense commission, re-named the Immediate Commission to Prevent Cholera. General Thile was given "almost sovereign authority to execute the decisions of the Commission." The commission was established to unify the entire administrative process and "prevent disturbances and a loss of time through correspondence and discussions between the ministries involved." The commission met for the first time on May 5, 1831.[3]

The Immediate Commission consisted of government and ministerial councilors. The most prominent was Chief medical officer, Doctor Johann Nepomuk Rust, who was responsible for formulating the medical and sanitary policies for the Immediate Commission. Other departments represented included the Ministry of Religion, Education and Medical Affairs, the Ministry of Foreign Affairs, the Ministry of War, the Ministry of the

Interior and the Ministry of Trade and Industry. The representatives from each of the Ministries were responsible for the cholera measures and communicating with their respective ministries.

Physicians from the "Technical Section" of the Ministry of Religion, Education and Medical Affairs included army staff doctor Chief Medical Councilor von Wiebel, Professor Wagner and Medical Councilors Horn, Klug, Koenen and Link. The main duty of the latter group was to develop cholera defense priorities and appropriate therapies. Sanitary police measures were the responsibility of the Ministry of the Interior.[4]

The principle powers on the commission were two strong willed men—Major General Thile, and Dr. Rust.[5] Thile was described as a man who "...issues cabinet orders in a military like manner ... as for the rest, he puts it in his piety and God's hands."[6] Rust was such a stubborn advocate of contagion that Provincial President Schön later declared that he did not just fight against the contagion policy, but also "Rust's insane cholera regulations ... [in] ... 1831."[7]

As noted previously, the official reason for the creation of the commission was the outbreak of cholera in Poland following the Battle of Iganie on April 10, 1831. The commission was expected to function as a central authority in responding to the disease. It was empowered to issue orders to the generals, provincial presidents and had the authority to establish a "strict military cordon."[8]

The first meeting of the commission took place in Berlin on May 5, 1831. The question before the commission concerned proposing quarantine regulations on the Russian border. These regulations were recommended earlier to police and customs officials following measures drafted in January 1831 by the Technical Medical Section, but not published until April 5, 1831. They were primarily for customs officials, consuls, etc., and included instructions for quarantine officials, disinfection procedures for persons, animals and commodities traveling from cholera infected regions and regulations for the introduction of health certificates. These measures had been originally drafted in the event that the cholera proved contagious.[9]

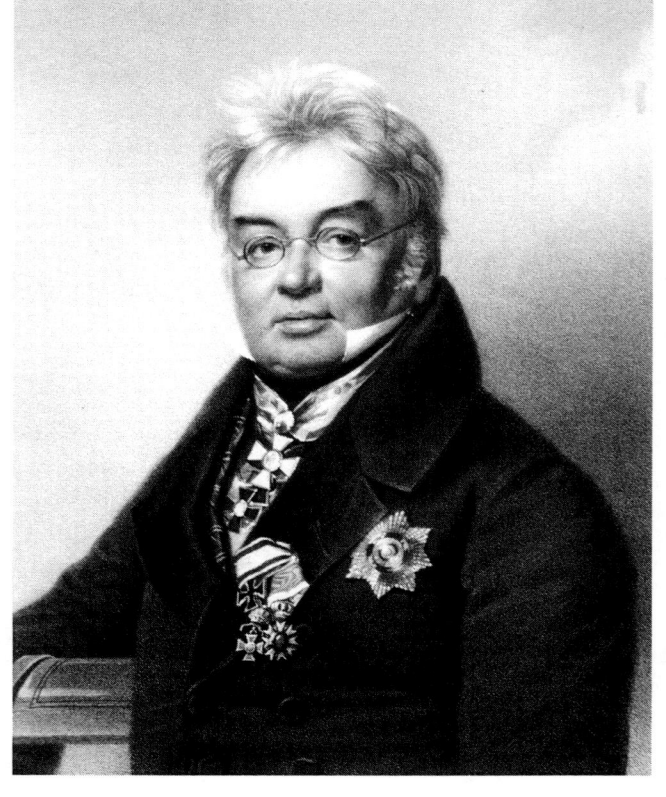

"Dr. Johann Nepomuk Rust." Lithograph by F. Krüger (Wellcome Library, London).

4. First Response to Cholera

The commission grappled with the question as to whether the two week quarantine between the Memel and Niemes Rivers on the Prussian-Russian Lithuanian border should be implemented. There had been no major outbreaks of cholera in this region. The hope at this early stage was that the area could be used to continue to communicate with St. Petersburg and remain open to couriers. Prussian officials were urged to be diligent. The minutes reflect that in the event of a cholera outbreak in Russian Lithuania, due to the "uncertainty that would follow ... traffic would be restricted, the area surrounded by a military cordon and passage would require 14 days through this area." The Prussian ambassador to Russia, General Schöler and the Russian ambassador to Prussia, Alopeus, were informed of this decision.[10]

The second major topic discussed was the cordoning of the Polish border. Earlier following the receipt of the unexpected news of the insurrection in Poland, there was much confusion in Berlin. General Grolmann was ordered to the Grand Duchy of Posen with 6,000 men. This was followed by the order to station the First, Second, Fifth, and Sixth Army Corps in the Grand Duchy of Posen under the command of General Field Marshall von Gneisenau to secure the Province.[11] The major purpose of the military lines along the border prior to the outbreak of the cholera in Poland was to secure the border and prevent unauthorized border crossings and the smuggling of weaponry and other military supplies.

Throughout May, the Immediate Commission became more concerned about cholera in the Polish areas adjacent to Posen. Major Thile ordered Field Marshal Gneisenau to impose quarantine on the boundary from Thorn to Silesia (sealing off Posen from Poland).[12] This action caused alarm in the Polish government. A Prussian representative in Poland forwarded a request from the Polish government, asking Prussia to be "less severe relative to the time of quarantine" as it would "impede and paralyze communications with all of Europe."[13]

The commission continued to receive reports cholera was spreading throughout Poland. It appeared urgent to establish a *cordon sanitaire*. By the third meeting, the commission had reports from sanitary officials that the cholera was "contagious" and a policy based on contagion was recommended. A policy of medical blockades was developed for the Prussian interior. Prussian health officials were ordered to follow quarantine precautions. Provincial President Flottwell of the Grand Duchy of Posen recommended the establishment of quarantine facilities in Posen.[14]

The commission discussed the communication of information to the provincial presidents and the level of information to be made available to the public concerning cholera.[15] On May 7, 1831, Karl Friedrich von Lottum, State Minister for domestic affairs, sent a memorandum to Thile suggesting official reports from the commission be placed in local newspapers and that unofficial reports about cholera be suppressed (especially once cholera crossed into Prussia). All cholera articles were to be regulated by the Minister of the Interior and Police. The provincial presidents were ordered to watch their local newspapers.[16] Provincial presidents determined how much freedom local newspapers and other publications had when discussing cholera. In the Province of Prussia, under the more liberal Schön, cholera policy was freely discussed. Soon after the Immediate Commission met and began issuing strict sanitary measures, it faced the first test of the medical effectiveness of these regulations in the port city of Danzig.

Cholera in Danzig

Cholera moved sporadically, occurring in individual cases along the Russian and Polish borders. Generally, cholera does not move easily overland, unless special circumstances allow it to move rapidly in armies (as in Russia and Poland) or by caravans and pilgrimages. These special conditions allow cholera to spread quickly outside of its water born environment. For cholera to become epidemic it requires a contaminated water source that supplies a densely populated area.

The first major outbreak in Prussia occurred in Danzig. The governmental region of Danzig was comprised of 11 cities and 1,984 towns, with 337,925 inhabitants. Cholera attacked all 11 cities, 220 towns and 5,343 inhabitants. Of the 5,343 people infected, 3,550 died and 1,793 recovered. Within the city of Danzig, out of a total population of 70,014, over 1,445 persons contracted cholera and only 291 recovered. For every 100 inhabitants in Danzig who contracted the disease, 79.86 died.[17]

The first cases occurred on May 27, 1831, when four workers in the mud-barges in the port at Neufahrwasser fell ill. Neufahrwasser is about an hour's travel time from Danzig. The dredgers returned home to their villages on May 28. On May 29, the physician of the Danzig district, Dr. Lenz, was told that four workers had fallen ill in Neufahrwasser. They were conveyed to their homes in the villages of Nickelswalde, Krohnenhoff, Einlage and Schnackenburg, on the Danzig Nehrung. Three of the men had died suddenly from a suspicious sickness, and one was still alive. Dr. Lenz found symptoms of "Indian cholera in the latter patient. He judged the other three had died of cholera." He reported the cases to the government. A meeting was held that evening with the *Regierung* president of Danzig, Johann Carl Rothé. It was decided to isolate the villages immediately and "to investigate the particulars of the mud-barges." The investigation was undertaken the following morning. The workers in the two mud-barges under investigation had been working on them since May 16. The two barges had crews of thirty-four and thirty-six men. The men all arrived for work on May 30 and were all in good health, except for one suspicious case and the four previously mentioned.

Although there were no other cases of cholera on the mud-barges besides the one noted, the "mud-barges, however, soon ceased to work after this." Cholera broke out on May 30, in the Danzig suburb of Schlapke a little more than one mile from the city. Cholera attacked several individuals in the Eimermacherhofe area of the city. The disease continued to spread chiefly among the lower classes. An English physician, sent to Danzig to observe the cholera, later reported cholera spread "without any marked order" and chiefly among the "destitute and poor." He reported between May 28 and July 23, 835 people were attacked by cholera and only 195 recovered.[18]

By May 31, eight persons had died of cholera in the city of Danzig. The Danzig authorities established a Sanitary Commission. This commission was unusual because it had no physicians. It was composed of Police President Baron von Vegesack—an old Prussian officer who had begun his career under Frederick the Great—Mayor Weikhmann, and a government councilor named Kries.[19]

The first question officials had to consider was how the disease entered Danzig. There were three opinions. First, it came through the harbor into the city by way of the Russian coast. Second, it came overland and was the same illness "that gripped Poland." Third, it was local in nature. Anti-contagionists supported the latter. It was this opinion that was articulated in a strongly worded report on the failure of the Government's severe regulations to arrest the epidemic. The regulations were blamed for creating more misery and expense than necessary. On July 3, 1831, the Danzig Sanitary Commission reported, "it does not appear likely cholera is spread by contagion."[20]

The Sanitary Commission issued a preliminary report questioning the post-mortem examination of one of the dredgers. It reported his death was not caused by cholera. Secondly, cholera broke out two days before the first Russian ship arrived in port on May 30, 1831:

> That ships from Russian ports did not arrive at Danzig before the 30th of May is ascertained by the list of arrivals here, which lies open to every one's inspection; at the same time it should be mentioned, that the earliest information of the cholera having appeared at Riga, was received on the first of June by Kitskats, the ship's broker, who had it from the Prussian Consul, General Wöhrmann, at Riga, in a letter dated 14–26 May.[21]

The Danzig Sanitary Commission had obtained the "list of arrivals" and reasoned that there was no compelling evidence that the Russian ships had infected Danzig with cholera because no Russian ships had arrived in port prior to May 30. No other vessel or boat from a Russian port had arrived. The report also stated that overland infection from Poland was unlikely because none of the dredgers had been in contact with either infected goods or recent arrivals from Poland.[22]

Upon a later independent investigation it was also shown that cholera had not been present in Riga when the ships sailed, nor had it appeared on board the ships, but it had appeared in Danzig before their arrival. The first four Russian ships to arrive at 5:00 am on May 30, 1831, were the *Minna*, captained by the aforementioned Brandt, the *Joh. Maria*, the *Stoffmung*, and the *Unga Neptunus*. The ships and crews were all examined by one Dr. Mathy and given a clean bill of health.[23]

Even with this preliminary investigation it was clear that the Danzig Sanitary Commission hoped to avoid the strict blockade of the city by emphasizing "cleanliness, determining the health of the sick and taking measures to prevent the infection from spreading."[24] Once cholera was confirmed in Danzig, the local government was forced to follow the strict regulations issued by the Immediate Commission in Berlin. On June 1, 1831, the Immediate Commission met to consider the Danzig outbreak. The commission ordered the establishment of quarantine facilities. It requested Danzig report how and in what manner the cholera was spread, the type of neighborhood it spread into and how it presented itself. Finally, as an additional precaution, a blockade of the city was ordered "to prevent the spread of the sickness." A *cordon sanitaire* made up of local militia was established around the city of Danzig. On June 24, 1831, Prussian army guards replaced the local militia. By June 27 the overland blockade was completed. Quarantine facilities were established in Danzig and Dirschau for land travelers and ships using the connecting waterways. Traffic from the interior with Danzig was only available by way of the city of Neustadt (for land travelers) and Dirschau (for land and water travelers).[25]

All communications with the Immediate Commission had to go through the provincial president of the Province of Prussia, Theodor von Schön. The Immediate Commission ordered a twenty day quarantine of Danzig. The harshest policy and one with the most serious effect on the Danzig economy and the region, was that all "shipping on the Vistula ... [was] ... halted." It was not re-established until a quarantine station was established at Dirschau.[26] However, even afterward, shipping was still inhibited along the Vistula. The government reported in August, that "traffic on the Vistula remains insignificant."[27] This lack of shipping prompted the Danzig Sanitary Commission to complain to Schön in August, that even after "cholera reached Elbing and Königsberg, no ships leave without quarantine. The cholera prevails in a suburb of Dirschau ... and yet, no ships move up the Vistula from Thorn or down the Vistula to Danzig. All ships have to undergo quarantine at Dirschau. Why? Because only here has a waterway quarantine station been established and there has been no order from the Government for its abolition."[28]

The dearth of trade led one newspaper to compare the situation to the Napoleonic blockade, "We are experiencing a period similar to 1807 to 1813. Although the shipping industry has not entirely stopped there are so many precautions and correct rules applied to incoming ships to avoid cholera that many ships are completely rejected. Aside from Russian and Prussian company staff in the harbors, no ships are chartered except with travelers, families, or those with urgent business because certainly no one else wants to go there." The harmful effect on the entire traffic along the rivers and in the usually busy Baltic ports was decried in this report.[29]

Description of the City of Danzig

In 1831, Danzig was a city with high dwellings and narrow streets through which two wagons could pass each other only with difficulty. Doctors were forced to conduct their practice on foot. Broad ditches and high walls surrounded the city. The city contained numerous canals periodically inundated by the Vistula.[30] In addition, one commentator later described the water supply in Danzig as "smelling badly" and polluted to the extent that the citizens were known for their "rotten teeth." People who moved to Danzig with good teeth would soon find them rotting. The polluted washing, cooking and drinking water contributed to the constant rash of fevers and ultimately cholera. For some doctors unsanitary conditions in Danzig contributed to the miasmic origin of cholera rather than proof of its contagious nature. Today we know the unhealthy water in Danzig was probably a contributing factor to the explosive outbreak and spread of cholera. There were many other intestinal diseases with symptoms similar to cholera rampant in the highly populated cities and towns in the nineteenth century.[31] In the past, physicians had treated fevers and intestinal diseases in Danzig severe enough to cause death.[32]

Dr. Wagner investigated cholera in Danzig for the Immediate Commission. He disagreed with the Danzig Sanitary Commission report of July 3, 1831. He attempted to prove that cholera was a contagious disease and that was how it had spread in Danzig. He theorized that cholera could have entered Danzig by sea, as it was the dredgers in the harbor who first became sick. The most likely origin of cholera was by the way of the "heavily infected city of Riga." Wagner thought it unlikely the disease had come from Poland because there were no cases along the Vistula. His shipping theory connected a Riga ship captain name Brandt, who died from cholera and a Danzig ship's captain named Lemm. Both captains had moored their boats next to each other. The day Captain Lemm was to leave port he became sick. Lemm returned to his lodgings near the Eimermacherhofe and died. Later, cholera was reported among the dredgers in the Neufahrwasser.[33]

Coincidentally, as Wagner reported, there was still traffic between Poland and Danzig even after trade was forbidden. He reported that on May 30, 1831, a Jewish peddler, Simonson Rambaum, who lived near the Eimermacherhofe become sick from cholera and died. In addition three soldiers and two other inhabitants in the same neighborhood died.[34] Still Wagner could not directly link the "shipping" theory or the "overland" theory to the introduction of cholera into Danzig. The one common element both theories had was the center of infection, the Eimermacherhofe area. The Sanitary Commission originally concluded that it was never proven that the infection was initiated in the Eimermacherhofe. The Danzig Sanitary Commission continued to hold the "miasmist" position and wrote that the introduction of cholera in Danzig was "never proven ... through commodities" or that it was contact through "someone from Poland or Russia" that spread cholera.[35]

Later, with access to other documents, Wagner wrote, in spite of the *cordon sanitaire* there were numerous illegal border crossings between Poland and Prussia prior to and following quarantine.[36]

Wagner believed the Eimermacherhofe area was the focus of the disease. Cholera spread rapidly throughout the city and this was probably due to its role as home to the many laundresses who received the washing of the entire city. The laundresses had frequent traffic with the Neufahrwasser. Wagner was not sure whether it was imported from Riga by Brandt or whether Lemm had become infected by Rambaum and then infected Brandt.[37]

Nevertheless, the fouled clothing and bed clothes would have been brought to this neighborhood to be cleaned. Even sporadic outbreaks of cholera can be dangerous if the victim's clothing and bedclothes are sent out to be laundered. In cholera's final stages the victim has nearly clear stools invisible on the clothing.

One can easily see how the laundresses, with limited hygienic standards and no knowledge of how the disease was transmitted, became unwitting vectors of the disease. In addition, careless food preparation, contaminated drinking water and infected clothing also spread the disease. Finally, sewage from a critical number of victims undoubtedly polluted the public water supply. Once this occurred the disease exploded and spread rapidly throughout the city.

Cholera first broke out in the older neighborhood of the city with its "great number of poor people." Conditions among the poor made them ready victims—poor health, bad hygiene, and overcrowded conditions with limited access to clean water. The anti-contagionists, a group with whom Danzig doctors identified, believed cholera was the result of environmental and nutritional factors. For example, cold foods, raw fruit and bad beer were foods the poor were most likely to consume.[38]

The anti-contagionists believed people with poor digestion, old people, children, and workers in proximity to damp areas were the most susceptible to cholera. They were also concerned about the poor who slept at night "half naked in unwholesome quarters."[39]

Initially, the upper classes saw cholera as a disease of the poor. As the anti-contagionists listed the conditions that made the individual susceptible to the disease, these conditions did not seem to apply to the wealthier citizens. There were fewer deaths among the wealthy because they were less apt to be exposed to squalid conditions, overcrowding, poor sanitation and lack of personal hygiene which contributed to contracting cholera.[40]

The first Civil-Hospital erected in Danzig for cholera victims was on the island of Holm in the Vistula. It contained 150 beds. Unfortunately, it was a great distance from the city and required a trip by ferry. By the time the sick were transported to the hospital, most were near death.[41]

Eventually two other cholera hospitals were established in the city. Hospital number II, for 16 patients lay in the middle of the old part of the city, in a "dismal old building, the so called jail."[42] Hospital number III, lay in the lower part of the city and contained space for 22 patients. Excluding the beds in number I, there were 38 beds within the city during the entire epidemic and they were left empty for only a few hours during the entire time.[43]

Numerous officials staffed the three cholera hospitals. Aside from a doctor and surgeon, hospital III had twelve male and four female attendants, four stretcher bearers, two messengers, four washerwomen, one cook and one administrator.[44] This would not have been unusual, because according to the *Instructions for Service in the Cholera Lazarets* for Posen (the instructions would have been the same throughout Prussia), attendants were instructed to care for the sick day and night. They were required to be "permanently quarantined in the lazaret." Each hospital was required to have a supervisor for the inside and outside of the facility. The interior supervisor watched over the sick and the attendants, the exterior supervisor watched over the needs of the hospital, especially the acquisition of medications from the apothecaries. The exterior supervisor was not quarantined. It was his responsibility to avoid the sick. The chief doctor was required to visit the hospital twice a day, once in the morning and once in the evening, as well as "in the course of the day as a new sick case was announced."[45]

The treatment regime for cholera recommended by Prussian medical authorities for Danzig was Dr. Leopold Leo of Warsaw's highly praised therapy for cholera. This included (what today is a homeopathic treatment for a variety of intestinal ills) the application of *magisterium bismuthi*.[46] Other therapies for cholera practiced in Danzig hospitals included the application of opium, bloodletting and the use of salts. Other treatments called for rub downs, water baths and steam baths.[47] The Sanitary Commission reported "all experiments proposed by various Russian and Polish physicians showed no significant success once the disease presented itself."[48]

In light of today's knowledge, few of these treatments would have arrested the course of the disease although some of them might have helped relieve the distress of the victims. That some of the victims received care which they might never have gotten in their own dwellings, may in part have contributed to the statement in the Sanitary Commission's July 3 report, that within the "lazarets the number of recovered was growing in importance and the sickness was appearing less terrible."[49]

The Prussian government and officials in the city of Danzig by establishing hospitals and strict quarantine measures appeared to be acting in the best interests of the people. However, the heavy handed means by which these regulations were initiated seemed to be psychologically and economically more damaging than the disease. The regulations required the forced quarantine of all the sick. Family members who could not be cared for in their own homes were forcibly taken to a lazaret. It is not difficult to imagine the emotional and psychological impact of seeing a child or spouse being removed. To make matters worse, the sick person had to be "placed in a basket, which was completely covered with an oil cloth" suggesting a "great black coffin."[50] The stretcher bearers wore masks on their faces. Covered and masked attendants escorted the "sorrowful transports and each was prevented from approaching the other with their fatal litters."[51] Those placed on the litters were initially taken to the lazaret.[52]

Objects that the sick had contact with were burned. After attending to the sick masked doctors underwent a complete disinfection. All persons in contact with a sick person were "confined and not until after a long quarantine were they permitted to communicate with others."[53]

People were forbidden to bury their dead who remained where they had expired until officials, lacking personnel, could come and remove the bodies. The corpses were lifted with hooks and placed coffinless on a hearse, transported to a special cemetery (originally on the Holm next to the lazaret) and "thrown into graves and covered with quicklime."[54] One observer, critical of the Prussian cholera policy in 1831, later wrote the lower classes were "upset by these barbaric methods and educated people were filled with loathing and disgust."[55]

It was quarantine of the city and individual dwellings, and the strict precautionary measures to avoid contagion that were deemed expensive and ineffective by the Sanitary Commission. On July 3, 1831, the Danzig Sanitary Commission sent its report to Schön who forwarded it to the Immediate Commission. The Sanitary Commission stated that it was "against the strict quarantine of the city." It maintained that it was unnecessary to prevent commerce with other regions.[56] Quarantine was "useless and undermined the prosperity of the city and the region causing misery." It had not prevented the spread of cholera. It was becoming impossible for Danzig to continue to support this level of public welfare.[57] It was especially concerned with the impact of the quarantine on individual residences and requested that it "reduce barriers as they are highly useless." Quarantine of individual dwellings contributed to a higher death, the "common people do not report the sick, but conceal their illness for fear of the quarantine."[58]

The criticism of official policy was not a new direction for the Sanitary Commission. On June 6 and 9 it had reported to the Danzig Royal Government that "in its view carrying out the ordered blockades was useless and most pernicious." It recommended the blockades be mitigated and the regulations modified. On June 13 the commission reported the doctors of Danzig had requested the Immediate Commission modify its regulations. The Immediate Commission stubbornly refused to reconsider its policies and the regulations remained in place.[59]

In an August 11 follow-up report to Schön, the Danzig Sanitary Commission reported that on July 30 it had decided it could no longer continue the strict regulations ordered earlier. There were too many sick and the city did not have the means or finances to build additional lazarets. It was feared cholera would continue into the winter and the cost would be more than the city could bear. The Sanitary Committee concluded that "extraordinary circumstances justify extraordinary measures, so we decided on July 30th to deviate on only a few points from the provisions of the Immediate Commission." The Sanitary Commission modified the regulations. Now once a sick person was removed, no one else was quarantined but the dwelling was fumigated. If the sick person could not be moved, then fumigation of the dwelling and quarantine was ordered. After recovering or dying from cholera, quarantine was reduced to ten days.[60]

Explaining these deviations from the Immediate Commission's regulations, the Sanitary Commission wrote that its decision was supported by the "opinion of our physicians," and that the new regulations were entirely "sufficient for the safety of the city and saved from 150 to 200 talers or over half of the catering and security costs, every day."[61]

The Immediate Commission continued to hold steadfastly to its policy of isolation, quarantine and contagion. The Immediate Commission fearful that its policies might be undermined by the persistent appeals of the Danzig Sanitary Commission and the anti-contagionist doctors in Danzig, recommended that a State doctor, Professor Wagner, also a member of the Immediate Commission, be sent to Danzig to ensure government's "measures" were being followed.[62] Earlier on June 25, 1831, Thile had written to Schön, in a strongly worded statement, that "in a few days Professor Wagner, medical councilor and *physikus* of Berlin ... (was) ... being sent to Danzig, with a commission, to review the local hospital, quarantine and other medical institutions, and where he to find it necessary to intervene."[63]

This action was precipitated by Provincial President Schön, who had made inquiries about modifying the strict policies in Danzig in early June. He based this on earlier reports he had received from the Danzig Sanitary Commission and the appeals of his own doctors in Königsberg. He also inquired whether the Immediate Commission was convinced cholera was contagious and "if the directed precautions are absolutely necessary."[64] The commission members discussed his requests at the June 21 meeting and concluded all the precautions were necessary and they were in complete agreement on this matter.[65]

On July 2, 1831, Schön wrote to Thile concerning the commission's insistence on strict quarantine. Thile had accused him of not listening to the people that were of a contrary opinion to his in the Province. He replied that this was completely inaccurate and that the descriptions Thile obtained from "... the Postmaster [who] has described shocking matters in Danzig ... [and] ... the Police President no less..." are not reliable reports as to what is actually going on.[66]

Schön complained that Thile had listened to those whose opinions "had no value" in the provinces. The Danzig merchants, he wrote, did not consider the cholera contagious. He countered that the disease was not the greatest threat—the greater danger was in "not suspending these excessive and troubling regulations."[67]

Thile replied to Schön, enclosing a letter from a "scholar" discussing the contagious and non-contagious nature of cholera. Schön's response was critical of the enclosed letter.

4. First Response to Cholera 69

The writer clearly had no experience with cholera. He wrote that in order to understand cholera one had to be like a "lieutenant who must go into battle" and there get to know "the enemy, the terrain, the army and the battle plan." He learns from the battle how to fight the enemy.[68] Schön knew the members of Immediate Commission and most of the doctors in Berlin at this point had no direct experience with cholera.

Schön had read the reports of Dr. Barchewitz, who since returning from Russia had published his findings. He had become an opponent of the official theory of contagion. He doubted police and military cordons would prevent the spread of cholera. Schön's doubts were removed in June when he sent two doctors to investigate cholera outbreaks abroad. Dr. Jacobi was sent to Poland and Dr. Burdach to Russian-Lithuania. Both returned and came to the same conclusions as Dr. Barchewitz. Schön was convinced cholera was not contagious.[69] He wrote to General Thile that the "big question of contagiousness and non-contagiousness has been decided for me.... All experience speaks against it."[70] Schön placed great value on the report of the Danzig Sanitary Commission. He pointed out that it was not written by doctors but by three "well trained officials" and urged the adoption of the less severe regulations they recommended in the report.[71]

Schön wrote, this "report provided a detailed insight into the state of the emergency which had been caused by the strict execution of the Berlin regulations."[72] It described the problems created as a result of the strict regulations of isolation and quarantine in which "husbands were separated from wives, mothers from children." The city had over "1,000 people to support and watch." It was not cholera that paralyzed the people but the "fear of isolation." On the streets, the "sick remained helpless, waiting for official assistance, no one took them in, no one tried to bury the dead, so they would not have to be quarantined." Some "drove the sick into the street." The sick would not ask for medical help until it was too late and they could no longer conceal [their illness]."[73]

The Sanitary Commission declared there would come a time "...in which the healthy would no longer be adequate, to watch the isolated and it would be difficult to meet their needs." The Sanitary Commission saw the "destruction of the well-being of a great city if the quarantine was not reduced and costs defrayed for doctors and the lazarets."[74]

The effect of the July 3, 1831, report from the Danzig government as well as other correspondence with the Immediate Commission forced it to examine its policy. Schön had by this time drafted a letter in support of the Danzig government citing Dr. Barchewitz's recommendations.[75] In the minutes of July 8, 1831, Immediate Commission meeting, Rust was forced to examine the question of contagion versus non-contagion. He refused to change his opinion on the contagiousness of the cholera. He added that as for non-contagion "he would not be held a prisoner" to an opinion he did not hold.[76]

As if to emphasize the legitimacy of the contagionist position, on July 8, 1831, the king decreed that Danzig must follow the Ministerial decrees of April 5, 1831, and the modified June 1, 1831, regulations. A question was raised as to what would be done if cholera reached cities like Berlin or Königsberg. The commission concluded the "quarantine and the policy of isolation were appropriate."[77]

Neither the Danzig government nor Schön was willing to let this matter rest. On July 16, 1831, Schön wrote to Thile that he had received a copy of the cholera instructions sent to the king. Schön requested the king "not confirm these instructions. Experience had shown and the Danzig report had demonstrated the ministerial arrangements are wholly deficient."[78]

Schön argued the cholera regulations were applicable to plague but their effectiveness had not been demonstrated against cholera. Further, these measures are alien to Prussia, more fitting for a country like Russia, which used the military for everything, including the policing of its people.[79] He added "What, in uncultivated Russia is entirely good ... is not the same for us."[80] Schön feared an uprising like the one in St. Petersburg, in Russia. He added, "military involvement is for us the greatest embarrassment in these cholera regulations." The military is unfamiliar with local police procedures, he wrote; unless something is done "much mischief must result."[81]

On July 22, 1831, the Immediate Commission received a request from the Danzig government that the "sick be allowed to retain their beds."[82] It also received information that cholera had spread beyond Danzig to Elbing. The strict quarantine instructions were repeated, the Immediate Commission emphasized its policy of exerting strict quarantine over Danzig and any other place cholera erupted.[83]

Nevertheless, for all the protests of the Danzig Sanitary Commission and the support of the city government Major von Below and Professor Wagner both reported back to the Immediate Commission on July 22, 1831 "they were satisfied with the situation in Danzig."[84]

The Danzig Sanitary Commission bravely faced local conditions, as well as the public's wrath, by supporting official policy. It worked through official channels to have the policy modified. Although the Sanitary Commission was not able to convince the Immediate Commission to reverse its policy, the reports it produced based on medical, and economic arguments, as well as experience, were used by Schön and others to support their arguments against the Immediate Commission's strict policy.

Even the king was beginning to have his doubts about the strict policy. He was deeply concerned about the situation after reading the Danzig Sanitary Commission's report. At a dinner given by the Crown Prince, the king spoke of his concerns and of criticism leveled at the Immediate Commission's policies found in the report. He spoke to Dr. Rust:

> I have read this morning that cholera is not of an infectious nature, obviously it does not respect the blockade, jumping over it, and all that the learned men have said about it ... is refuted by experience. The blockade cost much money and in the end I will be the dupe in this affair.

Dr. Rust respectfully answered the king by stating that he was convinced it was a contagious disease, that the best doctors in St. Petersburg were of the same opinion, and that to prevent it spreading further it must be contained. He answered the king's complaint on the overall cost and that he would be "a dupe of the affair," by replying that his "benevolence toward the people and the country" was worth more than the money. The king then "shut-up and walked away."[85]

The Prussian government was not willing to relent in its policy even after receiving the first full report of the effect of its strict policy upon a populated center of Prussia. However, public opinion and local resistance stepped in to relieve some of the pressure created by the strict regulations in Danzig.

Dr. Louis Stromeyer from Hanover traveled to Danzig in 1831 and reported that "in all infected areas, the public were completely ... of the opinion that the cholera was not contagious."[86] The public came to fear the regulations more than the disease. Officials carrying out these measures were unpopular. Stromeyer recounted how nearly four hundred houses had been quarantined and eight hundred guards had been posted. In some instances only "one person was sick from cholera and over twenty people were quarantined," in the same dwelling with no means of support other than the city government.[87]

Means were discovered to subvert official policy. Guards were easily bribed. Back doors and roofs were used to avoid the restrictions of the "house quarantine."[88]

Two Danzig playwrights were quarantined as a punishment for writing a comedy about the cholera and quarantine policies. The fictitious comedy concerned the fate of a young man who disguised himself as a doctor in order to go into a quarantined house to visit his mistress. When he arrived at her home he discovered that his mistress had been taken to a cholera hospital where she had died the previous evening. The real doctor was at the house and discovered the young man's ruse, "his lamentable complaints were disregarded, to the amusement of the whole city," and he had to "endure three weeks [of quarantine] for his now deceased sweetheart."[89]

The sympathy of private doctors, actions of the Danzig Sanitary Commission and passive resistance to official government policy allowed Danzig to escape the violent "tumult" that occurred in Königsberg in opposition to official cholera policy in the latter part of July. It was not coincidental that the Danzig Sanitary Commission with the concurrence of the Danzig City Council and Magistrate reported on August 11 in an addendum to its July report that on July 30 it had decided to modify some of the Immediate Commission's regulations. It was clear to the government and medical authorities that for health and economic reasons some minor modifications were imperative.[90] The fact that the recent "tumult" in Königsberg had caused Schön to unilaterally modify the Immediate Commission's instructions gave the Danzig authorities the opportunity to make modifications to prevent any chance of a riot in Danzig. Also, it should be noted that the Immediate Commission was coming under considerable pressure from other quarters by the beginning of August to modify its strict regulations.

Nevertheless, the area surrounding Danzig did not entirely escape unrest. There was local violence, especially around harvest time. When the doctors visited the sick, their patients invariably died following the visit. This was because the doctors were not called until the victims were in the last stages of the disease. To the peasants, however, this constituted a direct cause and effect relationship, and "the provincial people showed an acute bitterness" towards the doctors. In one instance, after a physician visited a peasant family, "he found it necessary to flee through a window, because the peasants wanted to kill him."[91] This was not an isolated instance. In particular, the lower classes were of the opinion that the "doctors were being paid by the government, to provide poor people an exit from this world."[92]

With the Danzig Sanitary Commission's July report the negative impact of the government's medical policy was recognized. The Sanitary Commission had to disinfect 285 dwellings as well as 1,076 persons, 576 adults and 500 children under age 14. All of this was supported at public cost by the city.[93] To compound the desperate economic circumstances of the population the report stated that, "[since] ... families of workers only have one bed, consider the poverty brought about by the removal of the beds, by the quarantine of these dwellings, and at the same time by the removal of a livelihood for those unlucky enough to be quarantined."[94]

The Danzig Sanitary Commission concluded this cycle of poverty was improved with the rise of a cholera service industry that had grown up around the tragedy. It reported that if it had not been for the "watchers," the "stretcher bearers" and "cemetery workers," the economic conditions of the working and lower classes would have been worse.[95] Normal economic activity had been halted, merchants could not sell their wares and workers who were not quarantined could not find employment. This had a negative impact on all the classes, and affected the city's ability to support the public welfare. The Danzig Sanitary Commission concluded its report by pleading for the Prussian government to relieve them of some of the economic burden.[96]

To illustrate the cost, on July 18, 1831, the Immediate Commission received an estimate that to continue its policy in Danzig and the surrounding areas, the cost would be, "eight to ten thousand talers" and this only referred to the military cordon surrounding Danzig, along the coast and rivers.[97] The cities were expected to pay for their own doctors, nurses, hospitals and related cholera costs (medicines and burial fees). In 1831, even for a municipality of 2,875 people a 500 taler debt was an excessive burden.[98] The epidemic lasted from May 28 1831, through October 25, 1831. The economic effect was immediately apparent. In little more than one month since the first cases, the Danzig Sanitary Commission had already requested financial relief from the central government.[99]

The situation in Danzig sent a message to officials like Schön that the government's policy did not work. It was more detrimental than beneficial. The first line of defense, the military cordon, was an experiment that had failed. If any good had come of the strict policy in Danzig, it had been the city's example of faithfully following the government's instructions, the result, "lives had been lost and the city impoverished."[100] The recommendations contained in the two Danzig Sanitary Commission's reports demonstrated this policy did not work in a large urban center for two reasons, the prohibitive costs and the non-cooperation of the population. The public had come to believe that the regulations were more harmful than cholera.

Designed only to stop the epidemic, the measures taken in Danzig inflicted a heavy burden on the people and economy. The strict medical policy in its harbors and on its borders ordered by the Immediate Commission faced its most direct protests not from Poland or other western powers, but from its erstwhile ally Russia.

5

Prussian Cholera Policy and the Russian War Effort

One of the first challenges to the newly implemented Prussian sanitary policy on the Prussian border and harbors occurred in Danzig in June 1831. The challenge did not come from the Poles but the Russians, originating in the need to supply food to Russian troops in Poland. In late spring, the Russian army in Poland was ravaged by cholera, "wearied and discouraged by the disasters of the campaign, posted in regions they had devastated and therefore suffering from scarcity ... and with the cholera ravaging their ranks, the army was in a most precarious position."[1]

As part of the overall Polish campaign, Nicholas had planned that Danzig should be the port of entry to receive the bulk of its provisions for the Russian army in Poland. The supplies were to be taken up the Vistula to the magazine in Thorn and made available to the army. Originally the army was also to be supplied overland by Russia. In the spring of 1831, Russian-Lithuania revolted and joined the Polish cause. Supplying the Russian army became more difficult. In order for his military plan to succeed, the czar needed the cooperation of the Prussian government to allow Russian transports to enter Danzig harbor and unload supplies for passage to its commissaries at Thorn. Unfortunately, for the czar and his war plans, the Russian transport fleet arrived from St. Petersburg via Riga on May 28, 1831, the day following the implementation of quarantine in Danzig.

In addition to the expected grain transports, the Russian Consul in Danzig, Count Ludwik von Tengoborski had been purchasing supplies along the Vistula River, spending two million talers on oats, flour and other provisions for the campaign in Poland. He also bought supplies to build bridges for the Russian army to cross the Vistula.[2] His agent, Imperial Russian State councilor Dr. Peuker, was sent to Prussia on May 1, 1831, to purchase rye, flour, and oats to be added to the supplies acquired by the Russian Consul in Danzig. Provisions were also purchased in Königsberg and Thorn. The supplies were purchased throughout May and June. These purchases provided badly needed income for local merchants and farmers, making up for the Prussian military line along the Prussian-Polish and Russian borders that inhibited normal trade.

Commissaries were established near Thorn and along the Vistula River. The provisions from Russia were scheduled to be shipped to Thorn via the Danzig port, while Peuker continued to purchase additional supplies in Prussia. He also established large bakeries to convert the raw grain into bread and biscuits.[3]

On May 30, 1831, the long awaited Russian fleet consisting of 30 ships filled with grain began arriving in Danzig harbor. The grain ships were accompanied by two Russian frigates. The ships contained badly needed food for the Russian army in Poland. Unfortunately for the Russians, the city of Danzig was placed under quarantine just prior to the arrival of the Russian fleet. General Graf Toll—interim Commander of the Russian army until Field Marshal Paskievitch's arrival on June 17, 1831—wrote that supplies had been arriving from Danzig regularly until the quarantine on May 27 and by June 18 there was "no less than a six week delay of provisions" due to quarantine restrictions.[4]

The Russian Consul General, Tengoborski, recognized the difficulties quarantine would cause for the Russian army and complained to the Immediate Commission about quarantine affecting supplies on the frontier. On May 17 he wrote to the Immediate Commission, "measures taken by the government of Prussia relating to quarantine will necessitate matters of much difficulty to transport the provisions."[5]

He acknowledged that he had collected provisions in Augustowo and inadvertently "violated the regulations" which were being "vigorously" enforced.[6] Nevertheless, "vagabonds and runaways" were avoiding the quarantine by crossing from Poland into Prussia even from places where the cholera had already appeared.[7]

The English ambassador in Berlin, George William Chad, enclosed a letter to the British Foreign Office describing the effect of quarantine on the Russian Consul in Danzig trying to obtain supplies for the Russian army:

> The merchant who delivers the provisions to the Russian army, with the Russian Consul General, [Tengoborski] departed from hence a few days ago, in order to have a conference with the Commissary at Thorn, concerning these deliveries. They were furnished with a passport from Mr. de Schön, Chief President of East and West Prussia, residing at Konigsberg, according to which they were to be treated as Prussian publick [sic] officers, travelling on service, and thus only to be subjected to a short quarantine on passing the cordon, however, they met with some difficulties at Dirschau, the quarantine port on the road which increased as they proceeded, and learning that they would be subjected to the usual quarantine at Thorn, they turned around and were glad to get back hither without being detained.

Chad's correspondent in Danzig was sure the new quarantine policy would not last, "after the proper representations were made" quarantine of important Russian officials would cease.[8] Instead quarantines increased on the borders. This led to an increasingly contentious relationship between Prussia and Russia throughout the course of the conflict in Poland.

The seriousness of the Prussian government's quarantine regulations was demonstrated by two highly public events. The first was the public notice and explanation of the czar's *aide-de-camp* Imperial Russian General Count Orloff's apparent transgression of the new cholera regulations. The second, the heated negotiations between Prussia and Russia over Prussia's strict quarantine policy. The Russian's demanded a quick resolution because Russian ships were lying in Danzig harbor under quarantine, preventing their provisions from reaching the Russian army in Poland.

The first showed that the king was serious about quarantine. When Count Orloff, wished to "be allowed to pass freely through Quarantine, as it was important that he should make his report of the state of the army to the Emperor as quickly as possible," the "request was referred by Express to the King, who refused to grant it, and said, that as the Emperor himself had submitted to a quarantine detention on his return from Moscow to Petersburg, he certainly would not wish that these regulations should be violated in favor of his *aide-de-camp*."[9] Field Marshal Diebitsch wrote to Nicholas on May 26, three days before his unexpected death from cholera and shortly before the cholera outbreak in Danzig, that Count Orloff "arrived on May 23 and told me of all [your] ... requirements."[10] In a few days, he thinks to travel to Petersburg back through Prussia, where our couriers now pass without quarantine and a simple disinfection."[11]

When Count Orloff arrived from Poland either "without, or only after a short quarantine," the king was "indignant," and "ordered a strict inspection of quarantine."[12] The incident was reported in the *Preussischen Staats-Zeitung* (*Prussian State Gazette*) that Orloff had arrived from Poland and not undergone the "prescribed quarantine." The article somewhat apologetically concluded "cases of this kind should not be repeated and fortunately there was only a remote risk of infection being transmitted over the Prussian border."[13]

Public criticism continued of the police officials on the border, and those in charge of the quarantine facilities and quarantine policy. People asked if these officials had a "special relationship" with the Russians. The "loyalty" of the officials in the quarantine stations was questioned (no doubt fueled by the general sympathy for the Polish cause). An explanation followed the king's request for an inspection of quarantine operations on the border. Orloff had crossed the border earlier at Wellenberg, in East Prussia and "stayed there the proper time allowed for couriers." He was "washed and disinfected" and proceeded on his journey. When he reached Strasburg, local officials knew he had undergone an earlier quarantine and disinfection in Wellenberg. They let him leave after only two days of observation. Local officials were unaware of the new regulations that now required twenty-days of quarantine. Next time, Orloff would be held to the legal limit. The public was also advised not to criticize local police officials in charge of the quarantine facilities and not to make "hasty and unfounded judgments" because these were "conscientious officials" who should not be "criticized."[14]

However, what gave Thile the most "worries and headaches" was the "matter of the Russian provisions" on the ships in the Danzig port.[15] As one Polish general wrote "to Danzig were brought huge stocks of ammunition and food, which were then transported further to the Russian army." Danzig was the main "source for the Prussian army to secretly support the army of Czar Nicholas." However there is no evidence that there was anything more than grain on the ships. A Polish newspaper, *Le Messager Polonais,* reported on June 27, 1831, two important observations; the Russian ships in Danzig harbor were "laden with grain" with no mention of ammunition and they were undergoing "quarantine" in the harbor following Prussian regulations.[16]

Even with the strict quarantine, one Polish writer managed to connect Orloff's mission with helping to obtain supplies for the Russian army in Poland. He wrote, Orloff was in Berlin he received assistance for Nicholas from the Prussian Cabinet. First, the cities of Danzig and Königsberg would be opened to supply provisions for the Russian troops because of the interrupted communication with Russia due to the uprising in Lithuania. Second, Russia would have to arrange for shipments by the Baltic Sea. Prussia would provide naval escorts and if necessary carry out such shipments on the Niemen and Vistula rivers.[17] Prussia did not forgo quarantine and open its two major ports to Russia, nor did it provide naval escorts for Russian cargo ships on the Vistula.

With the outbreak of cholera in Prussia and the strict quarantine measures, "provisioning the Russian troops in Poland suffered serious obstacles." The czar, his generals and government officials were surprised at the severity of the Prussian measures. They had expected more cooperation than they received. The strict quarantine regulations impeded all transport along the inland rivers of Prussia including the Vistula. This affected supplying the Russian army. It was observed at the time that the "fate of the Russian army in Poland" was contingent on it receiving the food on these ships and the only "natural entry to Poland was now closed by a cordon."[18] Given the outbreak of cholera and the quarantine, it was highly questionable whether the Prussian authorities would allow this transport to land and unload at Danzig. The crew, cargo and ships would then have to go through a long quarantine process, first in Danzig, then in Dirschau on the Vistula. Also, the transports had come from St. Petersburg via Riga. One Russian ship, the *Minna* entered Danzig harbor on May 30, 1831, and had stopped in Riga. It received a clean bill of health from the Prussian Consul General, Wörhmann, in Riga. Contrary to later reports, Schön received a confidential letter from Thile. It was from an eyewitness to a devastating outbreak of cholera in the interior of Russia. It was in regard to the location where the grain was loaded on smaller boats to be shipped to Riga to be loaded on ships for transport to the Russian army. This letter from Thile was probably used as evidence to justify the strict quarantine of the Russian ships in Danzig ordered by the Immediate Commission.[19]

The Danzig government did not learn cholera had broken out in Riga on May 25 until June 1, 1831, when the ship's broker received a letter dated May 14–26 from the Prussian Consul. Prior to the report from Riga, there was already much doubt that the government in St. Petersburg would have implemented an effective sanitary policy. Prussian officials had a low opinion of the Russian quarantine. When they were informed that St. Petersburg had prepared for a potential cholera outbreak it was said the cordons around St. Petersburg were considered a joke. Where cholera was epidemic, "in Moscow there was no noticeable sign of police regulations" and "a bottle of good spirits will get you through the lines."[20] Prussian officials realized that if these transports were permitted "to leave Danzig without disinfection and quarantine" and proceed inland along the river route the recently imposed cordon would have been rendered "useless."[21]

The problem for Tengoborski was that Danzig was already infected with cholera and surrounded by a Prussian military cordon to prevent any external contact with the rest of Prussia. For the Russian ships that eventually completed quarantine and disinfection in Danzig, the ships, crew and goods would have to pass through a second quarantine and disinfection at Dirschau. This would further delay the delivery of food to the army. One approach to avoid this excessive delay was to ask the Immediate Commission to reduce quarantine time and re-direct the ships to the Königsberg port of Pillau. By unloading grain in Pillau, the ships could avoid the second quarantine in Dirschau.[22]

Tengoborski also issued a serious of "pessimistic reports" to the Russian government writing that the "population deeply resented Prussian contact with Russians" and they saw this contact as the probable reason for the increasing number of cholera victims. In addition,

Tengoborski's agent, Councilor Peuker and his staff of office workers in Thorn had to suspend their purchasing operations because they were quarantined in a house there.[23]

General Paskievitch, after assuming command of the Russian army on June 17, 1831, was deeply disturbed by the insufficiency of the food supply and the lack of cooperation by Prussian officials and private suppliers. On his arrival he had his intendant calculate the amount of food available for his troops. The answer was that there were enough supplies for the main troops until June 27, 1831. Obtaining additional supplies from Russia was difficult because Russian communication routes continued to be threatened by the enemy. Obtaining food from Prussia was also difficult because, "the authorities continued to increase the safety precautions" and each day "ordered a new procedure for the delivery of supplies to prevent any contact between the suppliers and the army."[24]

General Paskievitch exasperated by this state of affairs wrote to Nicholas, "Prussia betrays us.... I am dissatisfied with their government and especially their agents because they only put obstacles in our way to stop our movement ... cholera serves as a pretext for them."[25] The Russian Minister of War attempted to calm Paskievitch, he wrote, "Tengoborski reports concerning the difficulties in Danzig about the unloading of food are very unfortunate, despite this, the material amassed on the border of the Kingdom of Poland is quite satisfactory and you can hope for the arrival of convoys from Danzig."[26]

These complaints caused Nicholas to demand support from Prussia for supplying his army. Nicholas received some modification of the quarantine for Russian vessels from St. Petersburg and Kronstadt. However, almost immediately afterward because of the cholera outbreak in St. Petersburg on June 29, 1831, the Prussian government announced on July 6, 1831:

> According to official news from neighboring foreign countries ... the disease [cholera] has shown itself in Petersburg" and because of this the "strongest measures of quarantine in relation to communication with Petersburg have been ordered."[27]

Nicholas wrote to his father-in-law, Frederick III, and complained bitterly about Prussian quarantine measures and the lack of Prussian cooperation in supplying his army. Count Karl Nesselrode, Russian Minister of Foreign Affairs, informed Paskievitch he had "written ten times to the Prussian Ministry to persuade them of the futility of quarantine."[28] As late as August, Nicholas was still complaining that he was not "satisfied with the attitude of the Prussian government."[29]

General Toll reported on June 23, 1831, a second serious development that could have affected the food supply, but fortunately for the Russians it was quickly resolved. The Danzig house of Soermanns & Sons was under contract to supply the Russian army with provisions. It was balking at obtaining additional supplies for them. The agent for the firm had purchased on credit for the Russian army two million *talers* worth of supplies. He had only received half the funds in payment. With the recent death of Field Marshall Diebitsch and then Count Alopeus, the Russian ambassador to Prussia who had helped arrange the transaction, and the Russian defeats in Poland, the agent did not know if his firm would receive the remaining payment. If payment was not forthcoming it would have brought the firm down. Tengoborski and Peuker calmed the agent and negotiated a settlement. The army continued to receive its much needed supplies. However, after resolving the latter issue they were still faced with on-going delays with the Russian supply ships lying off Danzig and on the Prussian-Polish border that continued to complicate the supply issue.[30]

"Fast Tracking" Provisions for the Russian Army in Poland

Resolving the supply ships quarantine was becoming critical for the success of the Russian campaign in Poland.[31] The situation quickly became highly contentious between the two friendly powers. According to the Head of the Department of the Interior for the Province of Prussia, Johann Ewald, Tengoborski demanded the government of Königsberg allow the Russian fleet to enter into the port of Pillau. When this was refused, "the Russians got on their high horse, struck an imperious tone and threatened violence." The Königsberg government in return urged the commander of Pillau to meet "force with force." Tengoborski withdrew his request. He asked the government of Königsberg if the ships could be unloaded in a remote and uninhabited area on the Frischen Nehrung (the Vistula spit between Danzig and Königsberg), thus avoiding the port. The cargo would "be transferred to internal waters and transported from there."[32]

According to Ewald it was on this basis, that Provincial President Schön approached the Central government and the Immediate Commission to mediate an agreement to supply the Russian army in Poland with its supplies. He announced the following measure in the *Official Königsberg Journal* on June 18, 1831,

> the Russian transports lying off Danzig, their ships and cargo will have to submit to a strict quarantine; for the disinfection of their merchandise; then be sent to a beach in an uninhabited area, first unloaded on river vehicles, then the entire Russian crew with the merchandise and the packing materials will be disinfected (some of the packing will be destroyed). By taking these appropriate measures, the transport of these provisions of food will not spread the sickness.[33]

Schön had of course obtained the prior approval of the Central Government in Berlin for this arrangement. During the negotiations, General Thile, had difficulty with the directives coming from the Central government and tried to reconcile them with his "rigid belief in the theory of contagion.[34]

One critic wrote that this agreement by the local Königsberg government was welcome by the Immediate Commission as a "speedy and convenient discharge" of the latter to have a "suitable landing place." The author closed by posing the question as to why the Prussian government "favored the Russians by lifting the cholera cordon in what was otherwise a strict observance at a daily cost of 30,000 talers?"[35]

In contrast to this view, this decision was not welcome by the Immediate Commission and was controversial between members of the Central Government and the Immediate Commission. First, the Russian government had threatened to use force to obtain supplies for its troops. Negotiations by Schön lowered the level of tension but correspondence between Schön and Thile illustrate that this was not an easily arranged mediation. Ewald wrote that there were "quite difficult negotiations [with Russian officials] due to the friendship between the two countries. Yet at the same time Prussian officials were deeply "concerned for the security of their own country."[36]

Thile referred to the "great war" between him and Schön over the strict conditions ordered by the Immediate Commission that compromised the negotiations.[37] On June 25, 1831, Major Thile wrote:

> Russian developments had come at an untimely hour.... The situation was delicate and even the King recognized the awkward situation that he had been placed in. He did not want to put Prussia in the position where Russia doubted her as a true ally but on the other hand he could not put himself in the position of giving the people "an occasion to rebuke ... [him]."[38]

Moreover, Thile wrote that the affair of the Russian provisions had given him "many worries and headaches," because the arrangements had to be changed twice "fashioned by different facts as they were given to me. I hope that for now all parts of this have been satisfactorily arranged."[39]

According to Ewald the reason for the on-going difficulty over the arrangements was because Thile refused to have "instructions given to him from above." In addition, he changed the instructions he received to "reconcile them with the rigid contagion theory." A final decision was delayed because of his "persistence in holding fast to the contagion theory."[40]

In his correspondence with Schön, Thile wrote, "You, dearest Excellency—in strict opposition to all the voices from your own province, seem to put on the latter too little weight" when your own support of non-contagion cannot "be justified."[41]

Schön was not pleased with Thile's letter and on July 2, 1831, he wrote "in your report to the king you accused me of having an opinion that is more important than the regulations that have been ordered" and that I have "completely complied with and connived with the Russians." He answered, any collusion on his part with the Russians was an idea "wholly offensive to my character." He did not think that Prussia would be "damaged by these measures" and if so, he would have sooner let the "entire Russian army perish."[42]

In addition, Schön was no stranger to acting unilaterally (as we will see later) and in his capacity as Provincial President he reported directly to the king. On this matter he appealed to a higher authority than the Immediate Commission and received the approval of the Central Government over the objection of the Immediate Commission. He wrote, "...in the report to the king you assume in my mind that I hold a higher opinion than the official regulations" the Immediate Commission enacted. Further that he was a "stickler for legitimacy" as long as it is not based "on a foregone conclusion" [that is the contagion theory the doctors and ministers in Berlin with no direct experience based their sanitary measures on].

He admitted that he had gotten major Prussian government officials to yield on the Russian transports, the king, Altenstein, von Brenn and the War Minister, Karl Ernst von Hake. He convinced Altenstein and Hake, that "if 20–30 people died near the Silesian Gate," as the regulations now stood "the city would be cordoned off and no one would be let out of Berlin or the Residence." For him, having the Russian ships unload the grain miles from any population center, in a deserted and uninhabited area was simply not a threat to Prussia.[43]

Schön had not acted independently in arriving at a compromise with the Russians. His actions and those of the Central Government were not without controversy.[44] Schön may have been influenced by Dr. Barchewitz's theories on anti-contagion but prior to the outbreak in Königsberg most inhabitants still believed the cholera was contagious. Schön was faced with a city full of inhabitants who saw the spreading cholera in Poland. This aroused "fear and terror in Königsberg." The city magistrates complained it was Russian ships (that would have had to pass through quarantine) sailing on the Vistula that caused the cholera that ravaged Danzig and its surrounding areas.[45]

However, even those few doctors who had become anti-contagionists prior to the outbreak of cholera in Konigsberg on July 22, 1831, feared exposure to the cholera poison, especially if it was released into the atmosphere. One of the earliest complaints of the Königsberg doctors was that non-medical officials were making policy without consulting physicians (especially, Schön, although this charge was later proven to be untrue).

According to Dr. Baer, writing about the initial plans that Schön had described to land and unload the Russian grain, the Russians also wanted to unload cargo and put it under shelters for one week exposed only to the wind. This was to occur in a deserted area on the *Frischen Nehrung*. For him, there were undoubtedly "other areas of the world more suitable to have the most crucial plague material evaporate safely." The public fear in Konigsberg was great. Even this solution was a threat to the public safety, despite the fact the area selected was far from Pillau, bordered on two sides by water, and the other side by a sandy desert with settlements miles apart.[46]

Schön was no friend of Russia but recognized the consequences of not allowing desperate and (potentially) starving Russian troops to obtain food. Not allowing ships to land with their supplies of grain for the Russian army was not worth a violent confrontation, especially when the Russian army was heavily infected with cholera and had recently admitted that since March 1831, 11,000 Russian troops had the disease.[47]

The Prussian agreement to allow the Russian ships to land on the *Frischen Nehrung* was not as controversial as the discussions being held by the Immediate Commission. For example, Tengoborski continued to look for a more permanent solution, hoping the government would open the port of Pillau. He forwarded his request. It was discussed by the Immediate Commission on June 21, 1831. He asked for a four day observation of the transport ships (they had been in the harbor and not allowed to pull into port) and that they be "directed to Pillau" because the "grain on the ships was not poisoned" or infected with contagion.[48] The Immediate Commission expressed a cautionary note and was concerned that a mitigation of quarantine would allow contaminated Russian grain to infect the sound port of Pillau and the surrounding area.[49] On June 24, 1831, the Immediate Commission recommended what it probably thought was a cautious approach permitting Russian ships to enter the port of Pillau. The Russian ships had to first undergo twenty-day quarantine at stations in the ports of Hela or Bresen, in Danzig harbor. After quarantine the transport ships could then be directed to the port of Pillau and "when the Russian ships arrive" as "a precaution maintain quarantine."[50]

The Petition of the Königsberg Magistrates to the King of Prussia, July 4, 1831

Following the decision of the Immediate Commission that directed the Russian ships to Pillau, rumors began flying that the Russians wanted to develop a permanent landing site near the port for Russian provisions. Schön had negotiated a compromise for the initial unloading of supplies but this had not resolved the problem for the remaining transport ships to avoid the double quarantine at Dirschau. The Immediate Commission addressed this and informed Schön that with the conditions they had set down that Russian ships after doing quarantine at Hele or Bresen (Danzig) would be directed to the port of Pillau. It was this directive that served as the basis for the complaints of the Königsberg magistrates. The magistrates thought the situation serious and they would be put "at risk from shipping traffic for the sake of supplying Russian troops in Poland."[51]

On July 4, 1831, a British merchant wrote from Königsberg,

> I have just learned that the Prussian government has it in contemplation to allow to land at Pillau harbor, part of the Russian provisions ships now in Danzig ... by which all inhabitants of this town are in the greatest alarm, and they are all about to petition and protest against it. It would certainly be shocking if a measure should come into execution that would endanger the security of a still sound Port.[52]

The Magistrates had received reliable information that the Immediate Commission was going to open the port of Pillau. The Immediate Commission's minutes show that Pillau would become a permanent port of entry for Russian army supplies like the Danzig port. However, it would require that ships undergo a preliminary quarantine in Danzig and undergo additional quarantine and disinfection in Pillau. This does not appear to have assuaged their fear:

> that the Government [Immediate] Commission appointed by Your Majesty to preserve us from cholera, has proposed to open the port to the Russians at Pillau and all communications with the Upper Vistula. This Government Committee will request that the [wrappings] that contain the flour for the Russians can cross our province, although these [wrappings] ... expose us most to the contagion.[53]

The *Petition* was used as evidence by the revolutionary Polish government to show that the Prussians were not neutral and violating quarantine in favor of the Russians. To the Poles, the *Petition* made it perfectly clear that the magistrates in Königsberg were offering written proof that for the Prussian government "trade was only one sided, not with Poland and without obstruction for the sole purpose of catering to the Russian army." Opening the port to the Russians would spread cholera to Königsberg and the surrounding area like the arrival of the Russian ships at Danzig. Also, a special bakery had been established to supply bread for the Russian army.[54] The petition began:

> The purpose of preserving our province from the cholera *morbus* resulted in significant restrictions on our business as well, it is only on the side of Poland that trade is not interrupted, for the sole purpose of supplying the Russian army. A bakery was established at Königsberg to provide bread for Russians. Russian ships sail on the Vistula and are the only cause of the cholera that ravages the city of Danzig and its environs.[55]

The petition also addressed the economic consequences to the city and its surrounding area. It requested that if this was done that strict quarantine measures not be imposed because these measures would be ruinous to the economy of the Province:

> Soon our city, the banks of our river will be poisoned by cholera, and foreign vessels will avoid us, our business will be reduced to nothing. What will happen to our city, our province?" They

asked, "How beneficial can trade with the Russian army be for us if we are deprived of any commercial relationship with other parts of the country?" Finally and somewhat belatedly, "But it is not only the trade, but the lives of all the inhabitants of the city if the Committee deigns to order that trade can now take place on roads already infected!"[56]

The British ambassador, Chad, became involved, writing "there is also at Pillau, [British ships]" and "I shall not fail to do what is possible, to persuade the Regency against the intended Importation."[57] Discussions on this matter were continued by the Immediate Commission in response to inquiries and petitions the king received from the British and from his own subjects in Königsberg.[58]

Initially, the fear of contagion was palpable in Königsberg on both sides of the question. Schön would have none of this. He was aware of the machinations in the city concerning the *Petition* to be sent to the king. He wrote to Thile (primarily because the thrust of the *Petition* was to blame the Immediate Commission) on July 2, 1831, that it was his opinion that there would be no question of fear of cholera, but it was more a question of economic and business jealousy. The forthcoming *Petition* was the result of "the cooperation of the city council in Königsberg with the intent to accommodate the firm of Behrend Lork that had established a special bakery at Königsberg to provide bread for the Russians. I know all of these things in the making and would if I had been healthy, destroyed the cabal."[59]

The Immediate Commission, the king, numerous officials and merchants were sensitive to breaking the *cordon sanitaire* and quarantine. This in turn caused innumerable delays to the Russian fleet because the vessels had to satisfy multiple quarantines. Russian ships were required to have health certificates, to undergo rigid quarantines, or prove they had come from cholera free ports. Foodstuffs and other supplies from Russia had to undergo inspection as well, while additional food and forage was purchased locally near the frontier. This is confirmed by the innumerable complaints cited by Russian agents, diplomats, generals and even the czar.

However, the fear of spreading cholera as a result of Russian transport ships potentially landing in Pillau was a legitimate concern on the part of the Königsberg magistrates and merchants. The magistrates were aware that Russian ships had to satisfy rigid ship, crew, cargo quarantine and disinfection. Secondly, Russian ships were not running up and down the Vistula with impunity. In fact, Russian river ships in the upper Vistula were under the military authority of General Lieutenant von Krafft and were not allowed to land or to pass without undergoing quarantine.[60]

The irrational fear and the cholera outbreaks on the Russian and Polish borders seemed to create a climate of fear and distrust. The fear was that the Central Government was not abiding by the strict quarantine. The merchants knew full well that if cholera did break out as a result of Russian vessels breaking quarantine, the effect on their city would be as harmful as that occurring in Danzig and they did not want to be ruined.

The *Petition* put the government and the Immediate Commission in an awkward position. Prussia had been following the strict contagionist regulations of the Immediate Commission, except for the recent exception to ensure that Russian food supplies were delivered to the Russian army. The Immediate Commission only authorized the landing after Schön appealed to higher authorities and the commission had to accept the decision.

5. Prussian Cholera Policy and the Russian War Effort

In some respects the *Petition* was successful because on July 8, 1831, Thile reported that the king had "not approved of Russian ships being directed to Pillau to unload their cargo, due to the possibility of cholera being introduced into the protected area."[61] However, the king was not sympathetic to the magistrates because the petition was public and embarrassing. Moreover, he was not pleased with this "disrespectful petition ... demanding that intercourse with Russia, whether by land or sea should be absolutely prohibited, the king's rejoinder being a cabinet order couched in very ungracious terms."[62] On July 11, 1831, Frederick William replied to the Königsberg magistrates. He accused them of impertinence and a lack of trust in the wisdom of the king and his officials. They had caused more alarm with their petition and he asked why they thought that he would promote a foolish policy to endanger the city. He pointedly stated they were "promoting a premature fear among the inhabitants of the city" and criticized them harshly "to suspect that the government [would] actively try to present danger to the city [or would] authorize an event that would have pernicious consequences."[63]

Meanwhile Chad discussed the matter of the landing of Russian ships at Pillau with Minister Ancillon, in the Prussian Foreign Office. He received the following assurances on July 13, 1831, "the King has forbid [sic] the arrival of the craft from Danzig at Pillau and has ordered that no provisions for the Russian army shall be directed to this last named Place."[64]

This *Petition* to the King also played into the hands of the Polish revolutionary government. It suggested that the Prussians were giving unconditional support to the Russians. It supported the Polish case that the cholera was merely a pretext to close Prussian borders to the Poles. It showed sympathy for the Polish cause as it was well known that public opinion in Königsberg was highly sympathetic to the Poles. However, the accusations by the magistrates that trade was one sided was simply not true. Quarantine restrictions were in place and the rules applied to everyone. The biggest problem in maintaining the quarantine was the smuggling and illegal border crossings out of the control of Prussian officials.[65]

As if to clear up any misunderstanding Chad wrote to Lord Palmerston in the British Foreign Office, on July 25, 1831:

> Mr. Chatfield states in his dispatch to your Lordship ... that when he passed through Konigsberg, he saw preparations made for landing the Russian stores there, notwithstanding the assurances which he had received here from the Minister of the Interior, that this landing should not take place.... I take the liberty ... of observing that the preparations seen by Mr. Chatfield ... at his passage through Konigsberg which must have been in the latter part of the month of June cannot affect the assurances given me by Mr. Ancillon on 13 July.[66]

Although no Russian transport ships had unloaded their cargo at Pillau, the Immediate Commission had approved Pillau as a port for the Russian ships. As a result of the local protest and complaints of the British, the king on July 8, 1831, said he had not approved of this measure. The matter was officially decided and settled by July 13, 1831. This was confirmed in a letter of protest sent by the Polish government on July 14, 1831, that pointed out quarantine policy up until then was a ruse being practiced "on our frontiers stopping all transports of objects which are indispensable to our defense."[67] And that, "non-intervention" had not been respected by Prussia because Marshal Paskievitch had obtained "provisions of food and war" from Danzig and Thorn. The complaint the Prussian government had supplied the Russians with food, purchased vehicles to transport food and other supplies, and established commissaries on the border was later refuted. As for supplies of food and non-military goods, Prussians, Poles and Russians did a significant amount of business. One historian wrote, "sales were so considerable in the border cities" that manufacturing and trade losses did not occur, but were simply "imaginary on the part of the Poles."[68]

Danzig continued as a Russian port with quarantine facilities. Pillau did not become a Russian port of entry. For Danzig, the seriousness of the sanitary policy being observed in Prussia with regard to Russian shipping is shown by the observation of the English doctor in Danzig, Dr. Hamett. He wrote, "on board the 110 ships from Russian ports, laden with provisions for the Russian armies in Poland, which arrived at Danzig between the 30th of May and 17th of August ... in the *Contumace* establishment at Bresen, only two seamen died of it [cholera]; at the unloading of the cargoes of these ships in the roads and harbor and on the Vistula, no one died."[69]

Prussia was serious about its sanitary policy. The king supported the strict policy of the Immediate Commission. For example, Field Marshal Grafen Neithardt von Gneisenau and General Carl von Clausewitz found themselves in a similar situation in Posen in July 1831. The Russians requested permission to cross the Vistula in the vicinity of Thorn to obtain supplies. Gneisenau wanted to give the Russian troops permission to cross. Clausewitz advised him that this was a "delicate" matter and it should be put before the king. The king replied that he could only "allow" the Immediate Commission's "orders" to be carried out and that the Russians could not cross the Vistula. Clausewitz wrote that the answer "gave him great satisfaction" and that he and Gneisenau had "been commended by the Immediate Commission ... for their actions."[70]

Under the leadership of the Immediate Commission, from May 5 to September 6, 1831, Prussia's medical policy was wholly contagionist and employed a closed border policy, strict isolation and quarantines. There were no continual breaches of the quarantine (on an official basis).[71] There is no overwhelming evidence to argue that the strict Prussian quarantine policy was an attempt to thwart the Polish rebellion.[72]

As one historian wrote, "...at the first explosion of the Polish insurrection, the Prussian government, and especially King Frederick William III, had with great energy helped to suppress it.... But at the beginning of May 1831, the friendly disposition of Prussia cooled off."[73]

If the cholera had not broken out in Poland, the free movement of goods and other supplies across the border to the Russian troops would not have been delayed to the extent that it affected the fighting effectiveness of Russian army in Poland. Prussia would have been freer to choose to support the Russians more effectively. The outbreak of cholera, the domestic medical response and Prussian public sympathy toward the Poles, inhibited Prussia from providing the expected aid.[74]

As the cholera spread to Prussia, the government was forced to concern itself with protecting its own population as well as preventing unrest in the country. Poland was upper most as a matter of Prussian foreign policy and Russian success a desirable objective on the part of Prussia. However, Prussian sanitary policy during the cholera epidemic should not be solely interpreted as an excuse by Prussia to limit Poland's options and extend aid to the Russian army during the Polish uprising.

6

Cholera Policy on the Prussian Border

One of the most controversial aspects of Prussian policy toward Poland during the uprising in 1831 was the Prussian government *cordon sanitaire* on the Polish-Prussian frontier. The imposition of this sanitary policy was criticized as a breach of neutrality by the Polish government and as a means to harass and impede the uprising.[1] Prussian support of the Russian war effort by this action continues to be debated, because supporters of the insurrection saw this policy as a contributing factor to the ultimate failure of the revolt. Entangled in this debate is the sincerity of Prussian cholera policy during the revolt. This chapter focuses on Prussian frontier policy. It will deal with the measures the government undertook to ensure that cholera policy was rigorously enforced on the border and how both the Poles and the Russians felt betrayed by Prussia.

As noted earlier, the measures imposed in Prussian Danzig, inflicted a heavy burden on its own population and were designed specifically to stop the epidemic. The medical policy on the frontiers between Prussia and Poland originated from the same basic contagionist assumptions applied in Danzig and were consistent with this policy.

The first major challenge to the Immediate Commission's strict cholera policy on the border occurred in late June 1831. The challenge did not come from the Poles but from the Russian attempt to obtain food and other supplies to relieve its troops in Poland. In late spring, the Russian armies were ravaged by cholera. "Wearied and discouraged by the disasters of the campaign, posted in regions which they had devastated, and therefore suffering from scarcity ... and with cholera ravaging their ranks, that army was in the most precarious position."[2]

Danzig was always to be the main port for the Russian army to receive its supplies and other provisions.[3] As note previously, the Russian Consul, had been purchasing supplies along the Vistula while he awaited the transport fleet from Russia expected in Danzig harbor in late May 1831.[4] General Graf Toll, interim Commander of the Russian army until Paskievitch's arrival on June 26, 1831, wrote that supplies had been arriving from Danzig until the quarantine. By June 18, 1831, there was "no less than a six week delay of provisions." This is a partial explanation as to why relations became so contentious between Russia and Prussia in June and led to Russian threats to land grain transports in Pillau harbor. Danzig had always been important to the Russian war strategy as a port of entry for food and supplies, when the strategy was changed in mid–April, Danzig become even more critical to the success of the new Russian war plan.

The strategy for the Russian campaign in Poland underwent a complete change with a new plan as a series of failures on Diebitsch's part led to a growing lack of confidence on the part of the czar in Diebitsch's abilities. After the battle of Grochów on February 13, 1831, Diebitsch failed to follow-up his victory much to the annoyance of Czar Nicholas. For ten days following the battle Diebitsch's troops were required to forage food from the local Polish inhabitants and pay in "hard cash." The supply shortage was worsened by a lack of wagons to transport the food. The army was suffering from the irregular delivery of supplies and was now "desperate."[5]

On March 17, 1831, he decided to march south and cross the Vistula at the town of Tyrzcyn, approximately 42 miles south of Warsaw and attack the city from the rear. When he began the march to Tyrzcyn, with the main Russian army, Polish forces attacked Russian General Rosen's advance guard. Although overwhelmed by a Polish force that was three times the size of the Russian forces, the Russians fought a battle at Dębe Wielkie and managed to escape a disaster when the "Polish commander failed to push his advantage." Diebitsch marched back to attack the Pole's from the rear. He was told by his commanders that there were not sufficient supplies and his troops "could not fight without food." General Rosen's troops held the main Russian stronghold at Siedlce. On March 30, 1831, Diebitsch entered the city. The Russians had averted a complete disaster but Diebitsch's plans to cross the Vistula and attack Warsaw were stopped.[6]

Diebitsch remained between Siedlce and Warsaw for approximately one month attempting to obtain supplies and confronting the outbreak of cholera. The disease spread quickly with 8,720 troops sickened and 2,800 deaths during this period. After the outbreak of hostilities with the Polish troops in mid–May, cholera spread to the Polish troops. After the first cases of the cholera in the Russian army, Diebitsch created a separate committee to look for signs of the disease and to propose preventative measures. The committee recommended good food, warm clothing, and advised the troops to guard against moisture on their legs. These recommendations were to be used as a "necessary addition to pepper vodka [used traditionally in Russia as homeopathic remedy for colds and fevers]." To make matters more difficult, the Russian army initiated a military cordon that interrupted communications and left a "great number of patients in the hospitals." As a result, the army "needed time to strengthen itself."[7]

Nicholas became more frustrated with his Field Marshal and his inability to complete a decisive victory against the Poles. While Diebitsch was in Siedlce, Nicholas wrote to him describing Russia's current position concerning the "unlucky course of events" during the campaign. The army, "needed to return to the Russian border, to find supplies ... [as Volhynia and Lithuania] ... were in revolt and this increased the danger." He feared for the army and complained about Diebitsch's plan to cross the upper Vistula at Tyrzcyn.[8]

Diebitsch was sent a new detailed plan on April 15, 1831. The new plan recommended the Russian army cross on the lower Vistula at Plock and not at Tyrzcyn. The new plan was based on "having secured food from the beginning by purchasing it in Prussia" and by shuttling food from Danzig down the Vistula to his army.[9]

For Nicholas, the plan was "daring" but "not a consistently adventurous plan of operations." It offered a "tremendous advantage in securing food, the enemy would be surprised, and it would break the "moral connection of the enemy with Europe that is made by way of Prussia." Nicholas expected "he [Diebitsch] and Toll would act according to their convictions, but that he in return required a written explanation for their decision."[10]

Diebitsch and Toll had their reservations about the new plan and believed it consisted of nothing more "than a parade from the Narew River to Plonsk." They would be marching "past the gates" of the Polish controlled Modlin fortress. The Polish army would attack the Russian army at will and return to the safety of the fortress. Yet, Diebitsch and Toll did not want to alienate themselves any more than they had already from the emperor. They had been harshly criticized for their past actions and neither really had a well thought out plan to oppose the new war strategy.[11]

In May, Diebitsch turned to the Russian ambassador in Berlin, Count Alopeus, to make an "unprecedented request" to obtain permission from the Prussian Cabinet for the Russian army to advance into Prussia and then return into Poland. The plan was to cross the Vistula on "the bridge situated near Thorn" then fall back into Polish territory and attack the Poles. Alopeus hesitated to bring this request to the Prussian king as he knew it would undermine Prussia's position on neutrality and set off a storm of protest in Prussia and among the western powers. Instead he brought the petition to Prince Wittgenstein who he asked to present it to the king. When the king received the petition from Wittgenstein he was "very surprised" and responded negatively to the Russian ambassador. He replied that it was an imposition, and that he would have to maintain a force of 400,000 troops in the Grand Duchy of Posen to "prevent the consequences of the entry of the Russian army" into Prussian territory or he would have to act as if he knew nothing about the entry of the Russian army into Prussian territory. Something he thought "extraordinarily" unlikely "when we know the friendship that unites the king to the emperor."[12] The position of the king was made clear, he was sympathetic to the Russian cause, but sympathy for the Poles "predominated among the population of the Kingdom" as well as among some high level functionaries in the government and especially among the Polish inhabitants of Posen.[13]

On April 10, 1831, Nicholas received the news of the Russian defeat at the Battle of Iganie. He ordered Field Marshal Paskievitch to St. Petersburg and planned to replace Diebitsch. He sent a new military plan to Diebitsch on April 15, 1831.[14] He continued to complain about Diebitsch's lack of initiative and follow-through. On May 4, 1831, he wrote "everything is conducted with the same irresolution and the same disorder. I foresee disaster and misfortune instead of almost certain success."[15] On May 26, 1831, thoroughly exasperated with Diebitsch, he wrote "I defy anyone to understand you!"[16]

At the end of the April, Diebitsch sent Russian State Councilor, Peuker accompanied by the supply Intendant Colonel von Dreyling to Thorn "to lead the provisioning of the Russian army, if the army should gain control of the Vistula."[17]

Councilor Peuker began purchasing and storing rye, flour, and oats along with supplies acquired by Tengoborski in Danzig, Königsberg and Thorn. Peuker was authorized to continue to purchase supplies in Prussia and to establish bakeries to supply the army.[18]

On May 9, 1831, Diebitsch received no news from Peuker. He heard that Prussia wanted to establish barriers to contain cholera. This gave him "great anxiety" because it would affect communications and supplies coming through Prussia. He wrote, Provincial President

Schön, in Königsberg, "sent a doctor here" to observe the state of the disease. Diebitisch made every effort to persuade Schön not to impede communications. He wrote to Schön and ambassador Count Alopeus in Berlin, "hoping" Prussia would be content with a limited quarantine that included "fumigation" and "health certificates" for goods and men from uninfected areas. He asked that supply depots be built on the other side of the cordon, as close as possible to the frontier, and in a neutral area. Finally, he requested that a neutral area be established along the course of the Vistula between Thorn and the frontier. He observed that the disease was heading west toward Warsaw and had not gone north toward the Narew River.[19]

On May 12, 1831, Diebitsch wrote to the emperor that the "uncertainty of Prussian aid causes me much embarrassment.... My persistence in being independent of Prussia for food and taking measures on the lower Vistula" arises from the fact that "even your Imperial Majesty has noted, in the case there is not sufficient help from Prussia, due to barriers because of cholera, we would be deprived of the possibility of operations on the lower Vistula ... [and thus] ... left to return to our earlier plans on the upper Vistula."[20]

In Diebitsch's final letter to Nicholas on June 7, 1831, from the town of Kleszczewo, in Poland, he complained about the unexpected obstacles to supplying food for his troops and materials to construct a bridge. He did not think he would be prepared to cross the Vistula until the middle of June. He expected to remain in the same area longer than anticipated. Additional food supplies were far away in Königsberg and Tilsit. He would have to depend on "local purchases." In addition the "shallowness of the Vistula River made navigation below Thorn difficult." Also, cholera had erupted in Danzig and other Prussian harbors which subjected the "army vehicles coming with grain to twenty-day quarantine." General Toll wrote on June 1, 1831, to the czar that Prussia was "placing many obstacles before them, especially as a result of very strict measures against cholera."[21]

Diebitsch's fears were not unfounded. With the quarantine of the city of Danzig, the Russian fleet arrived and was not allowed to land. Provisioning the Russian army was becoming more desperate by the day. A decision to land the ships was now of paramount concern to relations between Russia and Prussia.

Count Orloff's Mission to Prussia and the Death of Field Marshal Diebitsch

On May 18, 1831, the czar sent Count Orloff to Diebitsch to "verbally clarify, what the Field Marshal did not seem to understand from his letters." His mission raised a number of questions at the time regarding Diebitsch's sudden death, and Prussia's seemingly more favorable attitude in support of the Russian army on the Polish-Prussian border. The Poles believed a bargain between Orloff and the Prussian Cabinet had been struck on this mission.

In early May 1831, the original military cordon, was supplemented by a *cordon sanitaire* initiated by the authorities in Berlin. One historian has written, this would have been a legitimate initiative if Prussia had treated all travelers equally. But "historical facts clearly indicated that restrictions concerning the Poles" were harsher than those "used against the Russians." His evidence was based on a report in a Warsaw newspaper of May 10, 1831, the "closure of the eastern border of Prussia was largely political ... the Prussian government decreed a quarantine period at our borders against the cholera on the twenty-first day ... [of the month] ... and could give only the reason to Poland of "its ignorance of the nature of the disease." On June 26, 1831, the same newspaper reported when Orloff traveled from Poland to Prussia he "had not completed quarantine."[22] As mentioned previously, the latter was attributed to the border guards unaware of new regulations. The situation was quickly rectified and the Prussian government apologized.

The initial criticism and seemingly additional Prussian support for Russia was attributed originally to Orloff's mission. His mission has never been completely clarified. It was undoubtedly twofold. To impress on Diebitsch the czar's displeasure and to obtain more support for the Russian initiative in Poland. According to Theodore Schiemann, the pretext for his visit to Prussia was to discuss "the provisioning of the Russian army" but it was actually to find out how Prussia would feel about some "ideas developed by the emperor" concerning the future of Poland. Orloff visited Diebitsch at his headquarters in Poland, a couple of days prior to his death on June 10, 1831. Diebitsch was preparing to celebrate the anniversary of his victory at Kulivecha in the Ukraine, on June 11, 1829, against the Turkish army. Afterward, Orloff reported to the emperor that the camp was properly stocked and the army full of "courage and pride" following the Russian victory at Ostroleka. Diebitsch had complained of feeling sick on June 9, 1831. He seemed to be in good spirits the entire day and his health did not arouse any concern. He retired to bed and was awakened on urgent business. He appeared healthy but felt weak and refused to see a doctor thinking he had indigestion. Later the pain increased. The head physician, doctor Szlega, was called to attend him. He found him "violently ill." Other doctors were called. On the morning of June 10, 1831, he died.[23]

Rumors concerning his death began circulating immediately. It was believed throughout Poland that he had poisoned himself, because a Polish pharmacist named Zimmermann in Pultusk had been arrested by the Russians. Others believed he had been deliberately poisoned and suspicion fell on Orloff. This was fueled by Orloff's actions in Berlin where he appeared "mysterious and equivocal" when questioned about the Field Marshal's death.[24] However, General Karl Ernst von Canitz (the Prussian agent at Diebitsch's headquarters), reported to the Prussian Army Central Command in Posen on June 10, 1831, the Field Marshal "had all the symptoms of the most violent cholera." Later General Heinrich Brandt, of the Prussian General Staff in Posen, reported that Dr. Koch, on the Prussian Army Staff, treated Diebitsch during his sickness and provided a complete report of the event in Posen. Dr. Koch concluded "he had all the symptoms of cholera."[25] Nevertheless, Count Orloff was given the epithet "The Great Poisoner" and soon the most "evil rumors" went about as to how Orloff had poisoned Diebitsch. Other writers later insinuated a larger poisoning plot by Orloff. This included the Grand Duke Constantine, the de facto Viceroy of Poland until the Polish revolt, who also died from cholera on June 27, 1831.[26]

When Orloff stopped in Thorn on the Polish Prussian border on June 15, 1831, he showed little "regret" over Diebitsch's death. Also, his death "did not cause grief in St. Petersburg either." Nicolas immediately confirmed the appointment of Field Marshal Paskievitch to lead the Russian army in Poland.[27]

Count Orloff's mission to Berlin in mid–June engendered a domestic controversy in Prussia concerning his transgression of the quarantine. In Poland and among the western powers the greater concern was the idea of a secret arrangement negotiated between Russia and Prussia. The Poles later speculated that he had fully succeeded in his mission in Prussia to provide the emperor with both offensive and defensive capability. Danzig and Königsberg were to remain open not to simply supply the Russian troops, but Prussian territory was to form a basis for all operations of the imperial army. Finally Prussia would undertake to build a bridge over the Vistula River in the eastern part of the territory.[28]

When Orloff was in Berlin his statements were "vague and sometimes contradictory." He made no formal request to the Prussian government and perhaps had no direct proposal.[29] In addition, there is no documentation or record of a meeting that would have been comparable to the earlier meeting in May between Alopeus and the king.

However, Orloff did propose to General von Hindenburg, Commandant at Thorn, another partition of Poland in which Prussia and Austria would obtain additional land. For Prussia, it would include Warsaw and territory Russia had acquired in the partition of 1794. However, to be successful Prussia and Austria were expected to intervene in the Polish uprising immediately. Orloff must have found a sympathetic ear in Hindenberg. General Brandt wrote of Hindenberg, "I myself found the Commandant of Thorn to have a great self-conscious bias towards the Russians."[30]

Hindenburg informed Field Marshal Gneisenau, head of the Central Army Command in Posen, of this proposal on June 21, 1831. Gneisenau wrote to Bernstorff, the Prussian Minister of Foreign Affairs, about a confidential message Orloff had proposed in Thorn.[31] He wanted "no part in a new partition of Poland." Besides, "the conditions of the Poles to the Prussians over the past 36 years have been rancorous" and they are "incapable of being guided by a gentle and just government like ours." He concluded that if France attacked Prussia before the uprising was put down by Russia, then Prussia would have to put her troops in Poland and suppress the rebellion. Prussia would then move its troops against France. Bernstorff answered him on June 23, 1831, and agreed with his opinion.[32] Orloff's activities gave rise to the view that Prussia had agreed to "provide valuable help" to Russia. The chief of the Polish armed forces General Skrzynecki, complained in a note to the Prussian king on June 16, 1831, that Prussian "civil authorities on the border not only violate neutrality but show kindness to the Russians," but more specifically he accused Prussian officials of the following:

> Prussian authorities provide Russians subsistence stores from Thorn and surrounding areas; Prussian artillerymen were sent into the Russian army to be used against us; The Russian army receives ammunition from Prussian fortresses; The uniforms of several Russian regiments are made in Prussia; A Prussian engineer, from Marienwerder (Rwidzyn) was used to construct a bridge over the Vistula ... for the passage of the Russians, and the necessary materials were also provided by Prussia.[33]

The note was rejected by the king, who claimed he "could not accept communications from an authority whose status he did not recognize." The letter was later published in July in Warsaw and in a number of German newspapers. In response, Carl von Clausewitz wrote an anonymous note that appeared on July 21, 1831, in the *Zeitung des Grossherzogtums Posen*:

> nothing is true in these statements except that the Russians bought foodstuffs and supplies for cash from private dealers, in the Prussian provinces—mainly grain, hay, and straw—that they shipped their purchases on rented barges and wagons to the points where they needed them, that in addition they wanted to use the barges to transport troops across the Vistula, and now have in fact done so. Everything else is a deliberate lie.[34]

Cholera, Quarantine and the Question of Prussian Support of the Russian Army

Even before the change in the campaign in Poland, the Poles already considered Danzig as the main "source for the Prussian army to secretly support the army of Czar Nicholas."[35] However, the plan as previously noted was not to have the Russians supplied by the Prussian government but to have the supplies purchased locally by the Russian consul in Danzig.[36] In addition, other supplies were to be shipped from Russia and transited along the Vistula. When Nicholas decided to change the campaign strategy, as a result of his belief in Diebitsch's ineptitude and to have the Russian army cross at the lower Vistula it became imperative that it receive supplies through Prussian territory. If necessary he would have his army enter Prussian territory (i.e. cross the bridge at Thorn) as part of its strategic march on Warsaw.

The original intent of this strategy was understood by Diebitsch and his second in command Toll, although as I noted they had reservations. Indeed, as we saw earlier Diebitsch had attempted to obtain cooperation from the Prussians for this plan in mid–May, however, "the request, which brutally disregarded Prussia's difficult position toward the western powers, was rejected by Frederick William in unusually forceful terms."[37]

Meanwhile, with Diebitsch's death and the arrival of Field Marshal Paskievitch additional pressure was put on Prussia to allow needed supplies to reach the Russian army in Poland. As noted earlier, Russia threatened to use force and land their transport ships in Pillau harbor. Instead, a compromise was reached allowing some of the food to be landed in a "wasteland" area and after being disinfected it was transported along the Vistula to the army.[38]

With the outbreak of cholera in Prussia, "the provisioning of the Russian troops suffered serious obstacles." Prussia by issuing a series of strict quarantine regulations impeded all transport along the rivers of Prussia including the Vistula. This affected the provisioning of the Russian army. It was observed at the time that the "fate of the Russian army and the entire campaign in Poland" was contingent on it receiving "food and ammunition" on time. The only "natural entry to Poland was closed by a cordon."

The Russian council in Danzig was "convinced it was unlikely that they could force their way into Danzig."[39] According to all reports, Prussia was willing to allow food and other related supplies to come through Prussia. There is no evidence that munitions were permitted.[40]

Given the outbreak of the cholera and the quarantine, it was questionable whether Prussian authorities would allow this transport to land at Danzig and unload without going through a long quarantine process. As we saw previously, Prussian officials had little respect for the Russian quarantine procedures and described them as "mere shadow boxing, a bottle of good spirits will get you through the lines and in Moscow there were no noticeable signs of police regulations."[41] Also, General Thile had received the troubling correspondence that boats from the interior of Russia had brought both grain and cholera to Riga. This seemed to confirm his mistrust of Russian sanitary policy and justify the strict quarantine policy regarding the Russian grain cargo in Danzig harbor.[42]

General Paskievitch Assumes Command

General Paskievitch assumed command of the Russian army on June 17, 1831, and reached his headquarters in Poland on June 24. On arrival he had his Intendant General Pogodin calculate the amount of food available for his troops. There were enough supplies for the main troops until June 27. As previously noted, obtaining supplies directly from Russia was difficult because Russian communication routes were threatened by the enemy. Prussia also presented a number of difficult issues. First, there were "not enough wagons to transport food." Second, because of the appearance of cholera, "the authorities continued to increase safety precautions." Each day they "ordered a new procedure for the delivery of supplies to prevent any contact between the suppliers and the army." Pogodin complained the lack of supplies for his troops was caused by the Prussian mistaken view of cholera. The quarantine stations "were thwarting" his ability to obtain supplies. In addition, local Prussian merchants refused to honor their contracts to supply food (especially baked biscuits and bread) and used cholera as an excuse.[43]

Prussian officials continued to delay the delivery of food. Exasperated, Paskievitch wrote to Nicholas on July 31, 1831, "Prussia betrays us.... I am unhappy with their government and their agents because they only put obstacles in our way in order to stop our movement and concluded the "cholera serves as a pretext for them."[44] These complaints from Paskievitch caused Nicholas to object about this state of affairs. In early August he wrote, he was not "satisfied with the attitude of the Prussian government" and he had previously complained about this situation to "his noble father-in-law." Russian Foreign Minister Count Nesselrode had also "written ten times to the Prussian Ministers to persuade them of the utter uselessness of the quarantine."[45]

To complicate matters, on June 23, 1831, the previously reported financial crisis with the commercial House of Soermanns & Sons in Danzig under contract to supply the Russian army with provisions needed to be resolved.[46] In addition, by mid–June, Consul Tengoborski and the Russian government were facing a crisis over the landing of the fleet in Prussia. The compromise facilitated by Schön allowed some of these ships to land and unload their cargos. But a resulting cholera outbreak in St. Petersburg, on June 25, 1831, reinforced Prussian resolve and Russian transport ships were only allowed to unload their cargo after a strict quarantine in Danzig. Paskievitch would have to depend on the provisions in the magazines that Peuker and Tengoborski had acquired in Thorn. He would have to purchase supplies locally. One Russian historian wrote, when it came to purchasing supplies locally "it was only money that could counter Polish patriotism."[47]

Notwithstanding all the problems encountered by the Russian army adversely affecting the Russian campaign, the Polish government sent a letter of protest to the Prussian government on July 14, 1831. It pointed out that quarantine was a ruse being practiced "on our frontiers stopping all transports of objects which are indispensable to our defense." And that, "non-intervention" had not been respected by Prussia because Marshal Paskievitch had obtained "provisions of food and war" from Danzig and Thorn.[48]

Marshal Paskievitch may have requested that war materials enter through Danzig but the following shows that this was unlikely to have occurred. On July 27, 1831, Paskievitch requested "siege guns be sent to him promptly." The Minister of War, Count Alexander Chernyshev, in St. Petersburg replied, "The siege artillery which you speak in your letter, dear Count, has caused us a lot of trouble and inconvenience in Berlin. We first named Memel for unloading, then Pillau and finally even this place was not available to us. Also, taking into account the difficulties created by quarantines and that inevitably arise unloading artillery pieces, the emperor, in accordance with your proposal, gave the order to direct you to Grodno [located in Russian Lithuania in 1831 on the Nieman River]."[49]

Field Marshal Paskievitch Crosses the Vistula

When word was received in St. Petersburg of the death of Diebitsch on June 10, 1831, Field Marshal Paskievitch left St. Petersburg seven days later, on June 17, 1831, and traveled by the steam ship, Isara, to take command of the troops in Poland. He arrived in Memel at 8 o'clock on the evening of June 20, 1831. The Field Marshal and his entourage traveled with questionable health certificates from St. Petersburg, however, there were two Prussian doctors on the Isara returning from Russia who vouched for his health and that of his retinue. They were not hindered on their journey and Paskievitch arrived at Russian army headquarters on the evening of June 26, 1831.[50]

The army was spread across the right bank of the Narew River between the villages of Wkra and Orzyc. Paskievitch made an immediate decision not to cross the Vistula at Pultusk. He wrote, "I decided to act according to the plan approved by your Imperial Majesty, while recognizing the undoubted danger of this movement."[51]

The decision was made in St. Petersburg to cross the Vistula at the town of Osiek in Poland, close to the Prussian border in the vicinity of Thorn. Thorn served as the base for obtaining provisions and bridge building materials. General von Hindenberg, the Commander at Thorn reported on June 22, 1831, that Peuker had amassed enough food for 100,000 men and forage for 30,000 horses, enough for a two month period. The supplies were stored in warehouses and "secured on this side of the border." In addition, materials (including 70 barges) were also stored to build bridges needed for crossing the Vistula at Osiek.[52]

Paskievitch calculated he had only had enough supplies for two weeks to maintain his army in its current position. He reasoned that he did not have a sufficient number of wagons to transport the needed food from the warehouses. Also, Prussian officials were uncooperative due to the cholera regulations. When his army arrived at the crossing point on July 12, 1831, he had one-tenth of what he needed for his men and horses. A few cases of cholera were also reported.[53]

Paskievitch had a choice: was it better to stay near the bridge on the right bank in order to "wait for food convoys," or to move forward without enough food for the 14 days? He knew that if he did not move forward he risked losing his "military advantage" and "morale acquired over the enemy." As for moving forward, it "offered great advantages in limiting the Polish provisional government's authority" and deprived it of the "resources to strengthen its army." The army marching toward Warsaw, would be seen as a threat and would "produce a great impression on the Polish nation." Even though he lacked food for more than 14 days, it was for these reasons that he chose to cross the Vistula at this time.[54]

The chosen location was "at the Prussian border, two versts [approximately 1.33 miles] from the village of Szilno, where is found quarantine and there is piled up a significant portion of our food." According to the generals responsible for selecting the location, the "two islands marked on our maps as belonging to Prussia, in fact are included within the Kingdom."[55]

An advance guard crossed and took possession of the main island in the middle of the Vistula along with a smaller island near the right bank of the river. The entire span was about 5,400 feet.[56] On July 11 and 12, supplies for constructing the bridges were unloaded. On July 15, the main Russian army began crossing the bridge day and night. The bridge consisted of boats tied together at the masts, barges that included a pontoon bridge section. The main army consisted of 80,000 men, 65,000 were combatants, as well as 300 pieces of artillery and 6,000 wagons. The crossing lasted from July 13 to the 17.[57] When the army crossed the Vistula, it stayed within 2,000 feet of the Prussian boundary.[58]

As for the arrangements for the distribution of food and materials for this crossing in the storage facilities on the right bank, there was the "greatest confusion." Although the army lacked wagons to transport supplies the army was also "stingy with its money." No agreement could be made with the locals. The result, the food was "held in quarantine." Peuker said, the arrangements were "a mess, of which you can have no idea."[59]

Brandt's Mission to Thorn

Some officials perceived lax sanitary conditions at Thorn and with the Russian military build-up; there was concern by the Prussian authorities to maintain a *cordon sanitaire* to protect the public from cholera. On July 7, 1831, Schön wrote, that the "residents of Thorn were initially careless in the market place" and "on the Prussian border at Thorn there are approximately 8,000 Russian men who prior to the building of the bridge across the river, freely cross the Vistula from the left bank on barges."[60]

On July 17, 1831, a few days following Schön's letter, the Immediate Commission in Berlin reported that Gneisenau who was responsible for the military administration of the *cordon sanitaire* on the eastern border of Prussia ordered an officer to investigate the sanitary measures in place at Thorn. He requested that municipal officials and the military Commander in Thorn, report on the *cordon sanitaire*, the level of implementation and effectiveness of cholera regulations.[61]

This initiative was not only tied to the cholera measures but also to Russian troop movements on the border. Posen was the central headquarters for both the military and civilian administration and of quarantine measures on the eastern border. With regard to Russian troop movements. Throughout the conflict Field Marshal Gneisenau and his aide General Carl von Clausewitz, did not have good intelligence as to what was going on in the Russian army. "One day I was in the Field Marshal's room," and he remarked that he was only aware of the new positions of the Russians "from the rare reports of Captain Canitz, the newspapers and private correspondence." It seems, "the Russians saw no reason for keeping Gneisenau up to date, and on occasion even such elementary information as the location of Diebitsch's headquarters was not known in Posen." Communications with Poland were even more difficult. The situation did not improve with the arrival of Paskievitch.[62]

In an attempt to obtain more accurate information and shore up his troops on the border during the crossing of the Vistula by the Russian army, Gneisenau wanted to send additional troops into the area around Thorn. Clausewitz was opposed and thought that Prussia should not show a "strong position" but act in a "low key" manner as this would be better for Prussia's "relationship" with Russia. However, Gneisenau was uncertain and "decided to submit his reasoning to the king." Clausewitz crafted the letter to the king. Gneisenau received the following answer in the form of a cabinet order:

> I received your message of the 17th of the month about the progress of the troop movements on the frontier ... with particular interest. Your properly qualified judgment with such convincing reasons ... I can only agree and approve of the measures that you intend to execute....

Although Clausewitz was pleased, he knew he could not take credit for the warm answer from the king because of his position. He concluded, "Until now, we have received more praise from the Immediate Commission."[63]

Clausewitz had been responsible for organizing the "sanitary cordon on the frontier and around the main seaport of Danzig." He and Gneisenau had not until then received any recognition for their activities from the king until the latter communication. Clausewitz believed that he and his commander had been slighted by the king because the only recognition they had received for their activities on the border so far was from the Immediate Commission. At the same time, he knew that even Gneisenau had his doubts about the value of the cordon and quarantine restrictions. On August 10, 1831, Gneisenau wrote to a friend in Königsberg:

> It is perhaps permissible to doubt the absolute contagiousness of the cholera, but to say this in public and rely on the testimony of physicians that even now the public denies, was probably not the wisest thing to do. I agree with Schön that the barriers are an evil, perhaps greater than the disease itself, he has already lifted regulations on trade in Königsberg or mitigated them, and I hope that he might be right.[64]

Clausewitz disagreed and, though "regretting" the evils that the military cordon created, wrote "they reduce the evil, or rather its spread, so as ... [cholera] ... moves west, if there are always new ... [military] ... lines resisting it, it will spread into ever thinner points and at last disappear altogether."[65]

At this time there were still many military and civilian officials who agreed with Clausewitz. This was certainly true in the Immediate Commission. This explains why they were in complete agreement when Gneisenau ordered an officer to Thorn with orders to investigate the actions of the local subjects, ensure civilians did not intermingle with the Russian soldiers, monitor the Russian troops (intelligence gathering) and evaluate quarantine at Thorn. The Commandant at Thorn was to be made to understand "that these quarantine measures were compulsory."[66]

The mission was undertaken by General Staff Officer, Heinrich Brandt, who had just returned from a previous mission where he had obtained practical experience with cholera regulations. These included inspecting cholera hospitals and trying to arrange for a Russian doctor named Kilduscheffsky, sent by the czar to cross into Poland and assist the Poles in Warsaw to combat the cholera epidemic. The latter, was seen as a humanitarian gesture on the part of the czar. The offer was refused by the Polish Minister of Foreign Affairs, Andreas Horodyski, who wrote concerning the emperor "after sending plague and war, and after his armies have depopulated and devastated our country feels obliged to rescue us from the evils he has caused us."[67]

The basic responsibilities at army headquarters in Posen "was limited to maintaining the cholera cordon" according to statutory measures and oversight of the security lines on maps."[68] Brandt, in keeping with these orders, was sent by the Field Marshal to Thorn to gather military intelligence. He was also ordered to investigate the difficulties between Commandant Hindenberg of Thorn and the municipal authorities. The magistrate of Thorn had complained that general Hindenberg was too friendly with the Russians and through "all sorts of indulgences would bring in the cholera." Later Brandt wrote, "I found the Commander at Thorn biased with a greater preference for the Russians."[69]

Brandt's instructions ordered him to Thorn and the surrounding area to obtain information about the cordons there and review quarantine procedures. This included the erection of a *Rastell*, a wooden shed with three sections cordoned off. The first section was for those from healthy areas, a middle section for quarantine officials and a third section for those from infected areas. He was also to investigate the Russian warehouses including their supplies, security and administration. Gneisenau expected a detailed and accurate report on these matters.

Upon Brandt's arrival, Hindenberg complained about the municipal authorities and thought they were overreacting, while Brandt felt the truth lay somewhere in the middle. The complaint by the municipal authorities was primarily aimed at determining whether "avoidable or unnecessary dealings had occurred due to leniency ... [with regard to the strict quarantine measures] ... by the authorities" and if so, "how they should be remedied?" Brandt's instructions were dated July 17, 1831. He was ordered to orient himself to the situation in Thorn in an appropriate way and adhere to instructions sent to him from headquarters.[70] Brandt's orders were discretionary there was not to be any formal investigation or hearings. He was instructed to gather information from the local authorities and inform himself from what he heard from the public. He was also to put into writing to the Prussian agent, General Karl Ernst von Canitz, at General Paskievitch's headquarters, his instructions so that he would receive the cooperation of the Russians. He was also ordered to:

> "scrupulously prevent any associating with the Russian Troops" and in the event that "a ten day quarantine of the city of Thorn was arranged because the ... [disease] ... was suspected," Brandt "would submit ... [to the quarantine] ... as well."

Finally, Brandt was ordered to collect any news on the theater of war and this intelligence was to be sent to headquarters twice daily.[71]

With these orders Brandt set out for Thorn. After arriving, he reported to Commandant General Hindenberg. He handed him a letter with the instructions. Hindenberg read it with great attention and then, somewhat irritated, according to Brandt, said "Where does the Major command that I set up the chopping block?" He discussed the conduct of the magistrate. He said he done had nothing that was contrary to the old idea of the Prussian-Russian army being "brothers in arms." He complained that the magistrate's claims that cholera had broken out in Thorn and the surrounding areas were not based on any proof but his own "groundless accusations." Brandt, replied that he had no "opinion" but was only there to receive Hindenberg's report on the "state of affairs" in Thorn and report back to the Field Marshal. The Commandant later provided a report that Brandt thought too wordy and not appropriate. He wrote that in the end it was up to the Field Marshal to decide "what had taken place and who had overstepped their authority."

After several quiet expeditions, Brandt received permission to inspect the quarantine facilities and the *Rastell* on the frontier border. The general accompanied Brandt to the border. Brandt reported that he found everything in order. There was only one death, all transport regulations were being observed on the border; and any abuses of the ordered cholera regulations were removed by the general.[72]

Prior to Paskievitch's crossing the Vistula, he continued to have problems provisioning his troops. Paskievitch wrote to the emperor, "with the immense difficulty of supply, was added another unfortunate incident," as a result of the outbreak of cholera in the surrounding towns of Thorn, the Regency at Marienwerder ordered a quarantine surrounding this area for a space of thirteen and a half miles. Szilno was included in the quarantined area and "Prussian access was forbidden." According to Paskievitch, he wrote, "immediately to Berlin, as well as Königsberg, focusing strongly on the revocation of these measures as frustrating for us and that they may even stop our military operations." Further, the army did not have the means to sustain itself on the Prussian side of the Vistula. It lacked the means of transporting supplies. It needed 7,000 supply wagons and they barely had 2,000. They could not rent more in Prussia because even the one hundred wagons they had rented were difficult to obtain due to the difficulties resulting from quarantine. The solution for Paskievitch was simple enough. Men were sent by the marshal into every area with orders to buy wheat, oats and potatoes, all at high prices set by the sellers themselves. The food "flocked to the army, because they paid cash, which also contributed to maintaining peace in the country occupied by our troops."[73]

Brandt also confirmed that there was a brisk trade occurring at Thorn. He wrote that there were great warehouses on the border filled with "mountains of flour, zwieback and

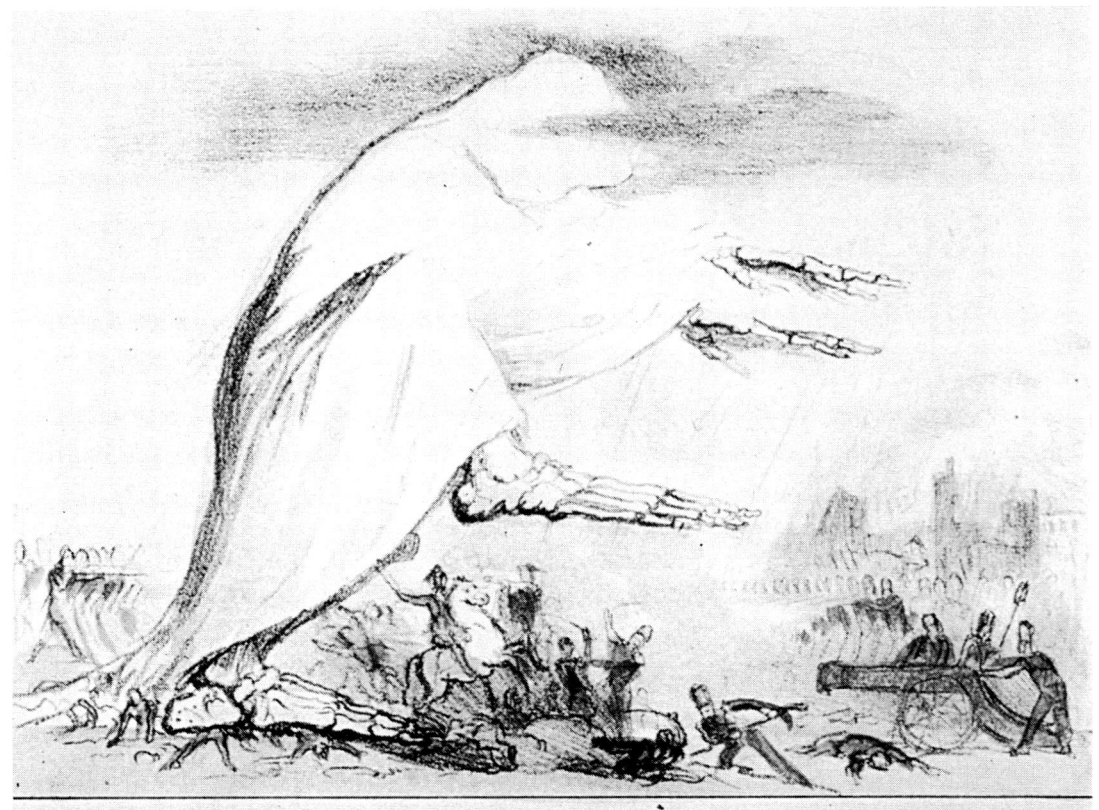

CHOLERA TRAMPLES THE VICTORS & THE VANQUISH'D BOTH.

"Cholera Tramples the Victors & the Vanquished Both," by Robert Seymour, *McLean's Monthly Sheet of Caricatures*, London, October 1, 1831. Cholera as a monstrous shrouded skeleton crushes Russian and Polish soldiers during the Polish uprising of 1831 (Courtesy U.S. National Library of Medicine).

groat sacks, material for building bridges as well as eighty large barges in the Vistula waiting to be deployed." Also, the Russians paid well for these supplies, and that much money had come into the area. So much so, that everyone was "cheerful," a situation that was not lost on the Poles who he said, "looked at all that was going on and secretly supplied their products to the Russians for a good price."[74]

Other evidence for Russian troops paying high prices for supplies to the locals and enjoying the goodwill of the population was noted by General Lieutenant, Hansen. He was detailed to obtain supplies for the Russian army. Major grain stores were purchased for cash and for reasonable prices. "The procedure was simple and practical." A commissioned officer went about looking for barns stored with "wheat, rye and oats." He paid a fixed price to the seller. Cattle were requisitioned from the estates and villages by the officers. The seller was well paid according to the size and approximate weight of the animal. Although the officer called them "requisition raids," the residents were not completely disadvantaged. He left it to the owner to decide what he wanted to sell. He claimed he had no reason to believe that other officers were not as "indulgent." The suppliers were all local nationals and the results could be seen by the quantity and type of food coming into the camp. Hansen wrote that he only mentioned these operations in detail to "refute the many allegations ... by the Polish side of "uncontrolled free requisitions." Hansen was honest enough to admit that he only referred to activity in the area of Pultusk, and that things might have been different elsewhere.[75]

As for Brandt, after concluding his business with the local authorities he sought out General Hindenberg for his report and left. When he reached the city of Gniewkowo (thirteen miles southeast of Thorn), he fell violently ill with cholera. Seventy-two hours later he was placed in an enclosed wagon and continued his journey. He stopped in Bromberg and prepared a report for Gneisenau on July 25, 1831. He gave a detailed account of the Russian army's crossing of the Vistula. Strangely enough, there was no mention of the health conditions at Thorn or in the Russian army.

Hindenberg sent his report to headquarters from Thorn on July 25, 1831. He provided specific information on the Russian army crossing the Vistula and a description of the condition of the Russian army. The Russian army was "somewhat tired and badly clothed ... [but on the whole] ... full of confidence in their new Commander." Then perhaps as a result of Brandt's visit, he added, "The health of the Thorn area continues to be very desirable. Count Pahlen assured me that in his corps there is not a single cholera victim and that ... [cholera] ... only occasionally shows when the troops remain in one place for a long time."[76] This observation was confirmed in a letter to the English ambassador in Berlin on the Russian army's crossing the Vistula, "the health of the Russian army is very satisfactory; there is only one individual sick from the cholera."[77]

When Brandt arrived back in Posen, there were already individual cases of cholera reported.[78] On his arrival he was treated as if he was still infected with cholera. The doctors prescribed a variety of treatments. He sarcastically wrote, "with their help I completely ruined my health," however, he was fully recovered ten days later.[79]

The Cholera Outbreak in Thorn and Surrounding Areas

Even with all the attempts to close the border near Thorn, the Russian army crossing the Vistula spread cholera into Thorn, the surrounding area and finally deeper into Prussia.[80] This was a result of the residents illegally communicating and trading with the Poles and Russians. One report attributed the cholera outbreak to "the Russian Commander ... [who ... created the greatest difficulties in the maintenance of the cordon and caused a breakdown of the laws and regulations in the prevention of cholera."[81] Paskievitch' s attitude toward Prussian cholera regulations and their interference in his fixation on obtaining supplies before and after crossing the Vistula is illustrated in a letter sent to Gneisenau on July 25, 1831. In this letter he made "all kinds of demands ... that extended to more direct assistance ... [Paskievitch wrote] ... because less fear of cholera existed, more lenient practices relating to the supply of food and other war needs could occur."

According to Brandt, receiving this letter was an unpleasant experience for Gneisenau who "believed he could not readily satisfy any of the demands."[82] Gneisenau later said that he thought that "his colleague appeared to want a great secure commissary in Silesia." He complained that the Russian army had crossed the Vistula on the 17 and 18 of July and "crawled like snails" to Warsaw. It took him thirteen days to settle in Lowicz, eighty-four miles from the crossing.[83] Gneisenau was correct in his assessment. Paskievitch wrote to Nicholas on July 31, 1831, that Prussian bureaucratic functionaries caused constant delays of food convoys from Prussia, where the purchase of supplies has become increasingly difficult. "The Prussians deceive us" Paskievitch wrote, "they regret giving us a bridge. [The Prussian government did not build or give Paskievitch bridge materials. All food and supplies were purchased by Russian agents]. "I am unhappy with their government and their agents especially as they put up barriers in order to stop us. Cholera is their excuse. I was thinking of buying food in Silesia.... Colonel Canitz, although he is devoted, gave us secretly to know that it will be very difficult, but assured me that I should only refer to the king on this matter."[84]

Paskievitch did not receive any supplies from Silesia. Count Nesselrode crafted a conciliatory message to the Prussian Cabinet. The Prussian Cabinet was visibly calmed by Count Nesselrode's dispatch still they continued to refrain from expediting the shipment of supplies for the main Russian army due to the strict cholera regulations.[85]

Faced with a stubborn Prussian government that refused to yield on this issue, the Russian response was a message sent by Minister of War Count Chernyshev, that his Majesty had ordered that large supplies be gathered on the western border of Volhynia (in the northwest corner of the Ukraine today) and shipped to the main army. The emperor informed Paskievitch that the matter of food, or rather, the transport of food purchased in Prussia continued to give him great concern."[86]

Paskievitch exposed his troops to the Prussian people along the route who were eager to engage in illicit trade with the troops. As a result of the outbreak in and around Thorn, this area became one of the main routes for the cholera to enter into Prussia and eventually infect two of the most populous cities in the Grand Duchy of Posen, Bromberg and Posen.[87]

When the Russian army crossed the Vistula near Thorn, the city did not expect to remain free of cholera.[88] The first diagnosed cholera cases occurred on July 19 and 20 in three districts near Thorn. One woman and two men from three different villages had illicitly crossed the frontier to sell food to the Russians, who a few days previously had crossed the Vistula. They sold their food at a site near a Russian field hospital where cholera was known to exist. A surviving son testified the three took bread from a sick Russian man and ate it. The woman and two men returned to villages on the Thorn side. All three died. Their dwellings were quarantined, their households and beds disinfected. For the moment the disease spread no further. More suspicious deaths followed, in the nearby village of Mosker—two soldiers and a workman who went to the frontier to deliver supplies to the Russians from a Thorn store house. There were deaths in Podgorze, a market town across the bridge from Thorn, on the left bank of the Vistula behind the cordon. Finally, more deaths began to occur in Thorn.[89] According to Dr. Weese, the district physician, the introduction of the disease was not easily detected. On July 21, 1831, a woman died under suspicious circumstances—she had not been to the frontier but her husband ran a public house that served many sailors. During the previous day there had been more suspicious deaths, the doctors did not diagnose cholera so as not to alarm the population. The first cholera case was not diagnosed until July 29, 1831. A woman two days before had presented with symptoms of cholera. She had eaten food from the border area and become sick. Her aunt and her aunt's mother became ill. It spread from there to other parts of the city. People fell ill one after the other and in some houses in the poorly built suburbs nearly everyone died. During the first thirteen days there were seventeen cases. Of those, thirteen were treated at the cholera hospital. Even in the cholera hospital ten employees became sick, two recovered and eight died. At the conclusion of the epidemic in Thorn 746 people became sick and 468 died.[90]

At the same time, smaller towns at some distance from Thorn because of their unusual circumstances had cases as well. In Strasburg on July 18, 1831, on the border north of Thorn, a man who had sold oxen to the Russian army became sick. When he returned home, he and his companions were taken to a quarantine facility where he later died.[91]

On July 25, 1831, cholera broke out in the city of Gollub on the Drewenz River, directly across from the Polish city of Dobrzyn. Five people died. Officials concluded "the cholera presumably broke out on the 18 of July in Gollub ... as a consequence of secret and illicit trafficking with the Russian army."[92]

The Cholera Outbreak in the Grand Duchy of Posen

Cholera more easily penetrated the Grand Duchy of Posen and had greater success reaching major cities because of two main rivers in Posen, the Warthe and Netz. Later it spread further into Prussia via the water transport system that connected them with the Oder River. For the city of Posen there were two routes that the cholera took into Posen, one down the Warthe River to the Oder. The other was from Thorn to Bromberg, along the Bromberg Canal and then in the Warthe and Oder river traffic.[93]

On August 1, 1831, the cholera broke out in the city of Bromberg, when a soldier fell ill and died. Then a woman who lived in a quarantined house in the suburbs of Thorn died.[94]

On August 2, 1831, a district physician reported cholera in the village of Zollendow north of Bromberg, a few miles away, on the left bank of the Brahe River. A ship's captain on the Vistula River had come into Bromberg. He fell ill and was taken to the local cholera hospital. Officials determined that the disease had come to Bromberg by shipping traffic on the Vistula and then to the Brahe River. It originated in the area surrounding Thorn.[95]

Perhaps what is most interesting about the Government District of Bromberg and in turn the city of Bromberg is the distribution of cholera cases. Primarily an urban disease, this area had an unusually high number of cases in the villages and small towns while there were substantially less in the city of Bromberg. On October 18, 1831, for example, the government reported that in the city of Bromberg there were 109 sick and 68 deaths while for the Bromberg District there were 209 sick and 175 deaths. General Thile privately wrote to the king on October 18, 1831, that the "the sickness was greatest" in the Bromberg Department. This was due to the explosive nature of the epidemic that had been reported to him for the counties of Inowrazlaw (821 sick and 460 dead) and Wirsitz (897 sick and 440 dead).[96]

Krehnke in his later study of cholera in the Bromberg Department reported more devastating statistics, for Inowrazlaw, 1,879 sick and 1,208 dead, giving it the dubious distinction of having the highest death rates per thousand inhabitants in Prussia of 29.73. The second highest was not found in Wirsitz (although it still had significant death rate per thousand of 18.01) but in Schubin with 1,040 sick and 704 dead at 21.12 deaths per thousand. Clearly the city of Bromberg fared somewhat better, with a reported figure of 847 sick and 595 dead and a death rate of 14.87 per thousand.

Overall the figures for the *Regierungsbezirk* of Bromberg with a population of 224,785, showed 7,779 sick and 4,592 deaths. The number of deaths per 1000 was 20.42. This was a high death rate when compared to the other districts. The two closest were the *Regierungsbezirk* of Marienwerder at 11.7 per thousand and *Regierungsbezirk* of Danzig at 11.76 per thousand. Take for example the city of Berlin with a population of 229, 843. Only 2,271 became sick and 1,426 died with a 6.2 per thousand death rate.[97]

The Inowrazlaw *Kreise* (county) for example, is located directly in the Bromberg district. It has a lengthy border with Poland. In the fall it contains high grain fields and forests that overlap the two borders. It was especially easy for "people to cross at night" including "deserters from Poland." The border could not easily be secured and thus prevent cholera from entering the district.[98]

What appears to be another critical factor is the role of the military. From May to October the district was the host to the ninth Infantry regiment and the first squadron of the third Dragoon regiment. In the last days of August, a "malignant form of cholera broke out in the district and spread quickly." The cholera had broken out again in Thorn only 22.5 miles from Inowraclaw. It next appeared in the village of Gross-Murzyno and spread to the village of Szymborze near Inowraclaw. The victim, a dragoon, was taken to an isolated saltpeter works building in Inowraclaw where he died on August 18, 1831. A few days later another dragoon died in Szymborze. The company surgeon treated the soldier and both died a few days later. From there the cholera spread throughout the entire village killing 60 inhabitants in a few weeks.[99]

Epidemic cholera broke out in a suburb of the city of Inowraclaw at the end of August and raged for three weeks. The disease first occurred in a house not far from the saltpeter works where the sick dragoon had been sequestered. A butcher who lived in the center of the city became sick. After September 1, 1831, the disease spread rapidly and was "exceedingly vicious," killing nearly 400 of 4,000 inhabitants in six weeks. Healthy soldiers who were "quartered in the homes" of civilians became sick. They appeared healthy in the camps but were found dead the next morning. The number of victims in the military-cholera lazaret quickly rose to 500. Because of the severity of the disease the military ceased quartering the soldiers with the civilians and the troops were dispatched to the city of Bromberg (where the disease seemed milder). The sick were sent to the three lazarets located there.[100]

A second district heavily hit by the cholera in Bromberg was the county of Wirsitz west of Bromberg. Official reports noted that the epicenter of the disease was the city of Sadtke. The cholera was probably imported there from Polish refugees and deserters who were hiding in Sadtke. The disease spread to neighboring villages in Wirsitz, then along the great military road leading to Berlin. From there it spread to the "highly trafficked" Warthe River, and then to Posen.[101]

The city of Posen was the central headquarters of the civilian and military authorities in Posen and for the military blockade of the border. Field Marshal Gneisenau had four corps under his command or about 145,000 men, approximately half the strength of the army. His forces were stationed in a "broad arc that curved from Tilsit to Königsberg in the northeast over to Danzig and Thorn west to Posen, and then to Silesia in the southeast."[102] It seems reasonable to assume that if quarantine measures were to be instituted here it would cripple the effectiveness of the agencies involved.[103] Nevertheless, the military was given its orders by the Immediate Commission and as we will see even the city of Posen was encircled with a cordon.[104]

In a suburb of Posen, St. Roch, the first case of the disease occurred on July 13, 1831, when a soldier named Jablonski guarding a lazaret became sick and died after fifteen hours. One eyewitness wrote, it is "impossible to describe the terror that the news has created among the inhabitants," that in the first moments the authorities had closed the city but realized their mistake and declared that the city was "not infected." The authorities believed it was necessary to "withdraw some of the troops from the city" and for good measure that it was "probable that the deceased were drawn to a dissolute life." Also, "seventeen soldiers quartered in the same dwelling" as the deceased soldier "were still well."[105] The soldiers and their commander stayed in quarantine for three weeks.[106]

The military took this first case seriously. Brandt wrote, even though Jablonski was the first soldier to die from cholera, a number of civilians had also died. These deaths had occurred under the cover of other diseases. With Jablonski's death, the Cholera Decree of June 1, 1831, was put into force. Cholera regulations prescribed that cholera dead were to be "dissected, carefully examined, and an autopsy recorded." When Gneisenau read his evening report he noted that this had not been done with Jablonski's corpse. He ordered the already buried soldier dug up and dissected. This was done during the night in the presence of an army doctor, and two representatives of the General Staff. None became infected afterward. The government put into practice all the "fearful measures with which cholera regulations were riddled."[107]

On July 16, a second case occurred in the suburb of Wallischei near St. Roch. A 13 year old boy became sick. The boy died that evening. On the night of 16 in the same suburb a third case occurred. A cooper journeyman named Mainda also died. On July 18, 1831, in the same suburb, but far from the house in which the cooper had died, the family of a Danish innkeeper, consisting of the father, mother, two daughters and a son, together with a maid became infected with the disease. The father, two daughters and the maid recovered. The mother and her son died. Officials investigating these deaths reported that the inn frequently received guests from Poland. According to the Royal Government of Posen, "it cannot be denied" that the Wallischei district "has the distinction of being the hearth of the contagion, it progressed into the surrounding areas and later out into other parts of the city."[108]

Though sentries died at their posts and an officer became sick and died on his watch, the people began to deride the cholera regulations as ineffective[109] Clausewitz wrote of the effrontery of the city authorities in Posen, who complained about the quartering of 50 soldiers in the city. He said their actions were "outrageous" and that apart from the "folly of their actions" they sent a courier to the king protesting the quarantine measures. They did this without following procedures by first making a complaint to the *Regierung*, the Provincial President or the Field Marshal. He wrote that the Mayor of Posen, Tatzler, a merchant, was asked to delay the courier by Provincial President Flottwell. He said he would "send the mayor's opinion to the Immediate Commission." Instead the mayor "hurried to the post office and demanded that the courier be sent at once, as he had paid for him and no one had a right to stop his courier." Clausewitz wrote that "if you consider the lack of trust, lack of support and also fear, you can probably add the behavior of this herring merchant as another opposed to the authorities." From this you get an idea of the "Polish spirit" among the local population."[110]

In their session of July 17, 1831, the Immediate Commission recorded that it received reports from Provincial President Flottwell, who described the spread of the disease into Posen. The order was given that cholera measures, including a cordon, in the "area surrounding Posen" was to be "forcibly implemented." General Field Marshal Gneisenau was "to take command and to use some of his troops for this cordon."[111]

Prior to these orders Flottwell had signed a number of public notices that dealt directly with how the medical and civil authorities were to handle the cholera victims. City authorities had organized prior to the Immediate Commission's cordon order. The following notice was dated July 17, 1831, and signed by Flottwell, entitled "Instructions for the doctors of the city of Posen." It said that the doctors had gotten together at the city hall because of the sudden outbreak of a sick case in the city. The objective was to organize medical help, determine the number of people needed for medical services and who to contact when someone became sick. Other issues concerned the logistics of medical services available and ensure the Central Government's lazaret regulations issued on June 15, 1831, were followed.[112]

A second notice, also dated July 17, 1831, had two objectives: to delineate the role of the chief district official in the city from the doctors, clarify areas of responsibility and notify the public of the penalties for interfering with the instructions in the notice. The district head was to obtain on a daily basis the local health circumstances of the inhabitants, investigate the circumstances of the sick and obtain the cooperation of the district doctor. It was his responsibility to notify the local Sanitary Commission, Police Bureau or the closest police official to arrange for the transport of the sick to the nearest lazaret. The military were to be relied upon as initial house guards where a sick person resided. It was up to the police to request a squad to quarantine a house. The district head was also responsible for the disinfection of a dwelling. It was his duty to report any infectious sites to the Sanitary Commission. The district head was not responsible for funding sanitary and medical support services. This was the responsibility of the Sanitary Commission. Anyone not obeying the authority of the civilian guards could be "imprisoned from 6 months to 2 years" and for anyone who disobeyed the military guards their punishment fell under the military code and they could receive "the death penalty."[113]

These measures were not sufficient for the Immediate Commission. A third notice much harsher and involving a military cordon on an interior city (as opposed to the cordon surrounding Danzig, a seaport), was ordered on July 18, 1831. This military blockade surrounding the city of Posen was the first to entirely surround a large area of the Prussian interior by a cordon that passed through seven towns. The use of the harsh military term *Cernierung* suggests not just an encircled area, but a blockade around a fortress to enclose troops to starve them out. Nevertheless, the intent appeared not to keep out the cholera but to contain the cholera in the infected area. The notice identified the fact that the doctors in the city agreed that cholera had infected Posen. To secure the rest of the area specific measures needed to be imposed. The city was enclosed by a 13.5 mile perimeter and could not trade with a non-infected area outside (unless quarantine restrictions were followed). The cordon line was to be imposed immediately by the military. No health passes were to be issued to avoid anyone trading with a non-infected area and trade with Posen required goods pass through the cordon. This was to occur at specific locations with the necessary *Rastell*. The entries into the enclosed area had to abide by fumigation and quarantine regulations. Trade between Posen and the outlying areas enclosed within the greater cordon was allowed to continue without restrictions. Punishment for serious transgressions would not to be suspended.[114]

Meanwhile one newspaper reported that Posen could not find reliable or sufficient guards. They left their posts when they needed to work in the day time. The overwhelmed police officers could not control them. The Posen Sanitary Commission declared that "to attempt to perform the isolation of houses" was an "empty formality." The authorities could "find no success in their efforts to obtain a consensus on the cordon." and "Police resources were insufficient to vigorously and promptly execute them."[115]

Flottwell feared "hostile acts" against the government, after all only three days previously an uprising had occurred in Königsberg. He requested additional troops from the border to maintain order in Posen.[116] The troops were not available because they were preparing to establish the perimeter line around Posen. The cordon line was initiated on the July 27, 1831, and lasted until September 11, 1831.[117]

Early reports and advice to the inhabitants of the city concluded that besides a good healthy diet good moderate behavior was also helpful. It seemed that some who died had a previous "fault in their behavior." Flottwell had not only given his imprimatur to an early pamphlet by Dr. Gumpert (the medical Councilor for the *Regierung* who advocated this, but had also written some general instructions for the publication).[118] It can then be imagined what the impact was when the cholera broke out at the Posen government offices housed in the castle. The castle also served as the home of a local noble family. The rooms housed 168 people and 18 people died within the first four weeks. The castle was cordoned off after the first cases and a private hospital was established there. The inhabitants were supplied via a *Rastell* with food.[119]

Cholera did not subside in Posen. There were many more victims. It spread throughout the neighborhoods, especially along waterways, swamps and lowlands. "Sporadic in some places and epidemic in others where it found a plentiful harvest of victims." As the cholera spread throughout August, there followed additional panic throughout more villages and towns of the Grand Duchy of Posen. Even the military troops were affected by the "sinister specter of the disease" that filled "brave men with horror." Entire "garrisons panicked and it took the best efforts of their officers to maintain order and discipline."[120]

High officials also succumbed, including the mayor of Posen and, on the morning of August 24, 1831, Field Marshal Gneisenau, who in his last few hours joked about his own death, saying that "in regard to Diebitsch and himself, the cholera would now be known as the Field Marshal's disease."[121]

Clausewitz continued to write about the cordon, stating that there was the greatest controversy in Posen concerning its usefulness. Just prior to his death, the Field Marshal had his doubts about its usefulness. Nevertheless, it was maintained even while making it difficult to obtain war news. Clausewitz wrote "the unfavorable cholera cordon robs us of all means to receive reports."[122]

The military cordon surrounding Posen was lifted on September 11, 1831. It had become clear its "effectiveness could not be assured" because as one physician observed, due to the "prevailing circumstances" the troops "often marched through the cordon" rendering it useless.[123]

As early as July 21 the cholera had "burst into Obornik (a city along the Warthe just north of Posen) eventually to Obersitke (a town also along the Warthe outside the cordon). A boatman had snuck out of Posen bringing the cholera to Obornik. From Obersitke the cholera spread along the Warthe to the Netze and the Oder rivers. From there the cholera branched out in three directions along the Oder to Stettin in the north, south along the Oder to Breslau in Silesia, and to Berlin along the Finow-kanel to the Havel and Spree rivers.[124]

The *Regierungsbezirk* of Posen included 17 counties with 92 cities, 3,887 rural villages and a total population of 721,695. In sum, 5,235 people became sick, 3,086 died and 2,149 recovered.[125] In the city of Posen the disease lasted 138 days from July 14 to November 28. Within a population of 25,211, 879 persons were sickened and 529 died. For every 100 people who became ill in Posen, 60.18 died and for the entire *Regierungsbezirk* of Posen, the figure was comparable at 58.94. The overall death rate per thousand for the *Regierung* of Posen was 4.27.[126]

By the end of October new cases of cholera subsided. On November 11, 1831, cholera broke out again when troops returned to the city and quartered there. They had been exposed to fellow soldiers who subsequently died from cholera. Two ill soldiers were taken to the lazaret. Later four civilians including one man (named Hellwing) who hosted the soldiers, his wife, son and another woman became sick. All five died. On November 15, 1831, Hellwing's maid servant and two others who had nursed him became ill with cramps.[127] Cholera continued in Posen until February 1832, when the last case was diagnosed in the city of Kemper near the Silesian border.[128]

The Controversy Over the Prussian Cordon Sanitaire *on the Prussian-Polish Border*

The controversy of Prussia's support of the Russian war effort in the Polish revolt and the *cordon sanitaire* is intertwined with a series of complaints to the Prussian government by the Poles initiated by General Skrzynecki, the Head of the Polish Army who complained to the king of Prussia that Prussia was not acting in a neutral manner as it stated. Prussian authorities were furnishing supplies from Prussian magazines in Thorn and the surrounding area. Prussian artillery men had been employed in the Russian army and the Russian army had received munitions from Prussian fortresses. In addition, uniforms of several Russian regiments were manufactured in Prussia, a Prussian engineer from Marienwerder had been "employed to construct a bridge on the Vistula near Zlotorya for the passage of the Russians," and materials for the bridge had been furnished by the Prussians [implying it was the Prussian government], and there had been a "great number of other circumstances that occurred since the beginning of the hostilities."[129]

As noted before, the king refused to accept the note because it had come from "an unrecognized authority" according to the official reply in the Prussian State Gazette.[130] The letter was published in the Warsaw Gazette in mid–July (probably to coincide with the Russian army crossing the Vistula). Other notes were also sent to the Prussian government by the Polish government on July 14 and July 16, 1831.[131]

The most provocative communication that seemed to require direct response was that of General Skrzynecki's. As noted earlier, the first reply was an anonymous article by Clausewitz published in the *Zeitung des Grossherzogtums Posen* on July 21, 1831. He wrote that the accusations except for providing food were no more than a "deliberate lie."[132]

Privately, Clausewitz wrote that the accusations that Prussia was supplying the Russians with ammunition and artillery were "absurd and silly." He claimed that these reports were being promoted by "French agents"[133] and that the purchase of foodstuffs in Prussia was no different than what the French were doing in Belgium. On August 20, 1831, Clausewitz wrote, Gneisenau had received a Cabinet Order from the king regarding his efforts:

> I read the article which appeared in the Posen newspaper on the 21st and in the Warsaw newspaper, asserting that the Russian troops were granted multiple concessions by the authorities from this side, I since learned that the article was drafted by Major General Carl Clausewitz in your command, I attest to my satisfaction with the entire content, Berlin, 15 August 1831.

Clausewitz was surprised that the king had lent his show of support in a formal cabinet order.[134] However he was pleased that it endorsed his answer to the criticism Prussia had been receiving from the Poles and the western powers concerning Prussian activities on its eastern border. According to the historian Peter Paret, the article also "struck a blow for Prussian raison d'état." Unfortunately, it was one of the last writings by Clausewitz. He succumbed to cholera shortly afterward in Breslau, on November 16, 1831.[135]

On July 31, 1831, the Prussian State Gazette published an official reply to General Skrzynecki's letter. This was a verbatim copy of Clausewitz's anonymous letter. Ambassador Chad's correspondence provided additional commentary on this official response by the recently appointed Secretary of State of Foreign Affairs, Friedrich Ancillon. The letter noted that the Poles used the term:

> neutrality, as it was sought to be applied to Prussia ... in too large a sense, that Prussia had been neutral in as much as she had never refused the Poles the power of purchasing provisions in Prussia, that Prussia had furnished neither arms nor ammunition to Russia, and had only allowed her subjects to sell provisions to Russian contractors—but that the Government had not taken

any part in the purchase or transport of these provisions which had been a matter of private agreement ... and that it would have been too hard to have denied to the Vendors the advantages of such Trade, as some compensation for the evils the war had entailed upon them.[136]

There is no doubt that the Prussian government was concerned with the various "violent accusations" made against Prussia in the western press and the greater effectiveness of the Poles in getting their message out.[137] Polish journals contained many accusations against the Prussian government including its breach of neutrality. The official answer from Ancillon was that the use of neutrality between states must be formally "declared between Governments fully recognized, no one will pretend that this is the case with respect to Poland."[138]

On August 11, 1831, the English ambassador, Chad had a further occasion to discuss Prussia's neutrality with Ancillon. He was told that it was an "injustice" to expect Prussia, who "never refused to the Poles the permission of purchasing provisions in Prussia should refuse that permission to her Ally Russia." Chad replied, "English Subjects and English goods were refused the transit through Prussia to Poland, whilst Russian Subjects and Russian Goods were allowed that transit." Ancillon replied that "Russian Subjects never applied to Prussia for permission to go to Poland ... and as to English Goods, they had already replied to that point by explaining the causes of their detention-namely-false declarations."[139]

Chad spoke about the fact that English travelers could not travel through to Warsaw. Ancillon said that he did not know about local travel restrictions but that at this time the "Russian army" might prevent travel to Warsaw. He said he would give passports to Posen, "but thence your Countrymen would neither be able to get forward into land, nor to retrace their steps further without performing a long Quarantine."[140]

Clearly questions of neutrality, trade and Prussian support of the Russian war effort was on the mind of General Skrzynecki. His letter set the agenda and the narrative that led to the official Prussian response. His main complaints were addressed, except for Prussia permitting food to be shipped to the Russian army at Thorn (although even this was not without controversy with the Russians). Even though most of these charges are without foundation, and were probably made to "defend Skrzynecki against his many Polish critics," they did not invalidate the main point that the Russian army was obtaining valuable help from Prussia."[141] However, from the Prussian perspective they did not recognize the insurgent Polish government. They rationalized that they had treated both sides equally regarding food and other supplies by leaving commercial transactions up to private agents. In addition, the Prussian government did not participate in this trade. However, the government did feel that Prussia's long term interests were tied to a Russian victory, or as Foreign Minister Bernstorff put it:

> Prussia did not profess or pretend to be neutral; that though inactive she wished for the success of the Russians, with whose success all Prussian Interests were connected.[142]

Although Skrzynecki did not directly mention the quarantine and *cordon sanitaire*, it undoubtedly came under the category "of an infinite number of other hostilities" and is prominently mentioned in the two complaints published in mid–July, including the Polish charge that Prussia established a "fake quarantine."[143]

The *Official Note of the Ministry of Foreign Affairs of the National Government of Poland to the Cabinet in Berlin* on July 16, 1831, reviewed all the complaints so far about

Prussian support for the Russian cause. It provided evidence that showed at the beginning of May, the Prussian government extended a *cordon sanitaire* along the Posen and Silesia borders. It said that closing the frontier would be "completely justified if it could be proven that the malady was contagious." Of course the reverse was also true, that it could not be proven that it was not contagious. Nevertheless, the "*cordon sanitaire* was most onerous ... [and] ... allows us to suspect the goal is political in fact, and to prove their affection for Russia at the same time."[144]

Prussia was serious about its medical policy and according to the evidence provided, to argue that it was an attempt to hinder the Polish rebellion would be incorrect.[145] Prussia's policy on the border was completely sanitary in nature. It employed a strict military *cordon sanitaire*, isolation and quarantines not only on the border but within Prussia itself. The unintended consequence of such a strict policy was that it affected both the Russian and Polish war efforts for medical and not for political reasons.

The outbreak of the Polish rebellion in November 1830 and the Russian invasion in February 1831 helped to facilitate the spread of cholera into Poland. This posed a medical threat to Prussia because Prussia disagreed with the Polish government's lack of a medical response. As we will see, not only did Prussia think of itself as preventing cholera from entering Prussia but also saw itself as a bulwark against cholera invading the rest of civilized Europe.[146]

Prussia did not supply any arms or ammunition to the Russian army. Even if the cholera had not broken out in Poland, the Prussians would probably still have limited their support of Russia due to domestic concerns resulting from Polish sympathizers and ethnic Poles in Prussia, the French threat and a fear of a two front war. On the latter, the French ambassador, Count Flahaut warned Prussia on July 20, 1831, that "he could state positively, that if Prussia aided Russia by force of arms to put down the Poles, the French government would make war upon Prussia."[147]

However, it could be argued that food and supplies would have probably flowed more freely than they had as a result of quarantine. The outbreak of cholera and the sanitary policy implemented prevented Prussia from effectively providing aid to the Russians during a critical period in the Russian campaign and caused much concern in the Russian government and among the field commanders. Perhaps too much credit has been given to how much Prussia supported Russia without looking at the domestic concerns of Prussia and the foregoing complaints of the Russians about Prussian support. When Count Nesselrode wrote the Prussian Cabinet, he noted it still "did not hurry food shipments destined for the Russian army."[148] As late as mid–August, the Minister of War wrote to Paskievitch that the "Emperor was worried" due to the "continuous obstruction in feeding his army and after all the problems and promises, it would be terrible if at this time we ran out of food." He attributed this to the Prussian quarantine.[149]

As a matter of Prussian foreign policy, Poland was of utmost importance, and Russian success was a desirable outcome. As cholera spread in Prussia, the government was forced to protect the public and prevent unrest in the country. The stringent sanitary policy in Prussia was beginning to be questioned. This would lead to a modification in the sanitary policy, however, this was due to internal factors independent of the Polish uprising or any Prussian support of the Russian war effort.

7

Cholera in East Prussia and the City of Königsberg

The outbreak of cholera in Poland and Russian Lithuania was reported by the Prussian authorities on May 1, 1831. The instructions to close the Prussian border and establish a *cordon sanitaire* were published in Polish on May 6. The notice was entitled "Closure of the Border to Poland and Russian-Lithuania due to Cholera." The border regions closed included the districts of Marienwerder, Königsberg, Gumbinnen and Memel. Border crossing was regulated and required quarantine, disinfection and washing people, goods and animals.[1] Travelers arriving from areas suspected of cholera infection were subject to ten day quarantine. For those coming from a cholera infected area, twenty-day quarantine was required. Travelers infected with cholera were not "passed though" but made to return. Travelers in quarantine who became sick were transferred to an infirmary. After recovering they were released. All costs were borne by the traveler.[2] Travelers who died in quarantine were sprinkled with quicklime and hastily buried deep in the ground."[3]

On May 10, 1831, yearly markets were cancelled (notably a large one at Königsberg) and on June 1, 1831, all "pilgrimages and processions outside churches were forbidden until the end of the threat of the epidemic."[4]

On the May 13, in the districts mentioned, military patrols were doubled. The new orders required that there be an officer, 4–5 non-commissioned officers, and about 30 soldiers every three quarters of a mile along the border. A military command of 30 men was ordered for each quarantine facility.[5]

On June 1, 1831, additional cholera regulations were issued. They consisted of fifty-one paragraphs modifying the instructions issued on April 5. This was due to the increased spread of cholera and to "protect the internal and western sections of Prussia, Posen and parts of Silesia bordering on the Oder River." Along with expanded areas of military blockades, stricter travel and quarantine restrictions were implemented. Additional latitude was given to the chief provincial presidents to administer the crossing points.[6]

The quarantine and border closing restrictions were criticized by the Polish government. In particular, the immediate closing caused numerous problems for Polish farmers located on the borders now closed off to the peasants. One historian wrote, "Prussian border guards committed many abuses against those that lived on the side of the border of the Kingdom of Poland.[7] In a number of cases Polish farmers had to pay the Prussians to recover their livestock. In other cases bridges in villages at border crossings were destroyed. In some instances, Poles complained they were only allowed to approach half-way across the bridge in their village. They were "forbidden to speak, except in German, and could only address soldiers or other persons in uniform." The strict *cordon sanitaire* also led to shootings and deaths on the Polish-Prussian frontier because of overzealous guards firing across the border into the fields and villages. The Polish government pointed out that in late May and early June there were a number of people wounded on the Polish side of the border. They were going about their business when Prussian guards fired at them. On May 19, 1831, the Polish government reported one shooting victim, Francois Trepka, who was returning home from his work in a Polish village near Posen. He was about 70 paces from the frontier when, without warning, he was shot and killed by a Prussian soldier. The charge was later proven to be true by the police during an inquest held on May 22. Other Poles were reported shot and killed well within the Polish border by Prussian soldiers in May and June.[8]

The instructions to the officials in the quarantine stations were specific: "the cholera contagion material" was the basis for the disease "in the neighboring countries." To prevent its introduction into "the Royal Prussian States, the establishment of quarantine buildings located on the threatened frontier at customs offices and the ports of the Kingdom has been ordered."[9] In addition, all those who interfered by trying to sneak through the cordon or threatened the "guards or the patrols" and did not immediately go back when ordered were a threat to national security. The "use of arms" was appropriate and guards could "shoot on the spot without any further consideration."[10]

The detailed regulations for travelers in quarantine underscored the threat that Prussian authorities believed they faced from travelers from infected areas. They were required to have an appropriate health certificate or provide other evidence in writing that the area they were coming from was not infected. Certificates issued for travel had to be obtained from consular, diplomatic or Prussian Police authorities and bear an official stamp.[11]

During quarantine, travelers had to undergo disinfecting baths with soap and water or bleaching powder. Their cloths were fumigated with potassium nitrate gas or washed with lye or bleaching powder. Craftsmen, merchants and Jews were watched closely. Goods that were especially susceptible to contagion, like feathers, fur, flax, wool, and linen, were "subject to special methods of disinfection" and had to be ventilated in a special shed. If the material was worn or the packaging damaged, the goods were destroyed. Depending on their type of fur, animals could cross the boundaries only after floating in water once or several times, and their owners had to certify that they had not come from an infected area. Dogs, cats and poultry coming from an area where an outbreak was suspected could not pass through the cordon.[12]

There were specific instructions for handling letters and other paper goods. Those that did not have "evidence of being entirely free from cholera, but from a suspected or known infected areas had to be fumigated." The first stage involved a wooden box divided into three sections. Letters and papers were placed in the top section of the box with a pair of pliers. A tight lid was placed on top of the box. In the middle section was "a pan with vinegar" and in the lowest section a "brazier with glowing coals. Scattered on top was one part sulfur, one part nitric acid, and two parts of bran. The box was closed and the letters and papers smoked for five minutes. This completed the external cleaning and disinfection, the letters and papers were removed. They were pierced with an awl and if they originated from a suspicious area they were placed to the side and put in a smoke machine and heated with vinegar fumes for an additional five minutes. After the letters were taken out they were stamped with an official mark, indicating they were "sanitary" and allowed to "continue on their journey" by post or courier. Couriers were only allowed to continue with their journey after they completed quarantine.[13]

Travelers generally wished to avoid quarantine due to the delay and the unpleasant experience they expected to undergo. One traveler on his way to England by way of Prussia complained of the fact that he would have to spend twenty days in quarantine in Strzalkowo, on the Polish-Posen border.[14] Doctor Alexandre Brierre De Boismont wrote, when a traveler from an infected area arrived on the border of a country where there is an "established cordon, he and his belongings must submit to a quarantine that varies from five to twenty days, and sometimes more." He described the living conditions in the lazaret in Strzalkowo. The hut that had once served as a customs station had been separated into three pine board sections that did not allow any communications among the sequestered people. He was "one among forty-two people crammed into one of those locations ... the haste with which this building was created, had not permitted the purchase of any furniture. They had to lie on straw, with no sheets, although a few of them had covers! The food was often appalling. When we addressed our complaints to the employees who were very polite, they answered us that they were far from the market, and lacked supplies." Although he was critical of the value of cordons, he wrote that under "the system of contagion all effects must necessarily be subject to cleansing ... but a lot of objects escape this action because travelers, convinced theses effects would be damaged by washing or gassing, are eager to have the objects escape the vigilance of the inspectors."[15]

More detailed information on the experience a traveler could expect while under quarantine was printed in an anonymous firsthand account printed in a Warsaw paper in 1831:

> "I'm already in a medical prison, where it is boring the entire day. I have to describe to you how it all looks. At the first barrier on the border stands a wooden hut ... [on the inside] ... in the corner is a fireplace with hot coals, at the other table sit the quarantine officials dressed in oil cloth uniforms and gloves, so that by their touch they do not embrace the plague. One puts forward passports, transit papers and money to be washed. After this operation, which lasts quite a long time ... the wayfarer delivers his other effects to the quarantine facility. Quarantine occurs in three buildings, each separated by a high fence. The newly arrived enter the first building, those in the first go to the second and those about to leave enter the third building. Except for bathing or the sick, the latter were sent to the infirmary, they did not go outside. There was a shed in the backyard that held all their effects and a barn for fumigating clothing and other goods.... Sadly here we eat without spoons, knives or glasses. Everything is thrown at us from a distance like animals. We sleep without bedding on straw mattresses. Worse provisions could not be had in purgatory. God grant us leave soon."[16]

The last few sentences may have been dramatized to play to readers in Warsaw. However, it does appear the experience for all travelers was extremely unpleasant. Some argued that the border restrictions "were targeted mainly at Polish citizens, and they were much easier on the Russians."[17] One only has to look at the Danzig blockade, or the initial restrictions in Königsberg to see that the Berlin central authorities were willing to hold their own subjects to the same standards that they imposed on the border. They did not give preferential treatment to the Russians.

For example, in Memel, as the disease advanced in Russia in May, the border was blocked by a military cordon. Two entry sites in Memel were established with a quarantine facility placed at both sites. Incoming ships and passengers had to undergo quarantine. If not, individuals could be arrested and the ships confiscated. Each time a fishing boat went to sea, it had to furnish an "identity card." All entrances to the city were guarded by the military. Citizens had to have authorization to be in the city, and new control bureaus staffed with citizens were established. In addition all letters were "pierced and fumigated" while "packets and money were not accepted."[18]

There was plenty of criticism not only of the harsh regulations, but their impracticality and cost. Some criticized their ineffectiveness at preventing the spreading cholera. Doctor Stromeyer while traveling to Danzig in August described the conditions at the Dirschau quarantine facility, established there because this was where the road divided and served as a transit point between Königsberg and Danzig. The facility was divided into three buildings, one for notables, one for the military, and the third for poor travelers. The latter were "cared for at State expense" and kept in an "old sheep barn." Yet, according to Stromeyer, the "conditions were very gratifying." However, when he later almost crossed the cordon mistakenly, he lamented that he would have had to endure another twenty days of quarantine without his servant and be "re-introduced to boredom, hunger and disinfection."[19]

Given the strict regulations concerning the cordons and the quarantines there was still much criticism the cordons were not effective. One reason, people believed the military guards and civil authorities were not as strict in enforcing quarantine and cordons as they should have been.

For some, the failure was explained by simple human greed. It was charged the "Danzig cordons were dominated by people greedy for a profit." The merchants and landowners did not always have proof that their goods came from uninfected areas and their certificates of health were not always authentic. In addition, village guards were not always the best trained and "travelers were often ill served and not respected." The government required that such "excesses be punished."[20] Other critics noted that when establishing cordons one had to "take into account the fictional boundaries that separate kingdoms" like rivers, or flat land with no mountains. Other boundaries consist of a "simple colored pole and sign that acts as a barrier that says you are moving from one country to another. The latter is the line that often separates a contiguous kingdom." This criticism was especially appropriate to the Prussian-Polish frontier, where it was observed, "if you move along this line a league or two, you are surrounded by farms, houses, gardens, groves, woods, yet all these places are filled with men who are all business and who are attendant to spying on the movements of soldiers" so they can avoid them. They speak the "same language and have the same costumes" and "protect" each other.[21] He clarified why the military may have been so quick to shoot into the border zone:

> What about the boldness of the smugglers? Does anyone believe that a gun stops them? At Strzalkowo on the frontiers of Prussia, where I was in quarantine, we heard firing on smugglers all

night, who passed from border to border, and I never heard that anyone had been killed, or at least the number of those who perished is infinitely small. How, indeed could the guards posted at one hundred and two hundred paces, and sometimes even further, in the middle of the night, reach individuals who enter clandestinely.[22]

Finally, what about the soldiers themselves, are they "free from corruption"? And if they are in touch with the people "can they be seduced?"[23]

As if in answer to these questions, a Prussian Royal Order was issued on June 15, 1831, listing punishments for officials who failed to report cholera cases, permitted illegal border crossings, or allowed people to leave quarantine facilities and quarantined villages prematurely. Neglect of duty was considered a "State" crime and anyone tried and convicted could be "imprisoned up to ten years or receive the death penalty." Obstructing the police or not reporting illnesses or deaths could lead to punishments from two months to two years imprisonment and for physicians the loss of a license to practice in Prussia.[24]

Despite the threat of punishment, in reports received by the Head of Internal Affairs of the Province of Prussia in Königsberg, Johann Ewald, there were frequent mentions of a lack of control on the Prussian-Polish border and especially of Polish Jews crossing into Prussia.[25] The Immediate Commission ordered Ewald to ensure transgressors were caught and punished. In addition, he was to pay close attention to travelers at the border and no one was to leave a quarantine station without a stamped passport or health certificate.[26]

On July 4, 1831, Ewald received reports of violations of the sanitary cordons around the border dominated by the people of Danzig. He again reminded his officials of the need for "proof of identity for travelers and evidence that their goods came from completely healthy areas." In Königsberg the "authorities had already confiscated large shipments of wool and flax due to a lack of relevant documents." There was doubt about the authenticity of the certificates obtained by some landowners and merchants.[27]

On July 21, 1831, Ewald wrote "sharply" to one magistrate indicating that he often "watched from the window of his apartment guards not checking travelers as they passed." Another official wrote to Ewald that he saw guards asleep while two travelers passed by and he had to "command them to stop." It seemed the police authorities had no control over the guards and he complained that this needed to be changed. Also, too many citizens were exempted from guard duty. In the same letter he also lamented that quarantined homes in Danzig were "often guarded from the street and the rear entrance was then used," even with the threat of harsh punishment. Dr. Stromeyer reported on conditions in the Danzig countryside that made it unlikely that even if officials wanted to enforce the strict regulations, to do so was nearly impossible. He observed that grain in the fields "was still on the plants for its reapers had a few weeks ago all died." In one village twelve workers had died, the rest of the "inhabitants remained in their huts and all field work had ceased." Finally in another village "all police regulations were neglected."[28]

Nevertheless, the Prussian government attempted to prevent cholera from spreading into Prussia at great cost to its own population and economy, and experienced social unrest in a number of cities. So it was not surprising that when the Polish government expressed its dissatisfaction with the Prussian government, and went so far as to publish their complaints in the French and British press, Prussian officials were incensed. Provincial President Flottwell was asked to reply to the various charges in the international press on Prussia's behalf. He argued that as long as there had been a possibility that cholera could be prevented, it was in Prussia's interest to do so, and that "nothing was done on the Polish side to prevent the disease from spreading." The accusation that Prussia established the cordon not to prevent the disease, but on "a political basis is so easily exposed and visible that it must be dismissed out of hand as absurd," he said:

> [B]efore the boundary cordon was imposed the inhabitants at the border were made aware of the rules and regulations and were granted a 48 hour allowance concerning the regulation of their business. Nonetheless, all the warnings were not upheld by the inhabitants at the boundary cordon, [especially] when proof was required.... A specific penal law was ... issued on June 15, [1831]. This law was made public knowledge by the Prussian consulate in Poland. The troops on the border were furnished with strict orders, to make use of their weapons, if and when there were unauthorized frontier crossings.... That unfavorable actions on the frontier were inevitable.... Exceptions to the frontier cordon could not be allowed and would weaken the entire system. Individuals were not allowed to come within 100 steps of the border.[29]

The regulations both on the border as well as internal to Prussia were highly restrictive and the Prussian government was convinced that if followed rigorously and backed up by harsh measures toward those who would ignore the regulations, it would be possible to prevent the cholera from entering Prussia. However, even with these restrictive measures the inevitable occurred. The first case of cholera in Prussia occurred on May 3, 1831, in the Stallupöner district near Gumbinnen, on the Polish border in the north. A journeyman, Carl Britt, returned from Poland to be with relatives following his mother's death two days previously. After returning to his village, he died seventeen hours later of cholera. District medical officials confirmed the cause of his death.[30]

Cholera moved sporadically along the Polish and Russian border in May and June. On May 27, 1831, in Dlottowen in the Johannisburger district near a quarantine station, a constable became infected with cholera. He had been in contact with Russian deserters from Poland and a number of Jewish peddlers who had likely been exposed to cholera. Another victim, a shoemaker in the Stallupöner district, had also just returned from the Polish village of Wystiten, where the cholera was "raging among the Jews." He developed cholera two days later. Strict measures were taken. The infected village was isolated to prevent the spread of the disease. It appeared at first the measures were effective.[31] Cholera next erupted on the Prussian border on June 17, 1831. A six year old boy, the son of a school teacher, died in the village of Lauken, parish of Bilderweitschen, Stallupöner district. On June 28, 1831, four more cases were reported, one-half mile from the border and two miles from the Prussian city of Memel. The victims became sick and died. The deaths had probably been the result of at least one of the victims crossing the border into the Russian (today Lithuanian) city of Krottingen and having "secret dealings with the Russian military."[32]

Meanwhile, in the village of Budweitschen, in the district of Stallupöner, another person died of the cholera on the June 28. From the June 29 to July 4, on one estate in the Budweitschen area, five persons became sick and four died. In the village of Gross Budweitschen and Publauken one person died in each village. On July 1, 1831, in the quarantine building in Shirwind in the Pillkallner district, a Russian soldier, who had fled from

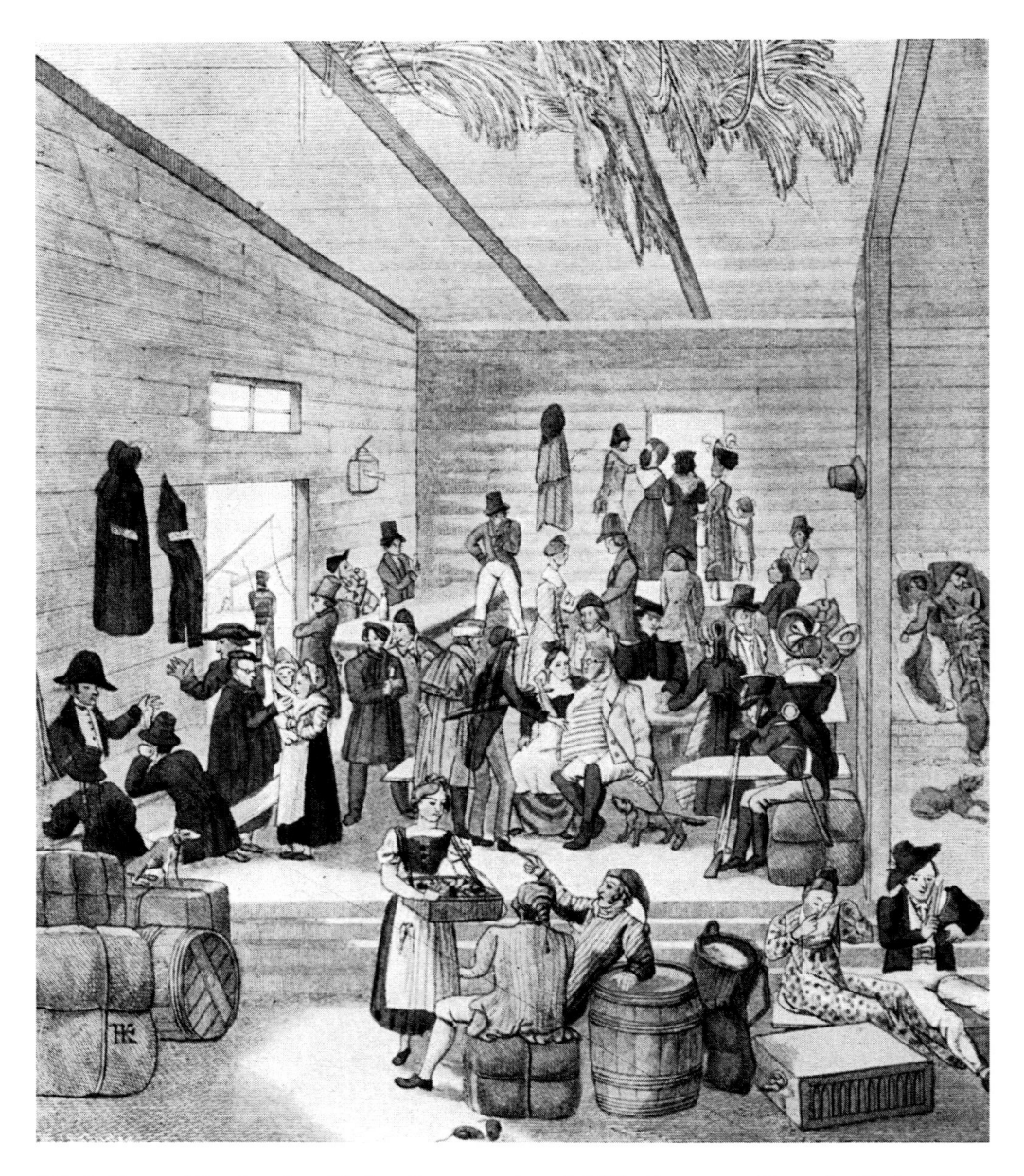

"Die Leiden und Freuden einer Cholera Contumaz Anstalt." (The Sorrows and Joys of a Cholera Quarantine Institution.) Early 1830s engraving, Munich. Indoor wooden structure, a public gathering place, most likely the departure room in the quarantine station. No disinfection or fumigation equipment is shown in the print. In the foreground, a female peddler sells merchandise to two men. People are gathered in groups, sitting on bales and barrels. This print depicts people from different social backgrounds together. As Stromeyer noted, this was not always the case. Reproduced from Eugen Holländer, *Die Karikatur und Satire in der Medizin, mediko-kunsthistorische Studie*. 2nd ed. Stuttgart, 1921, p. 182.

Poland as a prisoner of war, died. Shortly afterward, a nurse at the same quarantine station died.[33]

On July 3, 1831, in the villages of Coadjuten and Medischkehmen three miles from Tilsit, on the Russian border there were three deaths from cholera. From July 4 to July 9, there was one more death, a guard from Samlucken.[34] Wagner wrote, the areas of these limited outbreaks occurred primarily along the Russian border. He concluded the military quarantine was effective in preventing cholera from spreading further. This conclusion was to be expected since Wagner was a government official and, as a contagionist, supported the idea that quarantines prevented the spread of the cholera.[35]

Cholera broke out in Danzig on May 28, 1831, and spread to Elbing and the surrounding region.[36] From Elbing it spread to Graudenz by way of a ship captain named Schultz, who had arrived from Elbing on July 18, 1831. On July 22, he died in Graudenz and three days later three children from that city died. On that same day a night watchman hired to watch Schultz's boat contracted cholera.[37] On July 18, a serious epidemic broke out in the city of Posen.[38]

It appeared inevitable to the citizens of Königsberg that when cholera broke out in Poland and later in the neighboring cities of Memel and Elbing that it was only a matter of time before it would spread to their city. To understand the events that occurred in Königsberg during the epidemic some background on the city itself and the governing authorities is necessary.

The City of Königsberg

In East Prussia, Königsberg was originally a Hanse city, situated on the river Pregel which flows to the Baltic Sea. It has always been a commercial city with the harbor in nearby Pillau serving as its main port. In 1831, the city was divided into three major sections, the Altstadt or Old Town on the west side of the city, the Lobenicht on the east side and the Kneiphof on an island in the Pregel. In addition, there were extensive suburbs. The streets in the city were described as "long, narrow, dirty, ill paved and very often lined by lofty old fashioned houses ... which are not only inconvenient for the passage of carriages, but render that of pedestrians a work of real danger."[39]

Königsberg was a transit point between the Baltic Sea and the interior of Prussia and Poland. Its main port is Pillau, about 24 miles from the city. The Pregel River is too shallow for large ships. Königsberg imported grain, skins, oak, and fir timber from Poland by a canal that connected it to the Niemen River. Manufactures included woolen stuffs, flannel, stockings, ribbon, wax, soap and yellow amber. The city contained approximately 224 beer breweries and 135 distillers of brandy. The average number of ships entering and leaving the city annually from the Baltic during this period was 600 to 700.[40]

The approaching cholera alarmed the city fathers, who feared the central government would impose the same measures they had in Danzig. They could see this would devastate their city by disrupting domestic and international trade. The cordon on the Polish and Russian borders, as well as the sale of grain and meat to the Russian army, was already affecting food prices in the city and the surrounding countryside. One eyewitness wrote, "the provisioning of the Russian army and the threat of the disease getting even closer to our frontiers, the price of food, particularly meat prices has increased so much that the poorest can no longer afford it." Also, the lack of raw materials led to higher unemployment among the artisan and lower classes.[41]

The Governing Authorities in Königsberg on the Eve of the Cholera Outbreak

The local governance in Königsberg in 1831 was divided into four areas of authority. Each played a significant role in the cholera epidemic and the resulting "tumult" in July 1831. Königsberg was the seat of the president of the province of Prussia (formed by the merger of East and West Prussia in 1829). Theodor von Schön occupied this position and reported directly to the king. He was not trusted by many high level bureaucratic officials in Berlin. As result of his actions during the cholera epidemic, one senior official in Berlin referred to him as providing a "spirit of opposition to the capital" in East Prussia and Königsberg, by leading a "pernicious rebellion against the highest authorities."[42] The second area of governance was the *Regierung* or provincial government that was responsible for the cities, towns and villages in the province.

The third agency was the government of the city of Königsberg. The city was granted self-rule with Stein's Municipal Ordinance in 1808. The patrician class in Königsberg, as in other cities in Prussia including Berlin, resented the Municipal Ordinance. The citizens showed their unhappiness by electing opponents of the Ordinance to positions of authority in the various Prussian cities, including Königsberg. These individuals desired government by "corporate membership" and saw the Municipal Ordinance of 1808 as an attack on their "status." They did not want "residence or wealth" to determine political power.[43] The result was a group of officials and elites predisposed to resent any orders coming from Berlin. Also, they were fully aware of the "misery" resulting in Danzig as a direct result of these sanitary regulations and the potential severe economic impact that would come to their own city.

The fourth area of authority was the police. As a check on these "municipal patricians" the "police authority" in Prussia was not placed "under the control of its citizens but of the national government" as part of the central bureaucracy. In 1831, the police authority (which included the medical police) was headed by the Minister of the Interior and Police, Gustav Freiherr von Brenn. The police headquarters was housed in the Königsberg city hall or Schloss (castle) with the other government offices until 1831. It was moved to separate quarters in the Altstadt (Old Town) in early 1831. Its new location signified "its external source of authority."[44] In its new location in the Old Town section it could not be easily defended, unlike all the other government offices located in the walled castle. As a result, it would later serve as a convenient target during the cholera uprising on July 28, 1831, representing the central authorities in Berlin and the hated cholera regulations they had imposed on the city.

The Cholera in Königsberg

With the lessons of Danzig still fresh in the minds of officials in Königsberg, cholera broke out in the city on July 22, 1831, and lasted until January 4, 1832. The population of the city (excluding the military) numbered 67,360 inhabitants.[45] Cholera infected 2,221 people, 894 recovered and 1,327 died.[46]

In the first week of the cholera epidemic in Königsberg there were 71 cases. In the following weeks, the number of cases rose from 275 in the first week of August to 286 during the second week (the peak of the epidemic in Königsberg). New cases declined to 249 and finally dropped during the last week in August to 228 cases. During October the number of cases declined dramatically averaging just 100 per week. By early December new cases had dropped to 8.[47]

In most respects the course of the epidemic in Königsberg was not unusual. It struck deeply at the lower classes. Reported deaths were comparable to other cities in East Prussia. What set the cholera epidemic in Königsberg apart from cities like Memel and Stettin was that although they experienced some unrest, there were no lives lost and the damage was minimal compared to the unrest in Königsberg. In addition, the situation in Königsberg was exacerbated by the "blunders" of the local authorities "that initiated the disaster."[48] To understand why the "riot" occurred it is necessary to look at the situation in Königsberg before the outbreak of cholera there.[49]

The growing cholera threat in Poland aroused "fear and terror" in Königsberg. The public was certain the disease would come to their city. In Königsberg, travelers and their effects were subject to a detailed "investigation before they could enter the city." Entering and exiting over the city walls was strictly forbidden. Legislation was enacted to improve the cleanliness of the city.[50] When cholera first crossed the Prussian-Polish border a cholera hospital was established in the city. It was expected to house a hundred beds. Later two other hospitals were established. Special cemeteries were established, with restrictions on the burial of cholera dead and specific times set for funerals. To ensure the rapid transfer of the sick, special baskets and blankets were stored in various parts of the city to be used to bring patients to hospitals. The patients and their attendants were accompanied to the hospitals by armed guards.[51]

The public was fearful when the cholera broke out in Danzig, then they saw it approaching in the Elbing and Tilsit districts. Finally, the cholera fear in Königsberg and the strict regulations that would be imposed were raised to a fever pitch when a notification appeared, confirming the first cholera case in nearby Pillau:

> A Norwegian sailor became sick on the 17th of the month in Pillau ... he was removed from the city, completely quarantined, taken to a lazaret and treated medically; he regained his appetite and powers but died on the 21st of the month.... The man's nurse who had not followed precautions became sick on the evening of the 21st and morning of the 22nd of July. All connection with the city and lazaret was cut off. It is hoped that there will be no further cases entering Pillau. The necessary security precautions have been put into place. We bring this matter to the public.... Königsberg, the 23 of July 1831. Royal Prussian *Regierung*, Interior Section.[52]

The notification was posted for the public to allow them to take proper precautions. It indicated that the nurse who tended the first victim did not follow the prescribed regulations and that the local authorities acted immediately to quarantine the first victims. This suggested to the inhabitants of Königsberg that the government was acting to prevent the spread of the cholera from Pillau and to reassure the public the source of infection in Pillau had been effectively contained. At the same time, it gave the citizens of Königsberg a preview of what was to come in the event that cholera erupted in their city.

An article in the *Cholera Zeitung* (Königsberg), later gave an insight into the way the general public felt as they awaited the inevitable outbreak of cholera in Königsberg and what they expected would be the consequences of the Immediate Commission's regulations for their city. According to the article, prior to July 25, an individual heard rumors of a "horrible sickness in the land" and that death often came within a few hours. He was told by the government only "extraordinary police measures" could protect him from the ravages of this disease. He shook his head and said it was a "fairy tale and laughed nervously."[53]

Yet he heard the "wealthy console themselves." They said the "sickness befell poor people." With the quarantine regulations he felt certain these measures were to be applied "chiefly to the poor." As the price of goods increased, he knew this was a direct result of the quarantine of the city. He believed (as he did not see the sickness spreading) the regulations were a "pretext to bring about higher costs" to benefit the wealthy. Later, as the cholera began to spread, the sick were brought to a lazaret under an escort of guards. The streets near the lazaret were closed off by a wooden fence, guarded and inaccessible. He did not believe in contagion.[54] He knew the dead were taken to a special place and buried. Finally, the inhabitants of houses in which a person became sick were quarantined. A person's business and livelihood could be ruined by these measures and this would lead to "impoverishment and hunger." He finally came to the "insane conclusion" that the government intended "to get rid of the poor through poison and starvation."[55]

The article is a fairly accurate measure of how physicians and the middle class saw the impact of the cholera and the Immediate Commission's regulations. This is supported by statements that the disease "befell poor people," the anxiety expressed that a "person's business or livelihood could be ruined" and that the "disease was not contagious." Anxiety was raised among the poor by the idea of anonymous burial, "impoverishment and hunger" and what would later emerge as a wide ranging "poison" conspiracy. This all stemmed from the government's regulations. The author also attributed the bitterness of guild members toward the government, to the "violent acts against their traditional customs."[56]

General Thile wrote, to Schön, that "cholera seeks out for its victims the lowest and hungriest classes of mankind." Schön realized this was self-evident, but also knew that the upper and middle classes looked to the poor as a social danger (not only politically but also as disease carriers) and that they did not need more of these ideas being discussed by government officials. He replied, "this class is already unlucky enough and one increases this feeling toward the poor through pronouncements of such a dreadful nature." Thile remarked about the high death rate among the working classes. Schön replied, it is "horrible ... to prophesize more bad luck for men with little joy in life."[57] Thile's outlook was more common than Schön's. In the final analysis, the lower classes came to assume the doctors and police who treated the sick, quarantined and buried them were also responsible for their deaths. The Königsberg poor concluded doctors and the government were in league trying to poison them. This fear was not so "insane," as Malthusian ideas regarding overpopulation were filtering down to the poor and many of the German states were responding to their overpopulation problems with restrictive legislation that directly impacted the poor.[58]

More immediately, officials in Königsberg, especially Schön, looked to the hardship imposed upon Danzig as a result of the Immediate Commission's regulations. As the occurrence of cholera in the city seemed imminent, with anxiety and fear mounting, he turned to General Thile on July 16, 1831, with an urgent request, to ask the king not to enforce the instructions of the Immediate Commission. He wrote "experience shows from the Danzig report that the instructions established by the Ministry are imperfect, they are injurious, and these arrangements are for a different illness, the plague."[59] In St. Petersburg there had been a wild rebellion, and he made clear the danger of the current measures in Danzig. He asked that the instructions be completely rewritten, "the Medical Boards should be used more effectively rather than using military guards, and there should be a greater emphasis on medical measures." Referring again to the Danzig Sanitary Commission report of July 3, 1831, he wrote the current regulations will cause more misfortune, whereas, if "seriously and consistently handled, in a cultivated land such as ours, cholera ... can never cause as much misery."[60]

Schön's plea was futile at this time. The king ratified the Immediate Commission's new instructions." After all, Schön could look to the Danzig experience and read in the Danzig Sanitary Commission report, "if ever there was a quicker scheme to undermine the welfare and bring poverty to a city or region, it is by this current scheme." And then these harsh words: "it would be less evil, if a third of all the inhabitants of Danzig should ... die."[61]

The Königsberg Physicians Respond

The doctors in Königsberg, led by the physician Karl Burdach, resented the high handed manner in which the Central Government initiated public health regulations without involving the provincial medical authorities.[62] It seemed that all the "arrangements were made in advance by the Immediate Commission to Prevent the Cholera ... and their orders were only directed to the civil authorities." There was no discussion. They "decided cholera was as contagious as the plague," and "blockades were the only means to prevent the disease."[63]

Nevertheless, following the instructions published on April 5, 1831, the city government of Königsberg established a Central Sanitary Commission that included the mayor, five city deputies, the Police Chief, a police councilor and four physicians. With the blockade of the Polish-Russian frontier from Thorn to Nimmersatt (approximately 450 miles), and with only eight quarantine entry points along the frontier, Königsberg officials began checking all travelers and their goods before allowing them to enter the city. On June 14, 1831, eight district sanitary commissions were established within the city.[64]

On July 19, 1831, a representation of twenty-eight Königsberg private doctors met with Schön to ask why the Central Sanitary Commission was not functioning. They protested quarantining healthy individuals, trade barriers, and strict funeral regulations. They noted new funeral regulations only created "feverish phantasies" about cholera. They complained that experience had shown that cholera was not contagious. They insisted standard applications of "disinfection and covering the face" were the only measures required for treating the sick and dead."[65]

Doctor Burdach, who was also a Polish sympathizer, was certain the blockade of the frontier was imposed to prevent a successful Polish insurrection. He saw that provisioning the Russian army provided many occasions for the introduction of the disease. He decided to write to the Sanitary Commission with his own proposal, as both a "physician" and a "good citizen." In his proposal he wrote the "disposition to cholera was primarily a disorder of digestion" and good food needed to be supplied to the people. Unemployment caused by barriers to trade contributed to the disease. He recommended slaughtering and grain taxes be suspended. This would lower the cost of food (provisioning the Russian army added to the shortage of food and other supplies and increased prices). Because "fear and terror" are contributing factors to the disease, "horrible images" and descriptions of a plague like disease sent to the provincial areas should be avoided. The Sanitary Commission should educate the public about the disease. He concluded it was dangerous to adopt regulations so severe that there was little chance of the public actually following them. For example, the Police regulations of May 23, 1831, that required physicians to report all cases of suspected cholera before they even had an opportunity to diagnose cholera. In was also improper to initiate quarantine and barricades that would frighten the public, when the illness was probably not related to the new and deadlier disease of *cholera morbus*.[66]

Following his proposal, Burdach was asked to write instructions for the public. Among other things, he took a cautious approach to cholera and wrote that, like any illness, the Asiatic cholera could be contagious under certain circumstances, but the virulence of the Asiatic cholera was not yet sufficiently established.[67]

He later concluded cholera was not contagious and cannot be prevented with barricades. His opinion was endorsed by most Königsberg physicians. According to Burdach, Schön welcomed this opinion, because he was "provisioning Russian troops with the requisite transports to cholera suspected areas, and in the face of a bitter public, he could only justify it by the assertion that there was no existing danger of contagion."[68] Burdach added that Schön still had to play the game, that cholera was an infectious disease, like plague and needed the barriers. He added, the Prussian court was willing to pay the price of the ruin of their country for the love of Russia. Burdach was completely wrong in making this accusation against Schön and the Prussian government.

Schön's decision to provision the Russian army was based on the threat of Russian gunships sailing into Pillau. The Immediate Commission did not want the Russians to break their quarantine regulations. It was Schön acting in opposition to the Immediate Commission who had to convince the Prussian Cabinet Ministers to allow Russian ships to land. This was done to avoid potential violence that would have exposed the entire province to the unimpeded spread of cholera.[69]

Burdach also complained that Schön ignored the Königsberg Medical Society's requests for reports and articles on the epidemic. Schön allowed the Society members to have access to the files and reports in his office. They claimed this was not sufficient and they wanted to ask the Ministry "to order Schön to give them the necessary communications." According to Burdach, the Director of the Society was afraid of opposing Schön.

Burdach took his place and under his leadership the "private society" became the "medical authority" during the epidemic. It replaced the local medical board and the medical faculty at the University of Königsberg (which according to Burdach hardly mattered at all during this crisis). This new medical authority was composed of twenty-three private physicians and three pharmacists.[70]

Events began to move quickly. Shortly after Schön's meeting with the private physicians the cholera erupted in Königsberg on July 23, 1831. The Königsberg Medical Society, Dr. Burdach, and other members of the Society organized a medical response to the epidemic. They would participate in the development of a modified medical policy and recommended less severe sanitary regulations during the epidemic. They also founded the *Cholera Zeitung* (Königsberg) to provide accurate information to the public during the epidemic.[71]

The Outbreak of Cholera in Königsberg

On July 22, 1831, the sudden death of a man who was thought to have been suffering from cholera initiated a fright in the city. After his autopsy it was determined that he died from an "inflamed colon." The previously ordered blockade around the neighborhood was continued and no one was allowed to enter the neighborhood without a health certificate.[72]

The following day the cholera broke out in Königsberg in the Kniephof section at the far end of town, in the poorest area of the city, the *Deyschen Hofe*. It lay in a marshy area surrounded on three sides by water.[73] The section contained seven small boarding houses inhabited by 136 people, primarily day workers. The houses had two floors as well as three attics or lofts. The cobbler Meinert rented out two of the rooms and lived in the middle loft. One attic room was rented to the first victim, an "unmarried woman" named Malessa. The other loft was rented to a poor working family, the Brosches—a husband, wife and son.[74] Malessa was reported to have tuberculosis, was "mentally defective" and had spent time the previous year in a "mad house." She, like the Brosches, also received "alms"[75] On July 20, the Meinhert's visited the sick woman. She showed no change in her condition. On July 21, a doctor was called. She was reported near death and died that evening.[76]

The cobbler's wife and her neighbor, Mrs. Brosche washed and cleaned the dead woman's body and dwelling (as was customary).[77] The next day Mrs. Brosche became sick with cholera and died. The "boarding house lofts were quarantined and a guard posted." Mr. Brosche and his son did not become ill.[78] On July 23, Meinert's wife became sick. New cases followed on the first floor of the boarding house. Cholera began to spread to the other houses in the *Deyschen Hofe*.[79]

The police publicized the cholera outbreak and carried out the prescribed sanitary regulations. The entire courtyard was surrounded by the military. No one from the *Deyschen Hofe* was allowed into a healthy neighborhood. A high wooden fence was erected dividing it from the rest of the city. Food was supplied by the military.[80]

With the outbreak of the disease, the *Physical and Medical Society of Königsberg* began meeting daily. They invited other doctors to meet and deliberate on what actions they should take. They established an overnight medical watch of two physicians complete with a cart to take physicians wherever their assistance was needed. These activities were subsidized by the city communal authorities.[81]

Cholera Rumors in the City

As with previous outbreaks of lethal diseases, rumors of the cholera's origin spread rapidly and outsiders were usually blamed. As we will see later, the most dangerous and nefarious rumors that led to "mob" violence in Königsberg had to do with the fear that the doctors were poisoning the poor at the behest of the Prussian government.[82]

Schön ordered two doctors and a judge to investigate a number of rumors. The first attributed the outbreak of the cholera to infected hemp from Russia. The second blamed contaminated fish sold in the Königsberg market. The third traced the outbreak to a sea captain who had come from the port of Pillau.[83]

Of the three rumors, the contaminated fish rumor was the easiest to dispel: the Brosche woman had eaten the fish and died; but others had eaten fish and did not become sick. One investigator considered the idea of infected fish as a cause to be "laughable" to anyone who had lived in Königsberg and was aware of the quality of the fish sometimes sold in the market.[84]

The hemp rumor was taken seriously enough to lead to further action by Schön. On the previous day before the cholera outbreak he had received a deputation of merchants. They asked that a cargo of hemp that had come by water from Russian Lithuania not be permitted to be unloaded. They claimed they had a terrible fear of this contaminated Russian hemp and its potential horrible effects. Schön refused their petition. He did not believe cholera contagious and would try to prove it the next day.[85] A later investigation of the hemp rumor showed that the Broshes were too old to have worked with hemp. Besides, the hemp had undergone proper quarantine. Finally, it was probably confused with a flax shipment that was headed for Königsberg that did not have the proper health certificate. This shipment underwent twenty-day quarantine. The merchant produced a letter on August 22, 1831, showing that none of the workers handling the flax (over 200 individuals of both sexes) had become sick. Dr. Baer later wrote that at the beginning of the summer the border was blocked by a cordon. The people were so fearful of catching cholera from "infected goods," it was a "moral impossibility to commit fraud" by smuggling uninspected goods.[86]

Competing Investigations on the Origin of the Cholera in Königsberg

Investigating how cholera was introduced into Königsberg was an important question to be resolved because, for the doctors, it was part of a larger question about the trade regulations imposed by the government that affected the lives of so many people.[87] There were two important investigations. The first and earliest was by Dr. Baer, published in the anti-contagionist *Cholera Zeitung* (Königsberg). The second was undertaken by Dr. Wagner under the auspices of the Immediate Commission, and later published in the official contagionist report the *Cholera Archiv.*

The investigation of the Captain Hoffstädt rumor was the most difficult to dispel. This was due to the attack and plundering of the police building that occurred on July 28, 1831. Between the destruction of the police files and uncooperative witnesses, a detailed and accurate understanding of Hoffstädt's movements prior the outbreak of cholera was impossible to determine.

Dr. Baer concluded cholera "developed independently" in Königsberg. Dr. Wagner, with additional proof, concluded cholera was "communicated" by Hoffstädt and passed on from one individual to another.[88]

In Dr. Baer's account, he reported Hoffstädt was living in one of Meinert's lofts along with the Brosche family and the unmarried Malessa. On the morning of the quarantine following Malessa's death, Hoffstädt grabbed some boots and told the doctors that he had just come from Pillau to have his boots repaired. He did this to avoid being quarantined. The guard on duty was not fooled and refused to let him evade quarantine. Hoffstädt changed his story later saying he had not come from Pillau but had been in Königsberg since March. He also lied and claimed he had not been renting a room from Meinert.

R. Richter, the criminal judge appointed by Schön to undertake an official investigation, interrogated Hoffstädt, who told him he had been making a living repairing ships and selling small amounts of tobacco, amber and coral to sailors. He had been living in Königsberg since March 1831, but was actually a resident of Pillau. He was told by the police in April to return to Pillau. He did not return, but remained in Königsberg. He claimed he had arrived at the *Deyschen Hofe* on July 21, 1831, and slept there over night to the next day, when the deaths occurred.[89]

Richter said Hoffstädt had lied about coming from Pillau. He changed his story and seemed indifferent. He contradicted minor details and tried to take charge of the examination. In addition, Meinert had written on his door, "Hoffstädt aus Pillau." In short, he first claimed to have come from Pillau but when he realized that he was suspected of bringing cholera to the *Deyschen Hofe* he withdrew his statement. He said he had been in Königsberg since March and had worked on repairing ships that were no longer in port. He lived in places that he could not identify. Finally, he could not give details on how he happened to come to a house where the disease had broken out.[90]

Eventually Richter received further information concerning Hoffstädt's former landlord. Richter had not been able to locate him because he had the wrong name. The correct name was Cilly; he let Hoffstädt a room and was also good friends with the captain. Speaking with other acquaintances it turned out that Hoffstädt was somewhat of a vagabond and had different addresses from June 15 to July 13. Sometime after July 13, he moved to the *Deyschen Hofe.* Baer reported there was no cholera in Pillau (and that if he had gone to either Elbing or Danzig his visit would have been recorded). Baer concluded Hoffstädt could not have introduced cholera.[91]

Baer explained Hoffstädt lied about coming from Pillau because on the back of his passport it said the "possessor was a panhandler and therefore has to leave at once and return to Pillau." The passport was dated and signed on April 10, 1831, by the police president. He did not return to Pillau as ordered and this was why he said he lied and said he had recently returned from Pillau. This was also why his landlords were omitting to tell the police of his presence and explains why he "forgot" the names of his landlords. They were simply cooperating with him. He changed his story when he realized he was at the center of the contagion controversy.[92]

Baer concluded cholera developed independently in Königsberg. He described the unhealthy environment at the *Deyschen Hofe*, the dirty and damp surroundings, piles of garbage and other filth. The buildings were crowded and the residents "poor and unclean." These were all contributory factors to the miasmic cause of cholera.[93]

Dr. Baer described the Brosche family as so poor that the wife "engaged in collecting rags and bones" for income. Malessa could be seen "lying in her own filth." He described how the two women washed Malessa's corpse "with great disgust and loathing." Later Mrs. Brosche drank sour milk and that afternoon became sick. She died the following day. Afterward, the disease began to spread throughout the *Deyschen Hofe*.[94]

He speculated, the disease may have been caused by Malessa but it could not have spread directly to other inhabitants in the area. The lodgings were quarantined meanwhile the doctors, police and soldiers who went in and out remained healthy. Family members slept in the same beds with their spouses and remained healthy. Even Malessa on the day she fell ill had visited a neighbor and that family had remained healthy.[95]

Baer concluded that those who initially fell ill suffered from poor nutrition and an unhealthy environment. Other factors that accelerated "the onset of the disease" included drinking the sour milk and the anxiety producing consequences of quarantine.[96]

The evidence showed that on the July 23, Hoffstädt had stayed in an apartment in the *Deyschen Hofe* where cholera occurred. Hoffstädt insisted that he not be quarantined because he did not live there and had not been to Pillau since the cholera outbreak there. However, Hoffstädt did room with the shoemaker Meinert. Meinert could not say where Hoffstädt had been living prior to July 21. Neighbors agreed Hoffstädt visited Meinert at least eight days prior to the outbreak. Police records indicating where he had been between July 13 through July 21, had been destroyed in the riot on July 28. Richter and his investigators concluded they could not prove that Hoffstädt had not been to Pillau during the eight missing days, nevertheless, they finally concluded he had not been to Pillau and attributed the cholera outbreak to local unsanitary conditions.[97]

Based on Richter's evidence, Dr. Baer concluded cholera was not contagious and hoped that his investigation would quell rumors and assure the public that once pre-disposing conditions (poor sanitary conditions) were eliminated the disease would subside.

Dr. Wagner was critical of Baer's report. He later concluded with further evidence cholera had been communicated by Hoffstädt to the *Deyschen Hofe* and then throughout the city. There was no record where Hoffstädt stayed between the July 13 through July 21. But statements by witnesses and a note scrawled by the landlord on the door in Hoffstädt's room that read, "Hoffstädt aus Pillau" led Wagner to conclude Hoffstädt had traveled to Pillau. Why else would Meinert have scrawled it on the door? He also had new information: Hoffstädt had a colleague who was one of the first to become sick in Pillau. He believed Hoffstädt had probably visited him. Cholera appeared in Pillau two days prior to its appearance in the *Deyschen Hofe*. The living conditions in all the apartments in the *Deyschen Hofe* were basically similar. However, the only apartment where the disease broke out was the one where Hoffstädt lodged. The reason Malessa was the first victim was because there was no room for Hoffstädt in the Meinert or Brosche lofts. It fell to the single Malessa to let him room with her. Later the two women who washed and cleaned Malessa's body and her loft became sick. From here cholera spread to the other buildings in the *Deyschen Hofe*.[98]

With the knowledge today of how the cholera is spread, it is likely Hoffstädt may have infected Malessa through some manner of contact. Initially Malessa was diagnosed with tuberculosis but another doctor later claimed she must have had cholera.[99] She may have come into contact with Hoffstädt, who was likely an asymptomatic carrier. She then became the unwitting focal point of the epidemic infecting those around her who tended to her body following her death. As noted earlier, this could have occurred as a result of the common funeral practice of washing the body and the room after a person's death and distributing clothing (as well as bedding and other personal effects). Fluids from Malessa's body contaminated her bed clothing and bed with cholera. (Stains from the infected person would have been hard to see in the late stages of the disease. Bodily discharges dry clear and mix in with previous soiling).[100] When the Brosches, and perhaps other women cleaned the room (and distributed her belongings prior to the arrival of the doctors and sanitary police) they may have unwittingly carried the cholera back to their families or distributed it into the community. This could account for the somewhat sporadic outbreak in the immediate vicinity, although a common contaminated drinking water source cannot be ruled out. By July 27, 18 people out of 136 had contracted cholera in the *Deyschen Hofe*. From there it spread outside the sealed off area to the rest of the city.

The two investigations demonstrate two divergent positions concerning cholera. Königsberg was the center of the non-contagious theory supported by the Provincial President. As noted in the earlier article from the *Cholera Zeitung* (Königsberg), the government's regulations were seen by Schön, the city physicians and merchants as an impediment to trade and prevented the proper care of the sick. If the local investigation could prove cholera was not introduced in the city from the outside but developed from internal predisposing causes or local conditions, the need for interventionist government regulations would be lessened. The city's course of action could turn to locating breeding grounds of the disease and cleaning them up. On the other hand, Wagner set out to prove the disease was introduced from the outside and that there was direct contact from one victim to the next (contagion). This approach justified the Immediate Commission's interventionist sanitary policy during this time.

The Cause of the Königsberg "cholera riot"

The Königsberg uprising in itself was not a unique popular response to cholera. In Russia and later (in 1832) there were a series of popular uprisings in Paris. The causation and violence of these "riots" is similar in many ways to the uprising in Königsberg.[101] The "uprising" in Königsberg as well as lesser riots in Memel and Stettin represented some of the few examples of violence in Prussia during the stormy years of "rebellion" throughout Europe, as well as the other German states in 1830–1831.[102] However, the loss of lives and property in Königsberg was the most destructive and represented a rare example of unchecked collective violence in pre–March Prussia.

The immediate trigger of the Königsberg riot was a result of an overzealous application on the part of the police of the government's sanitary measures, following a modification of the policy ordered by the local Königsberg authorities. The riot demonstrated conflict and stress in a city under siege. What was unique about this violence is that that it was not initially instigated as traditional class warfare of rich against poor. The focus was on fear of the government in Berlin and the king creating policies that removed the poor from their homes and flouted their traditions (especially burial practices). Doctors were accused of being agents of the government, eliminating the poor by poisoning or starving them.[103]

On July 23, 1831, the police president of Königsberg, Johann Theodor Schmidt, after visiting the *Deyschen Hofe* on the same day dutifully ordered the implementation of the Immediate Commission's cholera regulations. Three houses were quarantined for several days and a wooden fence was erected. Head of Internal Affairs of the Province of Prussia, Ewald, wrote, he "saw what had been done," and agreed that it was a good idea. Then early Sunday morning he returned to observe the quarantine arrangements. He went to the Castle (or *Schloss* that contained government offices, including Schön's and the *Regierung*). He could not find Schön, but found members of the government assembled. They appeared "scared and helpless."[104]

Meanwhile, Schön, convinced by his medical advisors and local physicians that cholera was not contagious was determined to obtain his own evidence. He decided to visit the sick at the *Deyschen Hofe*. According to Ewald, he could have obtained the information he needed from his government medical councilor, Dr. Kessel (one of his medical technical advisors), but Kessel had been placed under house arrest by the "overanxious" *Regierung* President Meding. Dr. Kessel had previously gone to investigate a cholera outbreak in Elbing. He observed and treated cholera patients there. On returning he had not followed quarantine procedures. According to Ewald this was the first of the "blunders by which a disaster was initiated."[105]

Ewald located Schön and met with President Meding, Police President Schmidt and Councilor Hagen and other members of the government. At this time, the *Regierung* members showed no intention of disobeying the Immediate Commission regulations. However, Schön announced he would break quarantine and visit the *Deyschen Hofe*. He asked the other officials to accompany him on the visit. They looked as if they were setting out on a "journey to their deaths."[106] They followed Schön to the head of the stairs of the Castle. President Meding declared he had "an appointment."[107] The retinue proceeded with at least thirty people. At each corner "more of the convoy bolted." After arriving at the *Deyschen Hofe,* five of the original members of the retinue remained and included an official named Leibgard, Police President Schmidt, Councilor Hagen, Ewald and Schön. Only Schmidt, Ewald and Schön entered through the quarantine gate at the wooden fence in the *Deyschen Hofe*. When the three came to the door of the infected building, Schmidt declared "he had no duty" beyond this point.[108] Ewald entered the dwelling with Schön and saw a surgeon tending to the sick. The surgeon gave them a warning and "led his excellency into the sick room."[109] The room was filled with clouds of tobacco smoke from Dr. Jacobi who was smoking a pipe, as the doctor said, to protect him and his companions from contagion. Schön visited the sick, consoled them and remained there for about a half an hour. He ordered that a muddy ditch be filled in, that the *Deyschen Hofe* be cleaned and disinfected, that all apartment dwellings be cleaned and the quarantined be provided with good food.[110] After leaving the *Deyschen Hofe*, Ewald and Schön were met by two friendly doctors who washed them with chlorinated water and exclaimed that they had both been exposed to "infection." Both officials laughed this off but according to Ewald their public bath provided much "amusement to the street youth hurrying by."[111]

Schön was convinced cholera was not contagious and had been willing to break quarantine and defy the Immediate Commission to prove his point. By visiting the sick and ordering sanitary measures rather than a continuance of the "official quarantine measures" he had sided with the physicians of Königsberg and sent a strong signal that he was not going to allow Königsberg to follow regulations and become impoverished like Danzig.[112] This act was a "deliberate violation of regulations issued by the Immediate Commission and it made a big impression on the public."[113] It earned Schön the strong disapproval of the King, who wrote to him "that if indeed you did visit the sick beds you have been wrong, very, very wrong ... you have been an example of disobedience."[114] Schön had given his enemies something to use against him and had "disheartened" his friends.[115]

Meanwhile, President Meding and his cabinet were meeting all afternoon. Ewald arrived at the meeting at five o'clock. Ewald had a low opinion of the *Regierung* members. They seemed too easily frightened. He sarcastically wrote, "these wise men could not issue anything but an order ... to close all the bordellos."[116] When the order was delivered to him he tore it up and nothing more was heard of it again.[117] On the same day the *Regierung* and Police President Schmidt issued a notice to enforce the "quarantine of cholera infected houses."[118] This was still in keeping with the orders issued by the Immediate Commission.[119] Ewald and Schön had probably discussed the next course of action giving Ewald the courage to tear up the prior order.

A few days before Schön's visit to the *Deyschen Hofe* on July 19, the local Sanitary Commission received a proposal signed by twenty-eight physicians under the auspices of Dr. Hirsch, of the Physical and Medical Society, requesting the authorities focus more on "managing the disease, facilitating the acquisition of good healthy food and managing public opinion." They hoped these actions would help to decrease unfounded fear and terror, rather than focusing on the isolation of the sick and blockading parts of the city. The latter measures only excited and frightened the public.[120] The Magistrate did not dare to accept these recommendations "as they were contrary to the already adopted legislation."[121]

Once cholera erupted the authorities attempted to implement the Immediate Commission's measures. It became obvious there were patients whose houses were too small to allow them to be properly isolated and they had to be brought to hospitals by porters. The act of delivering these patients gave off a mysterious appearance. The patients were led along roads isolated by high wooden walls and anyone who fell ill from cholera saw his home surrounded by guards. The movements of all other people in the building were watched with suspicion.

Those who did not follow instructions could be fined 20 talers or put in prison for eight days on bread and water. Rather than the virulence of the disease frightening the public, it was the "lack of judgment in the measures" to prevent the disease. From this developed the "mad ideas" that the poor in the hospitals should be let out, that the police were hindering their fellow countrymen from coming into the city with food to prevent starvation and that physicians were poisoning people in quarantine.[122]

As a result of Schön's visit the day before and continued unrest in the city, at 10 o'clock, on Monday July 25, Schön called an assembly. It consisted of bureau chiefs, directors, military officials, members of the *Regierung* and two representatives from the Immediate Commission, Major von Below and Dr. Wagner. He proposed to lift the quarantine in Königsberg.[123] The result of the meeting was later reported:

> On the 25th of July, his excellency, the Chief President, Herr Schön, after having a conference with the Chiefs and members of different administrative departments, issued a decree to permit free trade in the city ... the stringent decrees of April 5 and June 1 was no longer advisable.... On the following day the Royal Government [i.e. Schön] declared that experience had shown that the quarantine in the interior of the country hitherto had appeared insufficient and that fear and apprehension had predisposed [the people] to the cholera; therefore the quarantine ... should be stopped.[124]

When the "notorious" proclamation of July 25 reached Berlin it was received with "horror." The president of the *Oberlandesgericht* (Provincial Superior Court) had written the document. Everyone who attended the meeting had signed it.[125] The proclamation stated cholera had made much progress in the whole province of Prussia and it was "pointless and impossible to strictly adhere to the instructions of April 5, 1831, and June 1, 1831." The military could not deliver a "sufficient number of soldiers who still were needed to guard the border from Memel to Thorn and maintain a cordon around Danzig." In "consideration for the good of the residents they were forced to relax the regulations to allow them to move more freely."

The following new regulations were issued:

a. Persons who lived in homes where the disease occurred were not permitted to leave the city;
b. All other persons who wished to leave the city had to report to a specially created committee to obtain identification stating they were not suspected of having the disease or did not live in an infected dwelling;
c. The pass entitled the person to leave quarantine and to travel to any town in Prussia;
d. Such cards to be stamped every night;
e. Individuals were allowed to export goods from Königsberg and to import goods and necessities, even from the most remote villages in the province;
f. Anyone carrying personal articles should have an identity card issued by the local police to show that the holder did not live in an infected dwelling;
g. Sellers of goods could use their stamped identification to return on the road at night but the identification had to be stamped every night;

h. The usual market was to be maintained;
i. The mail system is unchanged however travelers, coachmen and letter carriers must possess identification cards.

This was signed by order of Provincial President Schön. It was published on August 3, 1831.[126]

With this action Schön and his supporters on the council acted contrary to official policy. He later justified his actions to the king by arguing the Berlin instructions alarmed the people. When cholera broke out in the *Deyschen Hofe*, Schön could not obtain a good report from his officials as to what was occurring there. At the July 24, conference he decided to investigate the *Deyschen Hofe* himself. He wrote that many at the conference expressed "fear" and viewed the *Deyschen Hofe* as a "pest hole." Schön maintained he was doing his "duty" and that it was an "obligation" with which he proceeded with in good "conscience." He fully supported the anti-contagionist Königsberg doctors and the miasmic origin of the cholera. He demonstrated this by his visit to the *Deyschen Hofe* and subsequently ordered the removal of "garbage," had the area cleaned and ordered a "foul ditch be filled with chloride of lime." Schön wrote that positive measures like these were necessary from someone in his office. He expressed concern about the apparent certainty of the "Berlinische Theorie" believing that officials in Berlin did not really know the nature of the sickness or they would not keep insisting that it was contagious. He believed the physicians in Königsberg, who had experience with cholera, were in a better position to judge the measures that would lessen the impact of the disease.[127]

Schön wrote that he did not act in opposition to the king but to those officials advising the king, especially Rust, who had given orders "that cholera was ... wholly contagious."[128] Schön believed that certain officials in Berlin knew nothing about the sickness. Officials in Königsberg knew it was not contagious (as a result of their experience with the cholera) and the quarantine regulations would "ruin the whole country."[129]

Rust accused Schön of high treason as a result of his actions. Schön defended his position by stating that he generally went along with the opinions of officials in Berlin, but in this instance, where so many lives were at stake, he could not gamble on ruining the country. He referred to Danzig, as the primary example of a city which carried out the cholera instructions faithfully and as a result experienced the loss of many lives and the impoverishment of the city.[130]

The proclamation on July 25 may have set off a firestorm in Berlin, but as far as Dr. Burdach was concerned much of it was simply an opportunity to allow individuals to freely engage in commerce. The proclamation did not address specific medical measures that would put to rest the idea that cholera was infectious and had to be stopped by "plague methods." He got his opportunity the next day on July 26, when a "Select Committee" was called to provide additional medical instructions for the public and was asked to participate in this meeting. The end result was the "Regulations and Announcements of the Royal Government" to the public issued by the Interior Department of the Province under Ewald, on July 26, 1831. The notice explained changes were being made because cholera had reached the local Department, appeared in many places and in other cities including Königsberg.

The crowded cities and especially the unhealthy living conditions of the poor, was a concern not only for the cities but for the entire province. Military authorities no longer possessed the means to blockade or isolate the province. Experience had shown blockades were inadequate to halt the spread of the disease. The local government was left to make arrangements which it now felt could address the "worsening of the disease."

At the outset the notice indicated the disease was not considered contagious but it did caution those who had no "urgent reason" to approach the sick or the deceased should not do so. Conditions that made one susceptible to the disease included anxiety, cold and intemperance.

Additionally, the local government lacked the means to completely close the city and if it attempted to do so, it did not have adequate food and other necessities. The food shortage that existed would disappear in a few days as a result of the new regulations. Identification cards would be issued to regulate who was coming into the city to sell food and goods. One issue that the notice was expected to address was the quarantine or isolation of the sick and their dwellings. Of major concern was the notification of the authorities if someone became sick. The public was advised it was dangerous not to notify the authorities immediately when someone became sick so medical aid could be provided. This would improve the chances of recovery. Cholera hospitals were open to the sick, "whether rich or poor," and if their home was suitable, they could remain there.

The notice contained five separate paragraphs. The first explained what to do when someone "falls ill with diarrhea and vomiting." A doctor was to be called to investigate the situation, provide treatment and remove other persons as required. The most appropriate care would be recommended. If it was impossible for the patient to follow the advice of the doctor in the house, the doctor will recommend the cholera hospital. The second paragraph detailed what to do if the patient remained in the apartment. The house would not be isolated. A guard posted in front of the sick room at public cost would ensure that only authorized persons tend to the patient (on the doctor's authorization). A "yellow placard with the inscription 'Cholera'" is to be hung outside the front door of the dwelling. All residents will be able to come and go freely. Any food or other necessities must be placed on the table so that visitors do not have contact with the sick. Also, on the table is to be placed a "goblet with diluted vinegar" in which money is put to be used to purchase items for the patients.

Paragraph number three concerned the recovery of a patient. The room was to be scrubbed clean, white washed and fumigated with smoke for a few hours. The guard then removed the yellow placard. This would not to occur less than 48 hours after the recovery.

Paragraph four concerned the patient's death. The deceased should be buried as soon as possible. The body should not be washed but placed immediately in a "coffin that is to be nailed shut and covered with tar." If the body is brought to a "consecrated" cemetery that has already been selected to receive the bodies of cholera dead, the funeral will be at public expense. If the relatives wished to bury the deceased in their own chosen place, they could do so but the funeral must take place after 8 o'clock in the evening and before 8 o'clock in the morning. The funeral must be conducted at their own expense. In addition, instructions were given for the burial of the dead. These included the regulation that the grave must be six feet deep and completely filled in.

The fifth and last paragraph, that gave instructions for fumigating the dwelling of the deceased, was removed. Officials and physicians hoped these instructions would "calm the minds" of the public, help maintain health and to prevent the spread of the disease. They concluded by reminding the public that it was their duty to report any illness immediately, that not to do so "was a crime to their fellow citizens" and the "guilt" would also weigh heavily on their "conscience," especially if any person died as a result of their neglect. Finally, the authorities asked for the support of the public.[131]

An overriding question concerning these modified cholera regulations was that if they had been communicated sooner to the people it would have prevented the subsequent rioting. Hagen wrote that the modified cholera "Regulations and Announcements" notice was approved when Schön met with a representative from the Immediate Commission, Major von Below, Ewald and councilors in the Department of the Internal Affairs. Schön proposed less stringent local requirements for quarantining cholera patients because they did not have the means to completely isolate them. It was decided to issue a notification to the public. Hagen said he would prepare the notice that afternoon. During the afternoon, he sent messages to doctors and later consulted with Ewald, Dr. Kessel and others to produce an "improved draft." Around 6 or 7 p.m. that evening, the notice was sent to the printer of the *Hartungsche Zeitung*, to be published in the newspaper the following day. Hagen wrote that the riot could have been prevented if copies of the notice had gone directly to the public earlier. The "first collision over the funeral of a ship's carpenter" would have been avoided (see the following chapter).[132] However, Burdach did not agree with Hagen's version of events and blamed an unnamed government official who prevented the notice from being distributed. He wrote, "a member of the government, who supported contagion stood like a guard on the rampart ... and waited two days to deliver the printed notices." Meanwhile, "in indignation the people broke out in revolt."[133]

It is possible that if anyone had prevented the "Notice" from being distributed in a timely manner it was probably President Meding. Before Schön went to the *Deyschen Hofe* he had returned to the city to obtain information about the first cholera cases. When he explained what he proposed to do "he was confused because Meding had rebelled against him." Meding placed Dr. Kessel under house arrest after he returned from studying cholera in Elbing. He was also one of the first to offer the excuse that he had "an appointment with Dr. Elsner" when Schön was leaving for the *Deyschen Hofe*. Later, without blaming him for the missteps leading up to the tumult, Schön had President Meding removed from office.[134]

On the other hand, Burdach curiously did not name the official who prevented the announcement from being distributed. He did complain that the announcement did not go far enough. He agreed to some restrictions that he thought were probably not necessary, indicating not all the doctors were convinced the disease was not contagious and some were still taking a cautious approach.[135]

Schön later wrote the doctors advising him, Dr. Elsner (his private physician), Dr. Kessel and Dr. Baer all agreed with taking a more cautious approach with the announcement. However, Dr. Burdach and his followers wanted to suspend all the Berlin regulations and this was something Schön could not do at that time.[136] Burdach wrote that he had to agree to some "restrictions by which the present government council was giving the illusion that they were doing something against the infection; and these included placing the plaque with the word Cholera outside the sick room, posting guards, the goblet of diluted vinegar for the money for the patients, not washing the bodies of the dead and nailing coffins shut and sealing them with tar. To his knowledge no one was doing these things, but he agreed that if the notification of July 26, had been printed immediately and made available it would have "calmed the public" and the riot in Königsberg might have been avoided.[137]

Ewald wrote, Schön's "loyal disobedience was the beginning of a demonstration against the doctrine of the contagiousness of cholera, which was necessary if a reasonable treatment of the epidemic should ever be able to take place."[138]

Not everyone agreed with Schön. Other officials were no doubt fearful of the consequences of disobeying Berlin to their future careers. They inhibited clearer communication with the public. This miscommunication was combined with authoritarian police actions. Also, paranoia was rife among the poor. They believed they were being poisoned with cholera "germs." They also feared the consequences that would occur as a result of the imposition of "Rust's senseless regulations." All of these factors helped to contribute to the riot in Königsberg that led to a number of deaths, numerous imprisonments and the destruction of property throughout the city and suburbs.

8

The Cholera Tumult in Königsberg

One of the first reports concerning the "cholera tumult" in Königsberg appeared on August 2, 1831, in the *Prussian State Gazette:*

From Königsberg it is reported that the local authorities relocated a portion of the inhabitants of the *Deyschen Hofe* in order to administer good food and better medical services as significant measures to prevent the spread of the cholera. The sickness had since appeared in other parts of the city; on July 25 and on the morning of the 26th there were 5 new cases and 4 deaths that had come to the notice of the police. The houses of the victims were closed off. On the 28th of the month occurred an uprising in Königsberg. The cause of this is thought to be a general misunderstanding of the interpretation of the measures against the cholera and in particular the delusion that physicians instead of trying to heal people are trying to poison them and that doctors, in treating cholera by application of phosphorus ether and vitriol had poisoned several persons. Groups of people who did not agree with the cholera regulations assembled that morning at 10'oclock for the funeral of a journeymen carpenter who had died from cholera. The commanding general of the 1st Army Corps, Lieutenant General von Krafft at about 11 o'clock that morning attempted to move people along and disperse them by "friendly persuasion." When people refused to move and began to physically abuse doctors and police officers he tried to put what was a weak garrison under arms. The crowds invaded the Police building and threw files and papers into the street. The military fired on the crowd and eight people were killed. Gradually by the late afternoon order was restored. The citizens, students and others had assembled to help the weak garrison (as the greater number was assisting with the cordon). The night passed quietly. During the same evening 150 people from the lowest classes were arrested and some portion of this group was brought to Pillau.[1]

Wilhelm Leopold Richter, *Königlich Preussischen Criminalrichter,* later reported on the riot following an investigation and the trial of the rioters. He provided a description of the riot, select testimony, evidence about the actions of some of the more egregious rioters and their punishments. After the first cases of cholera, the Königsberg authorities ordered barricades in places where the disease had erupted. "Police and other sanitary officials dutifully carried out their orders."[2] On the night of July 26, 1831, a journeyman carpenter named Finkenstädt became ill. His wife tried to cure him with a household remedy of cow dung mixed in boiled milk. He drank the mixture and became sicker.[3] A physician, Dr. Vogdt was summoned at 4 o'clock in the morning. He found Finkenstädt ill "with diarrhea and cramps." He diagnosed him with cholera, and felt "there was little hope of his recovery" Nevertheless, he prescribed two medications. One made up of brown drops to be taken internally and the second, alcohol to wash his feet. Each medication had its own flask with clearly written instructions on each bottle. Vogdt handed the two flasks over to the wife. After he left, she gave her husband the medicine, "but probably agitated due to her pain and grief, she mixed up the medications, and gave him the alcohol instead of the brown drops." He died two hours later.

The widow later denied that she had confused the medicines. Her daughter stated that no one else had given the deceased medicine. Dr. Vogdt asked her what medicine she gave to her husband? She answered "the white." Dr. Vogdt said it was just alcohol and should not have injured him. However, since his "strength was nearly gone" it must have had an adverse effect.

A disaffected bookkeeper, previously employed by the pharmacy where the medicine had been obtained, arrived at the Finkenstädt home and was shown the prescription. Hearing that the man had died from drinking the alcohol, he said in a loud voice to the people on the door step "he must have died from that." The wife had spilled medicine on a book. The bookkeeper saw the yellow drops on the book and repeated his accusation to the crowd. The widow spread the rumor that "her husband was poisoned by Dr. Vogdt." The doctor tried to assure her he died from cholera. Police Commissioner Schmidt tried to convince the crowd that Finkenstädt died from cholera. His widow, friends and co-workers were not convinced. They demanded the doctor declare "that Finkenstädt had not died of cholera" and they wanted permission to take his body to the regular graveyard for burial with his fellow guild members. Dr. Vogdt refused to change the cause of death. He subsequently had to leave the city secretly because the mob became incensed and wanted to kill him.[4]

Following Finkenstädt's death, the police commissioner sent porters to remove his corpse for burial in a plot in the Sackheim graveyard, designated for cholera victims. His widow refused to allow the porters to take his body away. She wanted to make sure he was buried in the cemetery of her choice. A fellow carpenter and mourner named Sähm invited the other journeymen to help bury her husband. Twenty men remained at the deceased's house to prevent cholera porters from carrying off the corpse. Guards were placed in front of the house. The following morning, July 28, police commissioners declared "that due to the public notice published on July 26, the body could be buried in any cemetery." But the body could only be "taken to the cemetery by cholera porters." His guild members demanded they be allowed to carry his body to the cemetery. A member of the local Sanitary Commission and a city councilor asked whether the latter was possible. He was told to follow regulations "even if military assistance was required." When the Sanitary Commission representative returned to the Finkenstädt residence, cholera porters were waiting there with a military escort. The guild members said "if ... [cholera porters] ... were going to carry the body, then the police would be responsible for any violence done against the porters by a few hundred men."[5]

The police commissioner allowed the journeymen carpenters to have their way because the military escort was too small to be effective against the large crowd of people accompanying the body to the cemetery. After the burial (between 8 and 9 o'clock in the morning), the guild members returned peacefully to an inn. Other members of the crowd did not know what to do next. They went to the castle plaza (headquarters for all the government offices) just as a group of brewery assistants were coming out from the castle's inner court.

This crowd was coming from an inquest that resulted from another cholera demonstration the day before. The inquest resulted from a demonstration caused by the removal of a young girl from her home to a cholera hospital.[6]

On the afternoon of July 26, 1831, in the Löbnicht section of the city, ten-year-old Amalie Barz fell ill with cholera. She was taken to the lazaret at 6 p.m. As was common, a crowd assembled in front of her house. Soon the house was filled with people, the crowd was loud and more people tried to force their way into the house. The police commissioner was called; and the police tried to disperse the crowd. Many of them left but the brewery assistants remained, saying "they had to wait in the streets to get work." The crowd increased in size and was becoming rowdy. The police commissioner called in the military guard and arrested one of the "stubborn brewery assistants." The guards had hardly taken a few steps when other brewery workers came to his aid. They protested his arrest, surrounded the guards and put the prisoner in the middle. The crowd released the guards at the request of the police commissioner.[7]

Others in the house who had died from cholera were taken away. The crowd assembled again in front of the house. The people ignored the police and began to "sing, dance and cry hurrah." Meanwhile, between the nights of July 26 and 27, at least two of the more troublesome brewery workers were arrested. Their inquest was set for 10 a.m. July 28. They appeared accompanied by a few hundred of their companions, along with other curious onlookers. The brewery workers showed up at the inquest because a former overseer, the brewer Hamm, told them if they went as a group it would strengthen any demands they made. The brewery workers remained peaceful throughout the inquest held at the castle court and "left when ... [the two men] ... were cleared." During the hour-long hearing "a large crowd of both sexes from the lower classes" arrived at the castle court following the Finkenstädt burial. This crowd arrived just as the brewery workers were leaving to their own cheers."[8]

As the Finkenstädt crowd arrived at the castle gate, a policeman and a guard blocked the entrance to the inner courtyard. A boy insulted a policeman named Schumann. He beat the boy and brought him to a castle guard, which antagonized the crowd.[9] An unidentified person tried to strike the policeman with a stick and was arrested. After a second incident the crowd began to throw cabbages and other vegetables at the guard posts. Soon they began throwing stones at the guards. The guards tried to arrest the stone throwers. The mob turned and with shrieks people began to run through the streets toward the police headquarters building. Another boy was arrested for throwing stones at the windows of the police building. He was later rescued from the police by the mob.[10]

Police President Schmidt reported "the mob ... said the cholera sick had been poisoned."[11] Schön said, he communicated changes in the cholera regulations to the townspeople and the educated public. However, the "lowest classes had not acquired the full knowledge of the regulations."[12]

How did these incidents lead to a full scale riot? Ewald, Schmidt and Schön described their actions that day. At 11:00 a.m. on July 28, 1831, Ewald arrived at the castle on official business. Around 12:30 p.m. he went to the *Regierung* offices and noticed activity in front of the main guard box.[13] Schön wrote, "A small crowd had assembled over an unimportant criminal case in front of the Castle courtyard." He called Police President Schmidt to manage the situation and left.[14]

The Attack on the Police Building

Schmidt hurried from the castle courtyard after he received word that the Police building was surrounded. When he arrived the crowd was demanding less stringent cholera measures. He seized some of the rioters. He later wrote, they "were not bitter against his person, but against the Police ... [who] ... permit the doctors to poison them, deliver them to the lazarets and allow them to die there."[15] The crowd "wanted an investigation of the doctors, lazarets and all other institutions where cholera victims were treated."[16] Schmidt added, there were four companies of soldiers in the city, but they had been sent to guard the lazarets. He hoped that the military would be able to intervene because the rioters were becoming bolder.[17]

The passage to the street from the police building was blocked by the mob. The crowd became restive and then violent. After a few minutes not one window in the police building was left undamaged. The crowd continued to throw stones from all sides. Police officials tried to mollify the crowd but had to flee when the crowd became more violent. Mounted soldiers were summoned but quickly withdrew because their horses were frightened by the stones being thrown at them. The mob broke down the doors of the police building and "freed the recently arrested prisoners."[18] The mob split up, with some of the rioters heading off to the suburbs, breaking windows along the way. Physicians and their support services were especially targeted. For example, the Heubner pharmacy was demolished because it served as the place where doctors working the night shift met and obtained their supplies. The mob intended to destroy the cholera lazaret near the Brandenburg Gate. The fury of the crowd extended to plundering other businesses. There was an attempt to take the Fredericksburg Castle armory until the artillery corps stationed there put a stop to the rampaging crowd by firing on them. Several rioters were wounded.[19]

Meanwhile, the situation in the police building had become more desperate. Two guardsmen along with two police officers tried to hold the crowd back. Schmidt tried to remain at his post but he was forced "to flee from floor to floor" and finally to his apartment. When the crowd came for him in his apartment he fled to the rooftop and hid until the violence ended. The mob "completely demolished his apartment ... smashed all the furniture, broke precious mirrors, destroyed his pianoforte, cut up clothing and bedding, destroyed his library and stole easy to conceal items like silver spoons and jewelry."[20] The violence continued to haunt Schmidt and his family until his death. His "family had been sick with terror and fear" and in addition to losing his furniture and his library his daughter was nearly abused by the rioters.[21]

The crowd continued to throw stones, smash windows and plunder more of the building until they finally destroyed it. The military appeared but had no "orders to shoot." They left the infuriated crowd to finish its destruction of the police building.[22] The rioters tore up the police files and "threw documents and papers from the windows..." that pertained to quarantine and related matters.[23]

Richter reported that once in the police building the crowd cried "here is the cholera" and tore up papers, clothing, and bedding. The material was dragged away.[24] Schmidt wrote the crowd had cried out, "we want the cholera germs." The crowd broke into the building screaming "the doctors are poisoning the poor, the police drag them to the lazaret and close-up their houses, saying they have to go because they are poor." According to Schmidt, if an earlier doctor's report had not concluded that the barricades and the lazarets should be removed immediately, the people in their fury would have "demolished them" too.[25]

Earlier in the afternoon Ewald met with Schön and General Krafft. The General asked Ewald to accompany him to the old town market square where the rioting was occurring. No one could make sense of the crowd's complaints. The irrational screaming led to further disturbances. A group of militiamen finally drove the crowd away from the police building. According to Ewald, the riot could have been quelled at this point but General Krafft made a serious error of judgment. His men had fixed their bayonets and drove the crowd from the adjoining buildings. They could have easily overpowered the "gangs roaming the streets, smashing widows and mistreating the Jews and physicians they encountered." Instead of continuing with a show of force, Krafft rode into the plaza and "harangued" the crowd. "The defiant rabble addressed him in a loud voice.... Do you think we are the Devil, Sir! Who asked them to use their weapons? Thinking his "eloquence" had calmed the crowd and stopped the riot, he rode his horse provocatively through the crowd" and left the plaza with his escorts. As soon as he left the plaza, the people complained the "soldiers are allowed to do anything." The people now infuriated, "rushed to the right and to the left" and attacked a building they had earlier spared. With great joy they began to finish what they had started, especially the women. They broke windows and cut up bed clothing, which caused "feathers to rain down on the marketplace." The troops remaining in the market place marched unimpeded across the plaza and took up a position on the other side. Meanwhile, the noise coming from the Old Town center was so loud that when Krafft returned to the castle he felt compelled to take more serious measures.[26]

Escorted by a second company of soldiers and a small number of cavalry, he returned to the Old Town center. The enraged crowd began "to physically resist the advancing military and attacked them with sticks, poles and stones." Finally, General Krafft was assaulted and he gave orders to shoot, which led to some deaths and wounding of some rioters. The general was knocked off his horse. An attempted cavalry charge was unsuccessful, the horses turned back by a hail of stones. The small number of *cuirassiers* was not adequate to overpower the crowd.[27]

Ewald returned to the *Regierung* and attended a hurriedly called meeting. It included General Krafft, Captain Dankbahr, President Meding and the mayor of Königsberg.[28] Ewald later wrote that it appeared "they would not be able to quell the riot" and that a "plundering of the city would certainly occur." It was evident "that the local militia" was not adequate to contain the uprising. President Meding demanded that the army intervene. However, there were no regular army troops available because most of the troops were at the border due to the "unrest in Poland and the *cordon sanitaire*." There was only a weak garrison in the city. The reason the military did not fire on the rioters at first was because it was thought that they could appeal to their better instincts by not using live ammunition. This tactic was not successful, as the looting, destruction of property and the accosting of the "well dressed" showed.[29] It was then "put to General ... [Krafft] ... he had to ... arm the citizens so order could be restored." Only after long negotiations did he agree to distribute weapons to the citizens. However, too much time had passed for the citizens to organize. Meanwhile, the few students in Königsberg (only a hundred were available because the college was closed for summer vacation) quietly assembled with rapiers, sabers and any other weapons they could obtain. They were joined by the university rector, an officer named Major Ventzki and others. Ventzki was placed at the head of this group of students. They marched to the castle and asked permission to "clean up the Old Town center by force of arms." Krafft agreed.[30]

Other officials who participated in this operation included an *Oberlandesgericht* councilor, the university rector, and a city councilor. Ewald hurried to the town hall to assist the small assembly and to supply them with additional weapons. The citizens brigade composed of students, citizens and soldiers were given "swords and pikes" from the armory at the Fredericksburg fortress and white arm bands to identify them.[31] At 5:30 p.m. the citizen's brigade arrived at the police building with "orders to shoot."[32] The rioters initially greeted the students as allies when they arrived in the Old Town center. They thought they had come to help them. A city councilor named, Schartow, "exhorted the crowd ... asked them to remain calm and leave. He yelled out, "Long live our beloved King!" He was answered with a hail of stones.[33] The rioters and the brigade attacked each other. What followed was "carnage of gleaming blades, axes, hatchets and stones."[34] Several shots were fired into the mob, killing five men and one woman. Sixteen rioters were wounded (one would later die of his injuries). The fury of the crowd was demonstrated by one woman who was killed "clutching the stone in her hand that she wanted to throw at the commanding officer." The crowd was dispersed and order was restored in the Old Town. Some students were wounded in the attack but all recovered. One member of the citizen's brigade "the dyer Przettack, was separated from the others and mortally wounded in a back alley by the rioters." He died a few days later. The citizen's brigade took back the police building.[35]

Although order was finally restored around the police building, unrest continued in other parts of the city. This was directly related to the cholera regulations and to rumors of poisoning. In the Sackheim district, for example, a basket used to carry the sick was stopped by the rioters. The porters, police officials and soldiers were driven off and assaulted. The basket was torn into pieces and the doctors were beaten. Blankets and other utensils used to care for the sick were stolen. In the Baderstrasse section of the city, "women cabbage sellers and chimney sweep lads attacked a quarantined house and drove the guard away" and forcibly removed the barricades. In other parts of the city doctors were followed and in some instances stones were thrown at them.[36] Rioters unsuccessfully attempted to break into the cholera lazarets and save the sick from being poisoned by the doctors.[37] Schmidt reported, the "evil day was finally over" and more than sixty rioters and plunderers had been led away to prison in Pillau.[38]

That evening 300 citizens patrolled the streets of the city and arrested a large number of suspects, who were imprisoned in the castle. "Bound hand and foot," they went "quietly without resistance" under armed guard. They were not transported by soldiers but by sixty young citizens under the leadership of a Lieutenant Romans. They were turned over at the causeway to the military and from there the prisoners were transported to Pillau without incident. The next evening a larger group of prisoners were sent to a prison in Tapiau.[39]

A report on August 3, 1831, stated a total of 263 persons had been arrested. Twenty-eight were transported to Pillau and 76 to the prison in Tapiau. One hundred one were left in Königsberg. Fifty-eight prisoners were released after a hearing. After more denunciations, it was reported on September 20, 1831, that 559 persons had been implicated. The *Prussian State Gazette* reported eight people killed in the rioting and 150 people "of the lowest classes" taken to Pillau. The Hamburg correspondent for the *Allgemeine Zeitung* reported the number dead at between eight and 15 with many wounded. Private correspondence which reached the English Ambassador in Berlin, Chad noted "there had been several people killed" in the tumult.[40]

Following the July 28 riot, peace and order were not entirely restored and various actions broke out for a number of days following the tumult. The citizen patrols and night time security measures were continued until August 4.[41] A mob of journeyman bakers working in the "field bakery" near the Friedlander Gate attempted to free their imprisoned comrades from the artillery wagon house. There were approximately fifty of them who "with singing and much noise moved toward the artillery building" demanding the release of one of their leaders. A loaded cannon was moved into place in the event that the crowd became violent. Order was quickly restored. There were still other minor disturbances in other parts of the city, as well as numerous threats to the public order by the "lowest rabble." However, after few days order was restored.[42]

After the rioting, the police reported that none of the 44 soldiers and five officers involved were injured. Of the citizens and students who assisted in putting down the riot, 13 were hurt but all fully recovered. The damage to property was estimated at 14,660 talers (Richter noted this figure was an estimate because it was difficult to recover documents due to the destruction of the Police files).

The Trial and Punishment of Select Rioters

According to the police report about 500 persons who participated in the riot were arrested. One hundred twenty-three were released because there was no proof of their participation. As a result of the police investigation, 243 defendants received some punishment, while another group was acquitted. Based on the preliminary investigation, an additional 151 were remanded for further investigation. In the end, only 25 of this group remained in custody because they were considered "highly dangerous subjects." Their punishments were divided into five categories and fell under different penal codes: those who destroyed police files and records, took action against the military and citizen's brigade, and stole property or acted in excess; those who damaged goods and buildings; those who took action against the military and citizen's brigade; those who only committed thefts during the riot; and those who committed excesses in remote parts of the city. The punishments ranged from corporal punishment to imprisonment of a few months to 12 years.

Richter provided examples of the testimony and punishment meted out to some of the most serious defendants who committed crimes during the riot. These examples also give an insight into the events and demonstrate how the violence escalated, what type of individuals participated in the uprising and the punishments received.[43]

One of the most serious cases to come to trial was the workman Johann Ordner, accused of killing citizen brigade member Przettack. Ordner was 31 years old and born in Königsberg. He worked alternately as a chimney sweep and a *Leierspieler* or "hurdy gurdy player." He was bad at both jobs. Previously convicted of theft, evidence was given to the court that he had participated in the riot and mishandled Przettack. Police found a mirror and four books in his possession recovered from the destruction of the Police building. He claimed he obtained them from a boy in the street. A merchant's wife testified she saw him beating a citizen with a white arm band. She saw the victim take shelter in a shop. The rioters followed him in and beat him. When another merchant tried to help Przettack, he was struck by the rioters. Other witnesses gave similar testimony saying they saw the victim "struck with a wooden cudgel."

Przettack escaped with great difficulty and found shelter in a boarding house owned by a widow named Bartlau. His clothes were torn and he was "bleeding profusely." He spoke little and had been beaten unmercifully by unknown assailants and struck by stones. He had separated from the citizen's brigade and fell into the "hands of the rioters." He said his attackers had been drinking.

Przettack received medical treatment and lived four days following his beating. The prosecution tried to link his death directly with the blows he had received from Johann Ordner. Unfortunately, the medical evidence and treatment were questionable because various doctors and a surgeon disagreed over the exact cause of his death. One physician concluded he had died from a rock that had struck the back of his head while another from a "brain inflammation which brought about his death." Because his brain had already begun to decay, the court could not order an autopsy. The cause of death could not be determined.

The defense challenged the credibility of the witnesses and claimed they "were full of bitterness and hostility toward the defendant." However, the judge did not think challenging the credibility of all the witnesses made sense. Finally, because the victim had lived for four additional days and had even drunk brandy it could not be determined whether Ordner had actually caused the victims death. Under the law an individual participating in a riot near someone who was killed could receive a four to ten year prison sentence. If the individual was a ringleader and there was a death, the penalty was ten years to life imprisonment.

The conclusion of the court was the defendant had abused Przettack (but not killed him) and that he was more than a participant in the riot because he had thrown stones, helped in the destruction of the Police building, and threatened a merchant. Witnesses believed he was "one of the most dangerous rioters" and "suspected his mistreatment of Przettack helped lead to the former's death." This was an important factor in determining his punishment. Even though he was not a ringleader he was given a twelve year imprisonment. Richter concluded, the "punishment was fully justified."[44]

The next defendant was 20-year-old Johann Gottlieb Mehlpiz, a notorious thief who was born in Königsberg and who had already been charged with theft five times. He was imprisoned for striking Przettack with a sword. He denied participating in the excesses of the riot and said he was "just hanging around." However, witnesses testified they saw him repeatedly beat Przettack on the head with a sword and then throw the sword into the Pregel River. A shoemaker said he had been mistreated by Mehlpiz and also saw him throw the sword into the river. Because credible witnesses had demonstrated that the deceased had been beaten by the defendant, he was given 6 years of imprisonment.

The next defendant, Carl Bartsch, a 31-year-old shoemaker, belonged to the local militia and was accused of striking a military person. He confessed to being in the Old Town center among the rioters and hitting a soldier with his fists. He claimed he was struck first. Witnesses said that he went up to Lieutenant B. The lieutenant told him to return home. This infuriated Bartsch and he hit him with his fists. As he withdrew he yelled "you dog, I would hit you again." Later he returned home "bleeding heavily." A maid testified he said "the officer gave it to me good" and an hour later he said "Now I am going to pay the police back for everything." Bartsch was convicted of assaulting a person of "higher status" and breach of the "public peace and security." His punishment was 3 years imprisonment.

Carl Rebuschatis was a 30-year-old part-time night watchman who, according to the testimony, had thrown rocks at the soldiers. Lieutenant B. swore that the defendant had taken the reins of his horse as he came into the Old Town center. The lieutenant had to give the defendant "several blows to the head." This was why he was wounded. Another officer said he saw the defendant try to pull Krafft from his horse. The defendant said it was possible he grabbed the reins of the horse in a drunken state and received his wounds from the sabre as a result. It could not be definitely proven that he had thrown stones. He received 3 years imprisonment and 40 strokes.

Carl Riedel, a clerk from Poznan was only in the city for a short time prior to the uprising. He was under investigation for theft and the police described him as a dissolute person. Riedel admitted that during the turmoil he had hung around the Old Town center and neighborhood taverns. Witnesses said that he had participated in the "tumult" and thrown stones at the Police building. Sergeant P. said the defendant had been the culprit who seized the horse bridle of General Wrangel when he approached the Old Town center. He cried out "Hurrah" and called for the people to follow him. A merchant sitting near the defendant in a local tavern, heard him say it was "he who had grasped the famous General's reins and taken the legs out from under him." Witnesses said that on July 28 he had come into a local tavern making a lot of noise and said "that he had been one of the first to storm the doors of the Police building and thrown out the files. That he had participated in the Warsaw revolution and finally deserted." His statements were confirmed by other witnesses. They also reported when he was arrested he screamed at the police "they could go to the devil." He also made many threats against a police superintendent. He was charged with taking part in the "excesses of the riot by word and deed" and to "have taken an active part in the destruction of the Police files." He was sentenced to 3 years imprisonment and received 40 lashes.[45]

The Conclusions of the Prussian Provincial Superior Court

The question of exactly what happened to instigate the "riot" and the underlying causes was investigated by the Provincial Superior Court and later formed the basis for Richter's report. The court took a broader view of the events and wanted to assure the public and the government that the riot was not part of a greater revolutionary conspiracy against the government. This was not an unreasonable approach, given that Europe was rife with revolutionary movements. There was fear that Prussia, too, could become "infected" by the "plague of revolutionary ideas from the west."[46]

Based on events in France in 1830 and the Polish revolt in 1831, it is not surprising that the Provincial Superior Court began by investigating whether the riot had been part of a larger political conspiracy. When the July revolution washed over France, it did not overtake Prussia but it did revive liberal ideas in large cities like Königsberg.[47] In 1830, events in Paris were breathlessly reported in the German newspapers. The Königsberg post office was besieged by the public and reports were read aloud to the people as they were received. Cities in the other German states and in Prussia sympathized with the Polish revolt, including Königsberg. When sick or wounded Polish soldiers visited Königsberg, they were "invited to parties, balls and similar events."[48] Surprisingly, there is no mention of a conspiracy on the part of the rioters to support the Polish revolt in Königsberg, although there is some minor evidence that one of the rioters, Carl Reidel from Poznan, mentioned the "Warsaw Revolt" during the riot. However, no one followed him. If they had he might have been designated as a "ringleader" and received the maximum penalty. There is no evidence that sympathy for the Polish uprising contributed to the riot.

Other examples of a possible conspiracy occur in the transcripts of the trial. A watchman asked a brewery worker to come to the "Altstadt" on July 28 because there would be "food and drink there." A shoemaker a few days before spoke of a "tumult" and said there would be a revolution. The slogan would be "one for all and all for one." Finally, a crude broadside with a skull painted on it and a message was circulated among the rioters following the July 28 tumult. This has been suggested as evidence pointing to a possible political conspiracy. However, officials quickly dismissed this as the work of a "hack writer" trying to take advantage of the events. The broadside read:

> The top guys from the government and the Provincial Superior Court are the hidden oppressors of the people and the cause of all evil: the beasts have broken into the homes of the young people at night and in the same hour massacred and plundered them. We can now liberate our imprisoned comrades who have nothing further to fear, and at the same time something to live for.[49]

The broadside followed the riot and the subsequent arrests and could not have been a contributing factor to the riot. Finally, the court concluded that it could find no evidence of a conspiracy nor could they identify any "ringleaders" or anyone "agitating" to begin a riot. The tumult was neither political nor did it come from widespread dissatisfaction with the state government and there was no highly treasonable intention, and for this reason, even in spite of all the research, there is neither discovered a connection to a rioter, much less a secret leadership of this people's movement ... [the riot] ... is a consequence of the confluence of the excesses of various villains and the predatory rabble.[50]

In 1832, Richter published a report in the *Preussischer Provinzial Blatter* re-emphasizing that the rioting was not based on "political reasons or dissatisfaction with the government or the state. It was a "random sequence of events. It was an excuse to rob and steal." The immediate cause was "discontent with the cholera barricades." It was the "illusion of the intentional poisoning of a patient, due to the rashness of a woman over her husband's painful death." This was used as a pretext to damage the police building. Finally Richter dismissed the "talk of any conspiracy or revolution as not having being demonstrated by the evidence."[51] However, even if the court did not recognize it, there was a conspiracy involved in the riot but it stemmed from a "paranoia" that came from the bottom up. There was a public belief that the state and the doctors were trying to poison the poor. This was an update of the old belief that "plague" was caused by the Jews. After all, Ewald reported along with physicians, Jews were blamed and mistreated too.

In his public report of the cases he concluded that the crimes of the rioters had "filled us with horror and disgust." It was "good for nothings" and "rabble" that had committed these local crimes. He invoked the Achen uprising of August 30, 1830. He wrote there was "no comparison to the crimes committed in Königsberg to Achen as the crimes there were against the state government and a senseless imitation of what happened elsewhere in the wave of freedom, following the example of a neighboring Dutch province that brought about the sad events. But even as here, only the scum of the people committed the crimes."[52]

If the riot was not a political conspiracy could it be attributed to unresolved social and economic conditions. One historian concluded "The cholera was the occasion, not the basic cause of the Königsberg uprising."[53] However, it is clear from the events and eyewitnesses that the strict cholera regulations were entwined with social and economic conditions. There were also psychological aspects which contributed to the conspiracy theories surrounding the connection between the government and the physicians. Other individuals with immediate knowledge of the conditions in the city described two major economic factors that caused the unrest that led some journeymen and daily wage laborers, as well as the "rabble," to revolt. The Prussian government imposed strict cholera regulations which affected the economy, increasing food prices and unemployment. Local officials began forcibly carrying off the sick, barricading infected dwellings and imposing strict burial instructions on the public. These final actions became a flashpoint that caused individuals from the artisan and working class to directly confront the police, physicians and others in the service of the government's cholera apparatus.[54] This point was made by Police President Schmidt, who wrote to von Brenn, "it was the provisions against trade that truly agitated the working classes ... and the lack of adequate wages" to allow them to provide for their families.[55] The effect of this policy was undoubtedly more life threatening to these groups, as well as the very poor, than the cholera itself.

Adding to the unrest was the widespread belief in a fearful conspiracy that the doctors (as agents of the state) were not helping the sick but were poisoning them, especially the poor. The rumor circulating through the city was that there was no real epidemic but a plot by the doctors to poison people.[56]

Another important factor contributing to unrest was the initial overreaction of the police.⁵⁷ An egregious example of this was illustrated when a woman whose husband had fallen ill went to get help. The "overzealous" police, acting on old cholera instructions, removed her sick husband and her children too. When the woman returned home she went into a "wild rage," and became one of the chief instigators of events the following day.⁵⁸

For pre–March Germany, historians have traditionally focused on class conflict, economic necessity and traditional responses to state interference in the customary rights of people as causes of violence.⁵⁹ In many respects the tumult in Königsberg mirrored the pattern of pre–March violence in Prussia in two of the three elements: economic necessity and interference in customary rights. Citizens initially took part in demonstrations over the strict funeral regulations of the government. Once the customary rights issue of burials was settled, the artisans and workers returned to their homes and taverns and did not participate in the riots The "rabble" was responsible for initiating the rioting and plundering. The cholera combined with the government's strict regulations made the situation unique creating a latent fear among the poor.⁶⁰ This occurred because it was the poorest who found themselves immediately in dire circumstances when they could not easily move about because of quarantines. There was little or no work, the cost of food increased dramatically and, since they had limited resources to fall back on, they knew if they became sick they would be carted off by the authorities to die in a cholera hospital. Judging by the targets of their wrath—the police and the police building, physicians, cholera hospitals and a pharmacy—one could argue there was a distinctly rational response by the mob to those in authority who enforced the government's strict regulations during this crisis, coupled with the ineptness of the local government in stopping the rioting before it got beyond control.⁶¹

The Prussian people were not strangers to state attempts to regulate public health measures. However, not since the wars of liberation had the population faced epidemic disease and intrusive government regulations to keep disease from the healthy population, and regulate the economic and social life of the city. To complicate matters further, the basis for quarantine regulations were in dispute. Schmidt wrote there was a "spirit of insubordination" in the population of Königsberg and he traced this to the "blockade of subsistence items, the restriction of trade and industry ... the restriction of shipping and the suspension of the annual market."⁶² The government had interfered with the livelihood of the people. The "people were acquainted with the events in St. Petersburg against quarantine and lazarets," there was already great dissatisfaction.⁶³ As one would expect, there was little support for the central government's position when local physicians and the provincial president were openly critical of official policy. Schön later admitted that he knew there might be trouble. He blamed the authorities in Berlin who ordered the severe cholera regulations, disregarding "all moral and religious feeling for men."⁶⁴ By this time the people of Königsberg and Schön were well aware of the detrimental effects of the Immediate Commission's policy on the city of Danzig. The poor who depended on casual employment and ease of movement to find jobs realized the economic impact of these strict controls. They had already begun to complain about the increased prices for subsistence goods as a result of the quarantine at the main city gate.

The Doctor's Conspiracy and Poisoning the Poor

The day after the riots in Königsberg, the doctors tried to determine why physicians and other medical personnel were attacked. According to Dr. Burdach, the impetus had been a newspaper report that quoted Schön, who said there had been some deaths since July 23, 1831, but most of the "deceased had suffered, according to the doctors, not from Asiatic cholera, but an irregular lifestyle ... [it was this that] ... had caused their sudden death." Burdach blamed this article for propagating the "illusion that the cholera epidemic was a malicious fabrication by physicians." It gave additional credence to this idea and "encouraged the mob" to attack physicians. Burdach and his fellow doctors rushed to complain to Schön about this "dishonest notice." He accused Schön of evading their accusations by using "diplomatic phrases." Schön finally gave into their demands and a retraction was published July 29, 1831. In it Schön stated his information was based on the Sanitary Commission or doctors reports and the sick taken to lazarets had the Asiatic cholera. In order to counter incorrect reports from the authorities, counter false rumors and control the "exaggerated anxiety" due to cholera, Burdach and his colleagues established the *Cholera Zeitung* (Königsberg) on August 6, 1831.[65]

The fear of doctors and the state was more deeply rooted in the psyche of the people than a simple report in the newspaper. The deteriorating economic conditions and government regulations created by the epidemic at first gave rise not to fear of cholera as a disease but to the idea that no such disease existed. There was a greater fear of government policy in which the deaths "ascribed to that malady are produced by poison administered by the Doctors who are employed and bribed for that purpose."[66]

As an example of how this rumor could be seen as independent of the newspaper, we have the evidence of a poisoning conspiracy directly linked with the insult to the honor of the carpenter's guild (the traditional notion of the artisan's honor) when the authorities threatened to bury Finkenstädt in a dishonorable grave (common cholera grave). Ambassador Chad reported from an eyewitness in Königsberg who summarized the initial events and clarified how the combination of cholera and poisoning by the doctors was confused by the poor,

> A Carpenter taken ill of the cholera was poisoned by the mistake of his wife, who administered to him a draft of medicine intended for external application—His Corpse was about to be buried with those of the Victims of Cholera, but the populace resisted this measure, saying "this man was poisoned by the Doctors, and succeeded in causing him to be buried in the ordinary burying ground."[67]

This quotation illustrates that poisoning was suspected by the "Doctors," even though the poisoning was not done by the physician but by the victim's wife. The people were not concerned about the subtlety of whether the medicine was for "external application" or to be taken internally. Not trusting doctors anyway, as the *Prussian State Gazette* reported, the people were guilty "especially of the error, that doctors, in treating cholera by application of phosphorus ether and alcohol, had poisoned several persons."[68] To heap insult upon injury, the victim was scheduled to be buried in a common cholera grave. His fellow guildsmen would not accept this and concluded the victim was poisoned by doctors who were trying to bury the evidence. As we saw earlier, the crowd forced the body from the police and gave the deceased an honorable burial. On the following day when young Amalie Barz died from cholera, her coffin was filled with quicklime to prevent further infection. The people believed she also died by "foul means." The crowd not only cried "out that the Doctors were poisoning the poor," but added "and trying experiments upon them for the advantage of the rich."[69] This latter accusation has a modern ring to it. The contemporary literature is filled with experimental treatments performed on cholera victims. Many of these were undertaken in the lazarets and gave legitimacy to the accusations and rumors. In the case of cholera, the accusation of poisoning by the doctors is especially apt because "the observed gastrointestinal symptoms seemed to make it medically likely, and the recent economic theories of Malthus, which took a complacent attitude toward disease as a necessary check on population, seemed to supply a motive."[70]

The combination of strict cholera regulations and fear the poor would be poisoned by the doctors as a cause of the rioting in Königsberg and other cities is demonstrated in Memel, Stettin and other districts outside the immediate area of Königsberg. This also caused concern in Berlin, especially what would happen later if there was an attempt to impose strict regulations in a city as large as Berlin. After all, the rumor was rife the "Rich say ... that the poor are becoming too numerous to be conveniently governed, and therefore this plan of thinning out the population has been adopted it having been employed with success by the English in India."[71]

In Memel, as a response to the strict regulations stemming from the military cordon in early May, an even stricter maritime quarantine was imposed. By the time cholera broke out on July 18, 1831, conditions in the city had become deplorable. The people heard doctor's carts "rumbling through the streets at all hours. The doctors were dressed in wax covered robes and wore face masks. Cholera signs were placed in front of the homes of cholera victims and finally the dead were removed in tightly sealed baskets and taken to a cemetery to be buried." On July 25, the population in the Memel suburb of Vitte had enough and broke out in a "fierce rebellion" against "the doctors and the better classes." It was said that "only the poor were brought to the lazaret to be scalded in steam baths or poisoned by doctors on behalf of the rich" The military was called to put down the rebellion.[72]

On September 2, 1831, a rebellion took place in the city of Stettin when the lower classes came into conflict over whether a person had died of the cholera. Many people of the "lower sort gathered on a quay" and began to try to destroy some of the houses of the officials who were responsible for carrying out cholera regulations. The military was called to put down the rebellion but had orders not to shoot. Some of the military were wounded. They returned supported by a citizen militia, put the rebellion down and arrested many of the rioters.[73]

Fear that doctors were poisoning the poor in collusion with the government and the rich spread to the smaller cities and towns. Soon after the uprising in Königsberg, the lower classes there had the strange idea the nobles wanted to get rid of a portion of the poor. They believed the authorities had organized their poisoning by physicians and the state. They believed the doctors were paid 4 guilders per victim. This created an agitated state among the lower classes not just against doctors but local officials as well. The clergy felt the need to speak out against this "absurd prejudice." However, when the ministers spoke out they also came under suspicion. It was claimed they had negotiated an "agreement" with the doctors.[74]

The poisoning rumor was common throughout Prussia. Even the king was rumored to pay doctors a bounty for poisoning the poor. Ambassador Chad wrote he had heard that the King of Prussia "having humanly ordered a daily remuneration should be given to doctors who devote themselves to the treatment of Cholera-Patients, this fact has been distorted by these ignorant people into a bribe of two or, according to some, three talers a head to each doctor for every death caused by these means."[75] The poisoning conspiracy by doctors was not limited to one country. It paralleled the international "revolutionary conspiracies" feared by the ruling classes at the time. The poor saw the poisoning of the poor as part of an international conspiracy by "...foreign doctors who have been sent to Russia, Poland, and Prussia to observe the disease, according to the Hypothesis, the Delegates of a Central Committee consisting of 100 members formed in London, and who direct the whole proceeding." Ambassador Chad was not told this by one or two people but "these statements apply to nearly all the country-places where the Cholera reigns and to some of the towns."[76]

Aftermath of the Tumult

The tumult did not turn into a full-scale revolt involving a broad class of citizens but was limited to the "rabble" according to eyewitnesses. The fears which motivated the rioters were highest among the very poor. Schmidt reported the entire citizenry rose up "against the battle cry of the mob." The day laborers and shopkeepers did not support the riot. Whatever radical ideas may have been common in Königsberg, the "robbers found themselves deceived."[77]

A correspondent wrote to Chad about quelling the tumult, "the Mob not dispersing, the students, the Shopkeepers, and the Burghers joined the soldiers, and assisted them in re-establishing order."[78] With these two accounts plus the accounts presented at the trial of the rioters it appears the culprits were basically confined to the poorest elements in the city. The other classes supported the government because by now they were aware the strict quarantine regulations had been lifted. The regulations were no longer a threat to the economy of the city or the individual livelihood of most of the city population. Without the support of the other classes the tumult was doomed to fail. Even in the midst of the epidemic, when tensions should be exacerbated, a reasoned response by the government and the common sense recommendations of the anti-contagionist doctors and officials gave the lower-middle to upper classes the confidence to try to lead a "normal life" in the midst of the epidemic. In addition, "the property-less classes found themselves in business and not disturbed, and the property owners, as their property was no longer in danger, seemed to consider the cholera like any other epidemic" something that must be endured "like hail or thunderstorms."[79]

As for the city merchants, trade with the Poles and later the luxury good trade with the Russians that occurred after the blockade restrictions were lifted contributed to excellent profits for merchants (especially the trade in fine wines). The local butchers sold cattle to the Russian army and there was plenty of work for local freight haulers with the Russian trade.[80] For the very poor, tensions were eased when city officials under Schön's direction not only "brought a sudden calm" to the whole city with the elimination of strict quarantine measures, but also by beginning a public works program to employ the lower classes in road building and the leveling of walls between the "Steindammer and the Rossgärtner Gate."[81]

Even where one would expect disorganized mob violence, the sacking of the police building was not unorganized and had an objective greater than the random destruction of building.[82] The Police headquarters had been established earlier in 1831 in that building in the Old Town Center, outside the castle where the municipal offices were located, to signify that the police were not a part of the provincial or local government. By destroying the police building and the records, the rioters eliminated both the source of the disease and showed their displeasure with the measures of Central Government. This point was emphasized when a city official asked the rioters to desist and cheer for the king. Instead they began screaming and pummeling the officials and military with stones!

According to the official report in the *Prussian State Gazette*, the crowd complained of "maltreatment by the doctors and the police." The police were forced to carry out many of the quarantine measures on the doctor's orders. It was natural that there would be hostility toward the police and the Central Government because that was where their orders originated. The report went on to state that the "rioters entered the police building by force and threw documents and papers from the windows." These were burned as well.[83]

The rioters were not only looking for police records and other papers concerned with cholera and quarantine measures but according to Police President Schmidt, an eyewitness, "the plundering rioters screamed we want the cholera germs."[84] Many of the rioters believed it was the government that was importing the disease (this played into the conspiracy rumor that there was no disease but an effort in "thinning the poor") and the police building served as a distribution point for doctors to spread the seeds or germs to poison them.

Finally, the mob knew records pertaining to medical services for the sick and quarantined were kept by the police. The destruction of these records made it difficult for the authorities to track the movements of the inhabitants or to confine or restrict them. A good example was the inability of the authorities to confirm the movements of Captain Hoffstädt. Schmidt later reported to Minister von Brenn he had saved some important records in a rented room outside the police building related to the cholera, although he still had to depend on his memory to designate the houses that had been quarantined because those records were destroyed.[85]

It could be argued the riot was successful because with the destruction of the documents related to the disease the poor removed the evidence the doctors and the police needed to continue to interfere in their lives. The direction and organization of this tumult was not spontaneous. The object of the crowd's wrath was not a random target. The targeting of the police building was an intelligent choice on the part of the poor. After all, they were the most affected by regulations.[86]

No doubt there were others who jumped on the destructive band wagon by attempting to free their comrades or thought they could exploit the situation and riot. Not because they were against the cholera restrictions, but were simply trying to take advantage of the general unrest.

The altercation over an "honorable burial" for a journeyman carpenter eventually turned into a riot, and escalated for two reasons: most of the military were on duty at the border as part of the *cordon sanitaire*, and officials in Königsberg refused to call in the military, preferring the police. It should be noted that the next day, after the blockade measures had been repealed by Schön, there was "no lack of voices obliging that he had deliberately let the riot get out of hand to justify the [new] measures."[87] However, the government dependence on the police to keep order was not an uncommon occurrence in Prussia.[88] Prussian officials preferred not to use army troops to put down unrest because they were afraid of alienating the broad masses. They were aware of the harm that could be caused by relying on an "inelastic army" to put down unrest and preferred the "powerless gendarmerie."[89] Schön, especially, did not trust the military to handle civilian affairs and had earlier written to Thile that the army was unfamiliar with police matters and that "much mischief must result" if the army was used for general policing.[90]

Also, following the tumult, if Schön had wished to call in the army he would have had to obtain permission from the Immediate Commission because the army was under its command. Königsberg would have been subject to martial law and the strict quarantine policy of the Immediate Commission would have been re-imposed by the commission. Schön trusted his officials to handle the initial unrest. When the incident first began outside the castle, "The number ... [of people)] ... itself was not large and as I called the Police President, the crowd scattered."[91] Later, when the crowd re-assembled and attacked the police building, he wrote that "experience soon showed" the call up of the local militia had been enough to establish "peace and order."[92]

Nevertheless, Schön held Schmidt responsible for the "tumult" in Königsberg because he and other police officials had zealously executed the orders of the Immediate Commission in Berlin. "At the first outbreak of cholera ... husbands were taken from wives, children from their parents and brought to the lazaret."[93] In a January 8, 1832, investigation of the riot, Schön and the other authorities blamed the riots on "wine," but Schön also placed the greatest fault on Schmidt's lack of energy. He said Schmidt acted in an "incredibly naïve" manner. He was convinced the military had never been needed and that "Schmidt was not suitable for the position of Police President."[94] Schmidt in his first report on the "tumult" reported to Interior Minister von Brenn, that it had not been his fault. He had done his job conscientiously and fairly. In doing his duty, his family had also suffered. His apartment in the police building had been ransacked, and his family was without "clothing, beds, linens and a place to live." He expected reinforcements to be called out earlier (i.e. Schön had been slow to act).[95]

Another member of the government who would later have a "falling out" with Schön as a result of his actions during the cholera epidemic was *Regierung* President Meding. In a memorandum on August 11, 1831, Schön blamed Meding for the poor state of affairs of the local government. Schön's next step was to attempt to pension off Meding. His rationale, a "decrease in ... [Meding's] ... health and mental capacity was more noticeable." This excuse appealed to Schön, who "earlier had an appreciation of Meding, but now had become very dissatisfied since the fight that erupted with him during the cholera epidemic." Meding had completely failed in his official duties and left them to the already overburdened Ewald.[96]

Meanwhile, since August, the *Regierung* President of Köslin Graf Dohna-Wundlacken had been assisting the ailing Schön in his duties as part of an auxiliary force to undertake tasks related to the cholera epidemic. Dohna-Wundlacken succeeded Meding on October 31, 1831, as *Regeriung* President of Königsberg.

This was not the end of the affair. Meding would not go quietly, refusing to give up his post. His forced retirement had developed into a public scandal. He believed the Ministry had been misinformed about his health and demanded the right to transfer back to a less strenuous post as *Regierung* President of Marienwerder. The Ministry informed Schön that Meding's retirement due to health reasons was one of the "easiest shortcomings to overturn" and that he would have to take care of the matter. In order to contain the scandal, Schön was forced to backpedal on some of his criticism. He refused to praise Meding for any practical qualities but did enumerate "his good spirit" and otherwise praised his performance when he first took over from his predecessor. The Ministry agreed with Schön's revised opinion of Meding. Rather than retiring with one-half his salary, Meding was allowed to retire with five-eighths of his salary. Meding no longer opposed his retirement and the matter was resolved.[97]

Schön defended General Krafft's actions in the riot. He had not used force and thus did "not to compromise himself in the eyes of the people."[98] Schön was aware that calling in troops during the tumult or even after the riot to re-impose the quarantine regulations as the Immediate Commission wanted was not practical. Ewald estimated to do this would require an "army corps of 15,000."[99]

Schön and his officials did not want the army in Königsberg and did not trust the army to effectively manage the civilian population. Schön, like many of his liberal contemporaries, believed the army policing the civilian population was ultimately more trouble than it was worth, should not be necessary in a civilized country.[100] He believed the strict quarantine had caused the "tumult" in the first place. The educated classes and the upper classes had been aware that the quarantine regulations had been suspended. They had been willing to support the Königsberg government because they did not want to see the strict regulations imposed. Schön realized if additional troops were called during the tumult the army would have justified its presence in the city. The troops would not initially have been opposed by the citizens, since their property concerns came before quarantine fears. However, once the army had settled in it would have been easy for martial law to be declared (during this crisis the army was directly responsible to the Immediate Commission) and thus stringent quarantine regulations would have been re-imposed. In the end the city would have been at the mercy of the army and the Immediate Commission.

Fortunately, the local militia was able to control the situation in Königsberg. If the army attempted to re-impose the strict Berlin quarantine restrictions, it was likely that the poor as well as other groups would turn on the government and create a serious situation which could lead to more bloodshed and death.

When the first report of the Königsberg riots reached Berlin, there was "great excitement ... among the ruling circles." There was little coverage in the newspapers, which led to rumors. It was difficult to distinguish "truth from falsehood." Authorities in Berlin, especially Rust "complained of high treason" by Schön.[101]

There was great dissatisfaction with the raising of the cholera restrictions back in Berlin because of the fear of the disease spreading from Königsberg. In Königsberg the newspapers, and especially the *Cholera Zeitung* (Königsberg), supported the authorities in this endeavor. The cities of Elbing and Danzig that initially had the task of stopping the cholera, "voted" the Königsberg actions a "success." Still Rust remained "steadfast in his system of defense."[102]

The *Cholera Zeitung* (Königsberg) summed up the feelings of the people and reported on the "great benefits" which were received as a result of the city having been freed from the "many detriments" of the regulations. It was "thanks to ... Herr Schön, members of the Royal Provincial Government, as well as the administrative restraint of the city officials in regard to the police measures, that one breathes freely, that the pressure is lessened, and that the isolation policy which created fear and for a long time was pernicious on affairs, was turned about."[103]

Schön had initiated a challenge to the medical policy of the Immediate Commission. The tumult had confirmed his belief that the Immediate Commission's measures were dangerous and economically ruinous. The anti-contagion forces in Königsberg had predicted what the results of the Immediate Commission's policy would be and looked to the example of Danzig as a model of what could happen if a city slavishly followed the government's strict blockade policy.

However, while the Immediate Commission made some minor changes in its new regulations on August 5, it basically refused to relent on its most basic contagion policies. Public officials and doctors in Königsberg and elsewhere continued to challenge what they came to see as the commission's "senseless regulations." Nevertheless, the commission under Rust's medical leadership continued in its stubborn persistence of maintaining its strict sanitary policy as cholera approached Berlin.

9

Cholera Enters Berlin

Early attempts at modifying the Central State Cholera Policy can be said to have begun with the opposition in Königsberg, especially with the leadership of Provincial President Schön. Nevertheless the reversal of this strict policy occurred in stages as the failure of the centralized policy became evident to Prussian officials. Cholera continued to spread and the costs combined with the inordinate number of military men needed to maintain the cordons was simply too high.

The Immediate Commission admitted as much on August 5, 1831, and issued "Revised Rules for the Implementation of the Instructions on the Outbreak of Cholera, Procedures to be Observed after the Instructions of April 5th and June 1st" for the Provinces of Prussia, Posen and the part of Silesia lying on the right bank of the Oder. The justification for the revised measures stated that "the establishment of the great medical cordon" along the Russian-Polish national boundary, as well as in the interior of the country, and in Danzig and Posen had already claimed too many military resources. With the increasing spread of cholera in the provinces of Prussia and Posen the implementation of local blockades could no longer be carried out "in accordance with the ... [original] ... instructions." With the disease making further inroads, the strict "execution of internal blockade measures was no longer possible," as it previously had been "hoped" that cholera could be "limited to a few points of the monarchy." With this revision, the Immediate-Commission decided that it had to protect the western parts of the country as well as the provinces of Prussia, Posen and part of Silesia on the right bank of the Oder."[1]

The regulation of August 5, 1831, consisted of 13 paragraphs; most were not a major departure from the previous regulations. As a direct consequence of the lack of military manpower, paragraph six permitted villages and larger areas not affected by cholera to remain open to commerce. Travelers had to obtain "health passes" and those from suspicious areas or villages had to undergo quarantine. Larger districts could choose to isolate themselves, but only under the direction of the local governments and district authorities. Guards, quarantine stations as well as other health related institutions had to be available at the blockade line. They had to be paid for at community expense. Travelers had to be instructed on a different route to pass around the cordoned area. In addition, special accommodations for the post-office, military, and health officials had to be carefully enumerated for the enclosed areas.[2] On August 13, 1831, modified regulations stated holders of health passes should be able to pass through isolated areas. Local restrictions could not be more "stringent than the laws in force in the internal sanitary cordon."[3]

The most controversial of the regulations was the quarantining of entire houses and the forced transporting of the sick to cholera hospitals. These policies were major contributors to the misery in Danzig and Königsberg.[4] As a result, the August 5 regulations continued to exert a hardship on the population. The Immediate Commission relented somewhat by allowing an apartment rather than an entire house to be isolated, thus letting other residents go about their business. The sick were to be transported to the hospital. Those who had contact with the sick had to undergo a ten day quarantine. The other inhabitants in the building could go about their business, however, their personal effects and dwellings had to be disinfected. If a sick person remained in the house for treatment, the house was quarantined. Anyone who came into contact with the patient had to undergo twenty day quarantine. Those people who did not have contact with the patient in the building had to undergo ten days of quarantine. Their effects and residences had to undergo disinfection. Burial practices were also modified. Under the authority of the local sanitary commission, the dead could be buried in a regular cemetery so long as it was not located in a "built up area," and the attendants were required to use oil coated gloves. The burials were to take place between 8'o'clock in the evening and 7 o'clock in the morning.[5]

The release of these modified regulations had an immediate effect on the situation in Königsberg. As noted earlier, following the uprising, reports of what had happened in Königsberg circulated in Berlin and resulted in much excitement in the upper classes. Due to censorship little of this was mentioned in the papers (except a paragraph describing the events in the Prussian State Gazette). The public turned to "rumors and letter writing" for information. They did not expect to find reports in the daily press. The rumor mill was rife, and it seemed that even well connected individuals could not "distinguish truth from falsehood." According to Ewald, the usually well informed Count von Brunneck expressed the opinion that Schön had demonstrated "obstinacy" and "thus encouraged an anarchic state among the authorities."[6]

The "wrath" of the authorities in Berlin, especially Rust and his followers was according to Ewald excessive. They accused Schön of treason. This caused him to later write to the Crown Prince that it seemed if "one had a different opinion than those who serve the king, he is revealed as a traitor." Those in Berlin had no experience with the disease, yet insisted (like Rust) that it was contagious. The barriers according to von Schön that Rust had ordered "more than the disease would ruin the entire country" and he gave the example, Danzig.[7]

It seemed the extreme views were not changed because on August 5, 1831, the Immediate Commission issued the new regulations previously discussed. Ewald wrote that upon closer examination they only departed from the original regulations in few respects. In particular, he noted "the closing-up of the houses was maintained and their severity was at the same level that produced the uprising in Königsberg." Even Police President Schmidt complained about paragraph eleven in the new regulations of August 5. The quarantine of houses and the forced transport of the sick to the hospitals were essentially similar regulations, which originally "started the unrest on July 28" and "aroused the working class."[8]

As a result of the August 5 regulations, Schön called a Council of Notables on August

11 or 12 (Ewald was unsure of the date). The Council included Commanding General Krafft, the Head of the General Staff Colonel von Auer, the two commissioners from Berlin, Von Below and Dr. Wagner, the *Regierung* President Meding with several of his councilors as well other officials including Chancellor Wegern, Surgeon General Kranz, Dr. Burdach and Dr. Trotha, Mayor List and councilor Schartow, head of the city council. The August 5 regulations were placed before Schön. He was "asked how these modified measures were to be executed." It was a "painfully moving" meeting and the question received no response even the second time. When it was finally repeated a third time, Ewald said that carrying out the measures was "...feasible. The detention order can be arranged and executed, but in Königsberg this would require an army of 15,000 men. That would be a bloody act against these good citizens who a few days before had armed themselves to preserve order and tamed the plundering mob." He said "He could not do such a thing and asked to be relieved of his duties." The assembly then took a voice vote with no one opposed. When the same question was put to Commanding General, Krafft, he said was "unable to provide adequate military assistance." It was decided that a report should be forwarded to Berlin stating "it was impossible to follow what had been ordered there."[9]

According to Ewald the modified regulations of August 5 caused renewed disobedience and anger among the inhabitants. Following the uprising, general peace and quiet had prevailed. Even though yellow ribbons were still being used to mark houses where cholera was present, the public had become convinced that the disease was not as dangerous as previously thought. The situation was nowhere as serious as in Danzig with its cordons and house quarantines.[10]

Some cities did take up the challenge and sequestered themselves from travelers. The city of Brannberg for example, refused to allow travelers from Königsberg and Elbing to enter the city. It posted guards and even forced the post-office courier to drive around the city. No one was allowed inside the city unless they could demonstrate that they had not come from a place where cholera was prevalent.[11]

In Königsberg the blockade within the city was eliminated while the barrier outside the city existed only on paper. In order to move in and out of the city a health pass was required to authorize the guard at the city gate to allow people to enter and leave. Because the Königsberg physicians were vehemently opposed to the entire blockade system, they "readily signed these certificates" for anyone who requested them.[12]

To illustrate the value of these health certificates, Ewald used the example of the East Prussian city of Schippenbeil. The mayor, concerned for the welfare of his inhabitants, sent the city surgeon to Königsberg to study cholera in order to be able to return home and cure his fellow citizens. When the surgeon returned home he presented the mayor with two certificates. One showed he had worked in a cholera hospital and had learned as much as the doctors there knew about the cholera and the treatment of patients there. The second certificate attested he had come into contact with cholera patients, but it allowed him to pass through the city gates and the Schippenbeil gates as well. Since he remained healthy and neither the mayor nor anyone else he came into contact with became sick, calm was restored in Schippenbeil and it helped to bring towns like Braunberger and other "odd" places to see reason.[13]

This system of seclusion however was not seen by everyone as "odd" but as described by one physician it had a greater chance of success because it was based on self-interest. For example, unlike the Prussian military-sanitary lines along the border (exclusion) or the cordon around cities like Danzig or Posen (inclusion) where each measure was imposed by a distant authority, the inhabitants had little interest in obeying the rules. They felt inconvenienced by them and attempted to find every means to evade the "intentions of the government." With the system of seclusion (at the village, small city or commune level) these measures were established on a much smaller scale and carried out by those who protected them. Although they would be inconvenienced, they were invested in the decision and would take "good care that the regulations would be strictly enforced."[14]

The Effect of the Königsberg Actions in Berlin

Two factors caused immediate reactions in Berlin. In Danzig, the city that had suffered under "Rust's strict measures" the Sanitary Committee had followed the orders of the Immediate Commission and on August 11 reported that "it lacked all means to carry them out against the will of the crowd." It requested to withdraw the land cordon and replace the unworkable regulations with the measures which had come from Provincial President Schön and published in the official journals[15] The king who had predicted that Rust's strict measures would "cost much money" and he would "be the dupe of this affair" had even more reason to doubt the usefulness of Rusts' regulations, especially after receiving the Danzig request. On August 11, 1831, at the meeting of the Immediate Commission the king requested a joint meeting of the recently established Health Committee for Berlin and the Immediate Commission. The first order of business was to determine whether Berlin should be "encircled" with a blockade, along with other regulations thought to have a negative effect on the city and too severe to be effective.[16]

Following this meeting the king received Schön's report from the Council of Notables in Königsberg. The king became more convinced that Schön was probably right, and wrote privately to him on August 18 "you know I am not one who believes your criticism is based on error."[17] Naturally this report upset Rust's supporters who said Schön by his actions had committed "treason." They saw his actions as outright rebellion and blamed Schön for calling the second meeting. They demanded that a ministerial commission be appointed and sent to Königsberg to study the situation and hold tribunal there. The king gladly "appointed a commission" but ordered the members to present themselves to him at Charlottenburg before they continued on their journey. The king received them graciously spoke with them about their impending trip and "wished them a pleasant journey," and said dryly, "not much will come of it." He added, "Schön knew quite well what he was doing and was never wrong." The commission members were "thunderstruck" and quickly realized the trip would probably be useless and at the same time dangerous because of cholera. As a result, nothing ever came of the accusations against Schön.[18] Later it was Rust's turn to be on the receiving end not of official scorn like Schön but as the butt of the humor of the people in Berlin. By the time the cholera finally broke out in Berlin on August 30, 1831, the population of the city had become less convinced of the effectiveness of "Rust's fantastic regulations" and began to ridicule him. Even the Crown Prince, "who liked Rust" and later made him his personal physician, kept a "very funny caricature of him." The cartoon was displayed for a long time in the fashionable shop windows on the upscale *Unter der Linden*.[19]

The Approach of the Cholera toward Berlin and Its Effect on State Cholera Policy

However, when the epidemic and its high death rate first entered Prussia and it seemed inexorably moving toward Berlin the public was not so sanguine about the situation and the measures the government was prepared to take. The cholera of 1831 could be said to have led for the first time to "an organization of public healthcare in Berlin."[20] On June 5, the king established a Chief Sanitary Committee for Berlin. The committee was headed by the military commander Ernst Ludwig Tippelkirsch and the civilian Provincial President of West Prussia, Freiherr Magnus von Basserwitz. It included, the mayor, city councilors, physicians, the police chief and three military commanders.[21]

The immediate requirement was to prevent cholera from infected places like Danzig entering Berlin and its environs. The committee reviewed the general situation in Berlin and surrounding areas. It made preparatory arrangements for an effective public health response for the city to control the incoming traffic from infected areas.[22] On June 6, the Sanitary Committee for Berlin ordered the establishment of a *Kontumaz* in the "so-called castle" for all incoming travelers (from infected areas) before the Frankfurt Gate.[23] By June 28, the latter was made responsible for cleansing streets and buildings, it oversaw the purity of food and drink and had the authority to "inspect the dwellings of the poor."

With the outbreak of cholera, the committee ordered the establishment of shelters for the sick, which included using the *Pockenhaus*, associated with the Charité hospital. All administrative and medical matters were to be centralized once the cholera appeared. Nursing, transport of the sick, burial of the dead, and other administrative matters were also the responsibility of the Sanitary Committee. Later the latter formed a subcommittee called the "Administrative Authority of the Sanitary Committee for Berlin," composed of the military, police, medical and commune officials headed by the Police President of Berlin. This subordinate committee was divided into four divisions, military, police, sanitary and communal. This subordinate committee was responsible for coordinating the activities of Berlin's 61 newly appointed *Civil Schutz Commission*s (Civil Protection Commissions) organized along the lines of the 61 administrative poor districts in the city.[24]

The orders given by the Chief Sanitary Committee for Berlin corresponded to orders implemented earlier in Danzig (the result of the Immediate Commission's deliberations of June 1, 1831). Because the cholera had not yet broken out in Berlin, these regulations were preliminary. However, just as in Königsberg, the regulations caused concern among members of the city's commercial classes, city delegates, some members of the Sanitary Committee

9. Cholera Enters Berlin

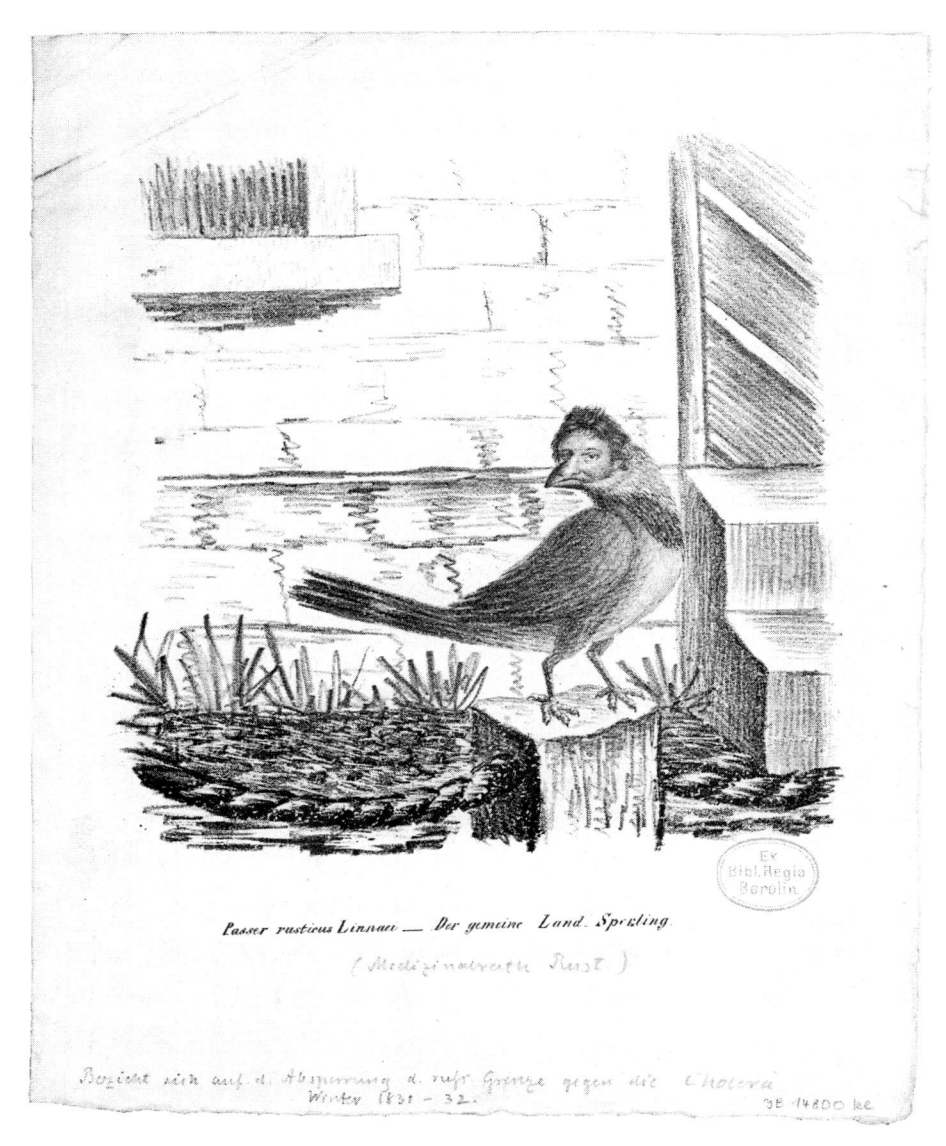

"Passer rusticus Linnaei—Der gemeine Land Sperling" (The Common Country Sparrow). Artist unknown. This black and white pencil drawing is a caricature of Dr. Johannes N. Rust, Chief Medical Privy Councilor responsible for the strict cholera regulations in Prussia and the 1831 blockade of Polish and Russian lands bordering Prussia. His face is drawn on a common sparrow. The key words are *rusticus*, a play on Rust's name (rural or countrified) in Latin and *Land-Sperling* or country sparrow. The joke occurs when a second "r" is substituted in *Sperling*, as a comment on Rust's policies. "Sperr" means an obstruction or barricade. At first the fear of cholera was real in Berlin but as time passed people began to weary of what they considered to be absurd regulations and turned to humor to criticize the government and, pointedly, the one official they felt was responsible. This caricature was said to have been prominently displayed in the best shops on the *Unter den Linden* in the fall of 1831, during the cholera epidemic. The Crown Prince, later Frederick William IV of Prussia, was also said to have displayed it in his lodgings. The caricature gave Rust no end of embarrassment. This caricature was much discussed in many subsequent histories of the time, and was embellished over time by different writers who had not seen the original. It was described as including a cage, with the bird draped in a doctor's cholera outfit. This may be the first time this caricature has been published (Staatsbibliothek zu Berlin, PK).

and high government officials. A prominent French doctor, after reading a circular entitled "Advice on the Means of Protection and Curatives Against Cholera," which was issued by the Sanitary Committee of Berlin, found it "incredible," that the "sick and the healthy were to be sequestered together."[25]

This French physician was an anticontagionist and was critical of quarantines and isolation which forced the sick to have continual contact with the healthy. His fears were well founded for this is what was occurring in Danzig. The greatest concern was whether there would be an attempt to quarantine Berlin similar to Danzig. Knowing the declining economic situation in Danzig, and the recent uprising in Königsberg, the working and middle classes of Berlin waited in terror either afraid of being a victim of the disease or "a sacrifice to the measures taken against it."[26] Still, Schön's actions, which were contrary to official policy, were not common knowledge outside Königsberg and higher official circles in Berlin. Ambassador Chad had not mentioned Schön's conduct in this matter until September 15. In a dispatch to Palmerston he wrote, "The President or Civil Governour ... Mr. de Schön, is convinced that the disease is not contagious and he is said to have acted upon this conviction in evasion of the orders of this Prussian Majesty."[27]

In early August, city officials in Berlin wanted a decision on whether Berlin was to be quarantined. Most believed that Berlin could not be effectively quarantined like Danzig. This controversy finally forced the king to act and on August 11 he ordered the Immediate Commission to meet with the Sanitary Committee.[28] This was the first meeting in which the commission met formally with another group and showed the strong support that the king had given the commission was wavering. The chief question under consideration for this meeting concerned the government's plans in the event of the outbreak of cholera in Berlin?[29] Both groups met in response to the quarantine instructions issued on August 1 and August 11. The issues discussed included whether Berlin would be quarantined in the event of an outbreak of cholera? Who would bear the cost of this outbreak? The arrangements for isolation and quarantine, the level and types of decisions to be carried out by the appointed administrative structure, the role of the newly formed protection commissions and the modification of instructions approved by the Sanitary Committee responsible for the sixty-one protection commissions.[30]

The Sanitary Committee argued the "isolation of Berlin was not possible." This argument was partly based on the need to "provision Berlin" not only civilians but for the military and the defense of the city. "Traffic with Berlin was so interconnected with the countryside that the interruption of the latter would constitute a great disadvantage."[31]

The Sanitary Committee for Berlin feared that the quarantine of the city would be too expensive and make it impossible to supply citizens with food and other goods, incurring a high cost to the population. The experience in Danzig showed the folly of the government's policy towards the people and towards trade. The "tumult" in Königsberg and rumors of unrest in Memel, indicated the danger to be found in the government's sanitary policy.[32] The members of the Sanitary Committee requested quarantine remain at the Elbe and the Oder rivers and that Berlin to continue trade with the surrounding territory.[33]

The second question addressed to the Immediate Commission was the policy of "isolation" of the sick and the "quarantine of entire houses." This caused great anxiety because not only were individual houses involved but also large multi-dwelling buildings containing many poor people. Sanitary Committee members argued it would be impossible to isolate these buildings. For example, officials could see the impossibility of "watching, controlling and maintaining at the public expense the great number of persons ... thus imprisoned and prevented from gaining their livelihood, and the temporary difficulties, and even financial ruin of many families whose social and commercial connexions [*sic*] were suddenly interrupted." If one included the "variety of exempted persons, such as medical men, clergymen, and even lawyers and police officers, whose intercourse frustrated the intended end." The objective "could only be accomplished in theory and on paper."[34]

City officials on the committee wanted the isolation confined to individual rooms. One city councilor requested the order to impose quarantine be decided at the local level.[35] This would have meant having the order come from the local protection committee. To allow the local committees autonomy (in interpreting the Immediate Commission's regulations it would have undermined the authority of the Immediate Commission's strict contagionist policy and given local authorities a latitude the commission could not allow if it wanted to retain its absolute control).[36] However, on August 22 the commission relented and modified quarantine regulations for houses. The protection committees could decide if an entire dwelling or an individual apartment needed to be quarantined but the detailed regulations left little room for local independent decision making.[37]

In the end the commission refused to modify the regulations of August 5 and end house quarantines or remove blockades as the non-contagionists advocated. It supported the view that the "isolation of dwellings and commerce restrained the spread of the contagion."[38] The members of the Sanitary Committee agreed in general with the measures but noted that quarantine of large buildings as a means to limit the spread of the cholera "was not possible in Berlin."[39] The two groups could not agree on this question.

A third issue concerned delivering cholera victims to a cholera hospital. Sanitary officials argued that this order could not be carried out on the scale which would be required if there was a general outbreak of cholera in Berlin. They also feared the consequences of using force.[40] The committee believed that the matter of who should be taken to a cholera hospital, the transportation of the sick, the means of transportation and which family members should be allowed to accompany the sick, should be left up to the members of the local protection committee. Local authorities supported this position because they believed if local control over the sick were demonstrated, then the "intent would be more acceptable to the public and the public would be more inclined to use the lazarets."[41]

The meeting then turned to questions of finance. The Immediate Commission informed the Sanitary Committee members that much of the funding to pay for cholera costs would have to be raised by local authorities. They could expect some financial support from the central government, but local magistrates were expected to raise and distribute money. In Berlin, the city assembly was ordered to institute a cholera fund. The costs for taking care of the "poor sick" were expected to fall on the traditional "poor law administrative" structure and funds raised at the commune level.[42]

The commission advised the committee that it was "necessary to hurry on these matters" as it would be an "unlucky fate if the city were taken unawares by the sickness." City officials (in conjunction with the local protection commissions) were expected to arrange "shelters to care for the sick and provide personnel to oversee these establishments."[43]

On August 13, the city deputies met and discussed the Immediate Commission's regulations with the members of the Sanitary Committee. They were not sure if they could enforce the commission's regulations, especially transporting the sick to the lazarets. The city deputies wanted to know what kind of support they could expect to receive from the central government.[44]

The fundamental question under consideration was how the public would react to the commission's directives. The city deputies realized they had better act quickly to ensure that when cholera broke out the city was prepared to "limit the infection." They had to develop a plan for transporting the sick to the lazarets, with the least amount of public disruption. They recommended that the lazarets be placed in remote parts of the city. They also discussed who would care for the sick and how to provide for those who lived alone.[45]

City officials decided that those taken to the lazarets should not to be required to pay the doctors attending them, nor should their families have to pay a burial fee in the event of their death. Doctors as well as other medical personnel were to be paid by the *Charité* administration. They estimated that the average cost to support 1,800 to 2,400 families would be between 60,000 to 80,000 talers or 34 talers per family. The deputies based these figures on the current number of poor families being maintained by the city. They also attempted to determine which streets might have to be quarantined and which communes would have to bear a higher burden of the cholera costs.[46]

The deputies believed that the city could not provide all the assistance necessary to the workers and decided it would be in the best interests of the business community to assist their own workers "outside their homes." The deputies feared worker unrest and that "business would come to a standstill" if they did not offer some support.[47]

The Formation of the Commune "Protection Commissions" in Berlin

While the Immediate Commission, the Chief Sanitary Committee for Berlin and city deputies were attempting to organize a response to the impending epidemic, the commune protection commissions previously established by order of the king and given the responsibility for the actual daily contact with the cholera sick and dying, were activated. The king ordered similar commissions in all large cities and in rural districts. Outside of Berlin they were generally called *Bezirk* (district) Commissions.

The commune protection commissions in Berlin were expected to follow the directives of the Sanitary Committee of Berlin (under the direction of a subordinate committee of the latter, the "Administrative Authority of the Chief Sanitary Committee.") This committee was headed by the Police President, who was the responsible authority for the "poor districts." He was appointed to supervise the sixty-one newly formed commune protection commissions. The latter were geographically comparable to the city's "poor districts."[48]

The members of the protection commissions were selected from the city council and confirmed by the city magistrate. The physicians and police members were given a commission received from the administrative authority. The police president was appointed as chief of the protective commissions and the deputies were elected by the members, confirmed by the magistrate and named by the administrative authority.[49]

The number of members of the commissions varied according to the number of individuals and houses in the district and the relative number of the poor in the different districts. In some districts of Berlin there were only fifteen members on a protection commission, on others there were from sixty to eighty members. Doctors were allocated to different commissions and if there was no doctor available a lower status surgeon was appointed. The physicians and surgeons were responsible for surveying the sanitary state of the individuals in the district, care for the sick and were required to inform the local commission of the number of sick patients they were treating. It was these protection commissions the people of Berlin came into contact with and represented the city's administrative structure to combat cholera.[50]

The sixty-one commissions were also responsible for collecting funds in their communes, establishing hospitals and subsidizing the needs of the poor. For those communes that could not raise adequate funds the Chief Sanitary Commission furnished additional monies.[51]

The individual commission members were appointed between August 18 and 20, the members as well as the administrative authority were announced on August 27.[52]

On August 22, the government under the auspices of the Immediate Commission issued a "Notice containing the revised regulations to be implemented and the procedures to be observed on the outbreak of cholera of April 5, 1831, and June 1, 1831" for the whole monarchy, with the exclusion of the Rhine Province, Westphalia, Fuerstenhümer Neuschatel and Balengin." The revisions consisted of 12 long detailed paragraphs ranging from the expansion of the sanitary commissions (protection commissions in the large cities) to regulations concerning travelers and health passes, trade, house quarantines, permitting the military to move more freely, and modifying burial regulations. The most contentious of these regulations in Berlin as we have seen was quarantine of houses and this revision was not much of an improvement over previous regulations. However, the commissions were given the authority to decide if a house should be partially or wholly quarantined and whether the patient could remain in the dwelling or needed to be removed. The Immediate Commission provided detailed guidelines for these decisions including requiring that if a patient was quarantined within a house that a "rope with guards" be placed outside the dwelling and that a warning plaque labeled "Cholera" be placed at the entrances of any dwelling in which a cholera patient remained in the house.[53]

City officials in Berlin attempted to dissuade the Immediate Commission from following through on a number of its directives. In Berlin, both the Sanitary Committee and the city deputies continued to complain that Berlin could not be effectively quarantined and requested more local control in the transportation of the sick to cholera hospitals and the issuing of quarantine restrictions. They were especially concerned with the isolation of individual apartments in large houses. They used as an example the situation in Berlin in the 59th district that included "four large houses in which between 2,000 and 3000 inhabitants, the most wretched population of Berlin live crowded together in a deplorable manner sometimes several families in a room."[54]

The Sanitary Committee had been ordered to draft measures for Berlin and submit them to the Immediate Commission. As we have seen in previous meetings the Immediate Commission was asked by members of the Sanitary Committee to modify its policies under pressure from the municipal and city councilors who had raised "their opposition against these traffic inhibiting measures."[55]

Nevertheless, on August 23, the Chief Sanitary Committee published "Regulations on the Procedures for the Approaching and Outbreak of Cholera," with a printing of 6,000 copies at a cost of 5 *Silbergroschen* each. Paragraph 30 of these new regulations "explicitly stated that the barricading of houses and quarantining the residents of the building" was necessary "without which they and others would have the highest risk of infection." Blockading Berlin was not specifically mentioned in the new regulations but in paragraph 20 the instructions that had been adopted for travelers and goods from infected sites where to apply "in general and for Berlin in particular will still be adopted."[56]

As noted earlier, there had been much discussion even in the Immediate Commission that Berlin was not to be blockaded. The decision was not communicated or at least we know discussions still continued. The concern was over the question what was to be done when the cholera "actually appeared." As late as the first days of September (see below) Police President Friedrich Wilhelm von Arnim, who served on the Chief Sanitary Committee and the subordinate committee, was still thinking about blockading Berlin in the days immediately following the outbreak.[57]

On August 29, the mayor of Berlin, Friedrich Bärensprung, reported the decision not to blockade Berlin along with an additional "surprising modification" that the house blockade was to be lifted and "only the apartments of the sick must be quarantined."[58] This ongoing challenge to the Immediate Commission's authority and its stubborn resistance on the question of contagion was beginning to weaken the king's support for the Immediate Commission's severe medical policy. This was derived from local officials, physicians and public opinion opposed to these regulations and the predicted economic results. These were some of the critical factors that led to a surprising shift in medical policy in early September. This was the situation in Berlin on the eve of the outbreak of the cholera epidemic.

"Berlin Gutters Stink"

The purity of the water and the drainage of waste in Berlin was simply not a factor in the discussions that we have seen for a host of reasons including the fact that the physicians themselves could not agree on the cause of transmission of the disease and did not at this time see water as a carrier of the "contagion." For the miasmists malodorous air was the culprit. However, the connection between cholera and the lack of good sanitation would only later be broached in Germany following the work of John Snow, who in an 1856 Parliamentary Report wrote on the importance of the water companies in Berlin. Nevertheless, for a contemporary reader I think it is of interest to briefly describe the sanitary conditions in Berlin about the time of the first cholera epidemic to determine what impact these may have had in 1831.[59]

Berlin did not lack for water; four rivers crossed the city. The water table was at a fairly high level. One could go down as little as six to ten feet to strike water. However, until the beginning of the nineteenth century the water supply was not a significant challenge because living close to abundant water, one could draw from the rivers or from the numerous fountains and water spigots in the various courts in the housing sections of Berlin.[60]

With the increasing population in Berlin, especially after 1815, the disposal of waste water was problematic "especially in the working class districts where hygienic conditions were becoming intolerable." Feces were transported in buckets to the bridges crossing the rivers and emptied there or ended up like the "heavy rainfall" in the gutters. Combined with this was household refuse that "merged with the muck" and the "unauthorized emptying of fecal buckets" to create a rotten and "smelly ferment" that bothered the city's inhabitants and led to the common expression: "Berlin gutters stink."[61]

Another contributing factor to health of the population in regard to access to water was the amount of work required to obtain the water and the opportunities to spread disease. For those not lucky enough to have children or other healthy family members to obtain water for them one could see the "sick staggering to the wells to procure water" or looking at it from a class perspective the honest and educated families, officials, teachers or single widows, wives and daughters on pensions" who could not afford to have someone else procure their water had to put up with "indelicate encounters in the dirty courts" to obtain water. Finally, even servants obtaining water for the wealthy could bring diseases into their master's homes.[62]

The smelly and foul gutters were a sore point among Berliners and this was found to be the case even in the best parts of the city. The lack of a sewerage system was recognized already in the 1820's as well as the urgent need to do something about it but was not implemented until mid-century in Berlin.[63] Given the importance of water as a vector in the spread of cholera it was ironic that when the physicians of Berlin as one of a number of their detailed dietary instructions to the public advocated "boiling water" the contagionist Dr. Becker wrote, "Even innocent cold water was prohibited."[64]

The Outbreak of Cholera in Berlin

The people of Berlin lived with anxiety and a sense of "confusion and fear" prior to the outbreak of the disease.[65] Initial orders issued by the Immediate Commission probably did more to scare the population of the city and inspire fear than the later effects of the disease itself. One foreign physician wrote that the orders of June 28, were "appalling."[66] The measures "threw fear into the population, each believed he would be designated a victim of the sickness, or sacrificed to the measures which would be taken against him." When the cholera did break out in Berlin on August 30, 1831 "terror seized the population, individuals locked themselves in their homes and isolated themselves, people hoarded food in their homes and for a short while the city lived as in a state of siege."[67]

There were other people who used the opportunity to profit for themselves. The following anecdote was common in Berlin at the time and illustrated the public's gullibility and the initial fear the epidemic created especially among the upper classes:

> A tailor managed to get himself carried into a different cholera hospital four or five times with the pretense of having the disease. In each case he had to pass four or five days in quarantine (according to existing regulations). He was comfortably lodged and well fed. It was discovered that he had been committing thefts while remaining in the clinic. Other persons extorted money by appearing under some pretense before those who were most afraid of the contagion. They stated that they had just come from a house infected with the cholera, where they were promptly satisfied in order to be rid of the alarming presence.[68]

The anti-contagionists and merchants believed that the government had over reacted and criticized quarantine measures as impediments to trade and travel. As one critic wrote about the government's quarantine policy, Thile had the "extraordinary foresight of providing a *table d'hôte*, for the pleasure of all travelers going through ..." the *Kontumaz*.[69]

Prior to the outbreak, the average person was more interested in making arrangements to prevent cholera. The fear and anxiety that greeted the initial outbreak of the cholera (at least among the general population) subsided once the people became accustomed to the sickness. Cholera related publications, medicines and a variety of devices whose advertisements filled the Berlin newspapers prior to the epidemic declined significantly by October. The unpleasant smell of chlorine gas originally found in most homes as well as ongoing disinfection procedures also became much less common.[70]

The Initial Response

On August 29 at 2:30 a.m., a barge operator, Johann Wegener died on his boat loaded with peat near Charlottenburg, a suburb of Berlin, from what initially appeared to be symptoms of cholera. He had been sick for the previous six weeks, suffering from "periodic diarrhea and vomiting." The previous day he returned from Oranienburg, 21 miles north of Berlin, where had visited a physician for the first time. He was well enough to continue with his business through the previous six weeks, but by six o'clock that evening he become violently ill and a doctor was called. Around eleven o'clock that same evening doctors Friedham and Grune arrived and found Johann Wegener, "his entire body was covered with cold sweat, his eyes sunken and cramps throughout his entire body." He died a few hours later.[71]

Two state medical councilors, Dr. Barez and Dr. Eck were sent to Charlottenburg that morning to examine the circumstances that preceded his death, to perform an autopsy on the body, and confirm the cause of death. On the basis of the autopsy and Wegener's appearance (as described by the attending physicians) the two doctors concluded that he had died from the "Asiatic cholera."[72]

It would seem that there was no question that cholera was the cause of Wegener's

9. Cholera Enters Berlin

death. Ambassador Chad was convinced by his physician to dispatch a letter to Lord Palmerston writing, "I was interrupted by my doctor who has been dissecting the body [of the boatman from Oranienberg] and he says there is no doubt of its' being a case of the oriental cholera."[73]

Officially there was still some question about whether Wegener had died from the "Asiatic cholera." Chad reported that a "Consultation of Doctors was held," on Wegener's cause of death and "of the 7 who formed the Council, 4 thought it the Asiatic cholera and 3 were of the contrary opinion."[74] Nevertheless the finding was sufficient for General Thile who shortly afterward, announced his death "with the symptoms of cholera" in a notice on August 29, 1831:

> according to an official report which arrived here yesterday a sailor on board a boat at Charlottenburg became ill and died with the symptoms of the cholera. The vessel was immediately sequestered. The town is yet unsuspected, and the usual communications between Charlottenburg and Berlin would only be able to be blocked with the greatest difficulty so a blockade of Charlottenburg will not occur ... shipping on the Spree between Spandau and Charlottenburg is prohibited.[75]

Even with all the preparations and regulations, we also have an example of what could go wrong due to a lack of official planning and experience when confronted with this first case of cholera. Chad reported "The Boatman who died of the cholera at Charlottenburg was to be buried further down the river near Spandau—three men pointed out by the Police as persons capable of undertaking what is considered a very perilous task, were employed to place the corpse in a little bark, and at midnight to convey to the appointed spot, and bury it. Their courage however required to be so continually supported by brandy that they became unfit to go through with it, they upset the boat and were all drowned."[76]

A second notice dated August 29 appeared on the same day in the *Prussian State Gazette* and stated for the first time "that the city of Berlin, Potsdam and Charlottenburg, in the case of an outbreak of the cholera, would not be subjected to containment," even though the city of Charlottenburg had its first case of cholera.[77] The relief and the expected consequences (if isolation was imposed) to the inhabitants of Berlin was reported in a Hamburg newspaper and demonstrated the public understanding of what was suddenly occurring in their midst. The correspondent wrote:

> suddenly yesterday morning a message arrived here, that a sailor had died of cholera.... The consternation here was not so great because the approach of cholera has been long expected.... There was some surprise because until Sunday evening we had heard of the outbreak of the disease in Stettin, [August 25] ... and did not to think that it would soon make such a huge leap. The former skipper had come here by way of Havel and the Finow Canal from the Oder River. It was at once arranged for a strict quarantine of all shipping on the Oder. Communication between Spandau and Charlottenburg are provisionally suspended and a military cordon of the Finow Canal has been established.... Barriers between the cities of Berlin, Potsdam and Charlottenburg will in no case occur to the great relief of the inhabitants who feared famine in the city of which we unfortunately already have a few traces, the rising price of meat, wares, and peat, everyone is acquiring as much as they can of these.[78]

On August 29, at 2 a.m., another sailor Johann Christian Mater died on his boat, on the river Spree near the Schiffbauerdamm at house number 13 in Berlin after showing symptoms of cholera for eight hours. Mater from Madgeburg, had been in Berlin for the past eight days and had stopped in the vicinity of the Schleusenbrücke. He seemed to be in good health but on the eighth day became violently ill and "was concerned that he would die." A doctor was sent for and Mater died a short time later.[79]

Rumors began and there was "great agitation, when the news spread that even here in Berlin at the barges, on the Schiffbauerdamm early yesterday morning that a sailor was suffering from cholera. This much is certain, the military is set up there and the returning doctors are disinfected. Whether the disease really is the Oriental cholera, and whether someone died, nothing is definitely known."[80]

An autopsy was performed on Mater's body on August 30 by Dr. Ratorp in the presence of several doctors. According to him the "findings were analogous to those found in the barge operator Wegener." He concluded "Mater had died from the Asiatic cholera." The authorities immediately took measures for the burial of the body, the isolation of the boat and people who lived in the area.[81]

Soon after, Dr. Ratorp was called to a house near the Schleusenbrücke, to a shoemaker named Radack, who died on August 30 with symptoms of cholera. He performed the autopsy and reported symptoms similar to those of the other two victims that preceded him.[82]

However, there was still doubt about this diagnosis. Few physicians had actually seen real cases of cholera and the diagnostic ability of the doctors at this time was not sophisticated enough to positively confirm the disease by the symptoms, besides there were many common illnesses that presented symptoms similar to cholera. Some physicians were convinced it was not cholera at all. But as government officials knew, an accurate diagnosis was important, because if it was "Asiatic cholera" the strict security measures would be implemented in Berlin.

As a result of the previous two cases, the police president of Berlin, Count F. W. Karl von Arnim, went to the Chief Sanitary Committee for Berlin to obtain a professional opinion on the two recent cholera deaths. On August 31, a meeting of the doctors of the Chief Sanitary Committee was called to obtain their opinions on the Mater and Radack cases. Had the two presented "symptoms of Asiatic cholera" and if so was cholera responsible for their deaths? After much discussion the commission made the following statement, "on the two cases of the disease of Mater and Radack ... the Commission ... cannot confirm them as cases of Asiatic cholera because the data was incomplete" and without definite proof they could only "suspect cholera."[83]

The confusion over the diagnosis of cholera is indicative that even among the medical "professionals" at the highest levels of government they simply did not have sufficient experience with the disease to be able to certify a diagnosis at this early stage. Cholera's symptoms were similar to a host of other diseases at the time that commonly afflicted the poor and arose from bad food and an unhealthy environment. Today we know the unhealthy living conditions exposed the poor to more bacteria and viruses than those in the upper classes who lived in more hygienic circumstances and were better nourished. Alternately, the doctors at that time at least realized the dire consequences of their actions if they misdiagnosed a case of cholera and the quarantine machinery was put into place.

As of August 31, there was no denying the outbreak of cholera in Berlin. A roofer named Bobach became ill and a policeman took him to the Charité hospital in Berlin. On his arrival the doctors recognized the basic symptoms of "Asiatic cholera." He was treated with "hot drinks and wrapped in a woolen blanket." In the beginning he seemed to be improving but later took a turn for the worse and died that night. It was determined by the doctors in the Charité that he was the first proven cholera patient from a specific location in Berlin. On his admittance into the hospital he was the "image of an Asiatic cholera" patient.[84]

Dr. Kluge along with five other physicians performed an autopsy on Bobach on August 31. The results were similar to the findings in the previous three autopsies. Kluge declared that Bobach "had died from Asiatic cholera." In the Charité the prescribed sanitary measures were immediately implemented in the room that the patient had stayed in. Now with all the facts, the members of the Chief Sanitary Committee no longer doubted the existence of the cholera in Berlin. The committee arranged for the first public announcement on September 1, 1831 "so the public could be subjected to the sanitary measures that had previously been announced."[85]

Police President Arnim also attended this meeting and made sure the doctors understood the severity of the situation. He informed the doctors what the consequences for Berlin would be if the city were blockaded as a result of the announcement that cholera was in Berlin. He warned that a cordon surrounding Berlin would lead to disease and famine within fourteen days.[86]

Following the official announcement of the Chief Sanitary Committee, the number of sick increased considerably. There were three new victims in the first two days, twenty by the September 4 and 5, and sixty-three by September 15.[87]

Once cholera appeared questions about the quarantine of Berlin rapidly surfaced. In previous discussions at the highest levels including of course the Immediate Commission, a policy of totally isolating Berlin was deemed "impractical" by officials connected with the administration of the city. In a closed meeting of the city council on September 2, the "council made a proposal to lift all blockade measures, quarantine facilities and all house barriers" because as they saw it "no cases had occurred in Berlin that even had the suspicion of direct infection" and anyway the "sickness was caused by diet, and against this no obstructive measures can help." They had also received reports from areas already attacked by the disease, that the sickness had only affected a "fraction of the population, whether blockade measures had been applied or not." In order to "protect the small percentage of the population against the alleged infection, it would not be responsible to put in jeopardy the livelihood of the remaining 97 percent or 98 percent." The city council unanimously supported this request.[88]

Nevertheless it appeared the situation concerning quarantining Berlin was not completely settled at least in the mind of Police President Arnim. Early in September following the cholera outbreak in Berlin, he invited nearly all of the practicing physicians of the medical department to his residence to hear for himself their opinions "about the contagiousness of the disease." There were approximately fifteen doctors in attendance including Doctors Rust, Horn, Eck, Kluge, and Heim. The first three doctors agreed "at the outset for absolute contagion." Kluge was in "doubt and said he could not decide whether it was contagious." Privy Head Medical Councilor von Könen said, "As a medical official I say the disease is contagious as a practicing physician I say it is not." According to one eyewitness this elicited much laughter on the part of the physicians, but Arnim was not amused and rebuked the doctors and said he invited them with the intent on hearing their opinions on the contagiousness of the cholera and that he would listen to their judgments and treat all their opinions fairly.[89] If all of them "unanimously pronounced that the disease was contagious he knew he would have to surround Berlin with a cordon." Even Rust when asked directly would not take responsibility for the consequences of a cordon of the city. As a result Berlin was not cordoned off and according to one eyewitness "a great evil was prevented."[90]

With the outbreak of cholera a minimal shipping blockade was imposed on the Spree, but Berlin and Charlottenburg were not closed to land traffic. What is significant is that there appears to have been developing a piecemeal modification of the original directives of the Immediate Commission. This previewed both a coming shift in official medical policy and the undermining of the role of the Immediate Commission as a consequence of practical considerations confronting higher government officials and city authorities in Berlin.

Cholera Policy Modified on the Eve of the Berlin Epidemic

The beginning of the shift in official cholera policy can be seen in the notice issued by Provincial President Bassewitz and confirmed by Thile on August 29, and published in the *Prussian State Gazette* on September 3, 1831. With the outbreak of cholera, Berlin, Charlottenburg, and Potsdam would not be sequestered.[91] This was a departure from the Immediate Commission's current policy which was being employed in East Prussia and especially in Danzig. In the August 29 meeting of the Immediate Commission it was even suggested there should be a blockade between Berlin and Spandau (however, this was not implemented). At the time, the commission received further information from Provincial President Flottwell of Posen, that the commission's directives were not being followed in some places. Nevertheless, the commission continued to assume that its policy would continue because there were ongoing discussions concerning the cordons and quarantine stations along the Vistula, Elbe and in Danzig.[92]

Other matters were raised with the commission that required answers or resolutions. There was for example, a suggestion to quarantine the Elbe, to protect those areas and countries in the west which had not been attacked by the cholera. It was in this meeting that the king inquired as to what was the basic reason for securing Prussia with a cordon? The answer given was to prevent the disease from entering Prussia. The expense, and the fact that the disease was already in Prussia, raised further doubts as to whether the strict policy was effective and even necessary.[93]

By September 5, matters concerning the general cordon in Prussia, especially in the East and around Berlin, had reached a crisis. There was open disagreement among members of the government over how to fight cholera. The *Augsburger Allgemeine Zeitung* reported on September 3, 1831 from Berlin, the "Provincial commissions had carried out few of the cholera regulations" and there was "disunity among the members" (doctors, government officials and city officials) because some had "denied the contagion." Even Mayor Bärensprung, of Berlin, a member of the Chief Sanitary Committee of Berlin, was quoted as saying that commerce in Berlin had not been interrupted even though the disease had broken out there and he hoped that it would not be "stifled" by a blockade of the city.[94]

The Intervention of the King

As we saw earlier in the case of Schön the king began to have his doubts about continuing the Immediate Commission's strict policy under Rust and was even less willing to support it as he gained more experience with the disease. A report by one physician who visited the king shortly after the outbreak of the cholera in Berlin gives a good indication of his state of mind. The physician reported that after the first public declaration of the outbreak of the cholera in Charlottenburg he visited the king to attend to him. When he first entered into his presence the king asked him, "How did things stand with the cholera?" He replied that he had just come from the third victim (see above) and had actually seen all three. They were not his patients anymore. All had "died within hours of contracting the dreadful disease." The king replied "and you come to me?" The physician replied that it was his duty and swore that the disease was not contagious. The king replied "No, Your Majesty does not believe it is either." But nevertheless the king had to follow the regulations authorized by the head of the medical department, Dr. Rust, and had to set an example because so many people were frightened.[95]

The king had been setting an example. At the residence at Sans-Souci one could only enter the community through a nearby house after passing through a cloud of chlorine gas. This had lasted for weeks on end because Rust and his colleagues persisted in their opinion of contagion. In addition, the king and his family had to avoid everything that was forbidden and follow a strict diet as well.[96]

The king was determined to remain at Charlottenburg to be close to his ministers and to be able to visit Berlin and "comfort the local inhabitants."[97] This would mean that in order for ministers and other persons to have access to the king at Charlottenburg a "disinfection station would have to be built." The palace was "separated by fences and palisades from any intercourse from without." When the cholera broke out in Charlottenburg the people were sure that the king would retire to Potsdam. However, as the newspapers reported, he remained in Charlottenburg, near Berlin where he took measures to "alleviate the distress" and gain the "confidence of the people" of Berlin. This policy was to avoid actions similar to those that had occurred in Königsberg and Stettin and to help suppress the "absurd illusion" that the lower working class was "being poisoned by the doctors."[98]

The careful preparations and the high cost of these restrictions were gradually taking a toll on the king. Following all these precautions suddenly a "menial" servant in the castle at Charlottenburg became sick and died from cholera. This may have shown the king the futility of the more extreme measures of Rust and his colleagues.[99] Initially, when the servant became sick with cholera the anti-contagionists "were triumphant in the evidence afforded by this case." It was later "ascertained, however, that the person alluded to had found means to quit the palace at night, and visit her relations in the town of Charlottenburg."[100]

The latter provided the background to help reinforce the king's interest in questioning the purpose of the cordons and the strict cholera policy in general. This was apparent at the Immediate Commission meetings, especially the meeting on September 2, 1831. Dr. Rust realized the king himself was questioning the strict contagionist policy of the commission and he found himself defending both the contagionist view and the overall quarantine policy. He stated that all the previous policies had been predicated to "impede the communication of the contagion" He warned that "not observing the strict measures would lessen the possibility of limiting the spread of the sickness."[101]

However it is clear from the king's actions he remained within the bounds of the recommendations of the Immediate Commission. But there is little doubt that the economic and social consequences were weighing on the king's mind as well as others. In the same September 2 meeting of the commission, the members discussed the issue of the possible effects of strict cholera regulations on the government of Frankfurt on the Oder. The local merchants requested modifications to the strict regulation because they saw these measures as a distinct "disadvantage" to their commercial trade.[102] The Frankfurt district government by its geographical location and topographical characteristics was more than any other portion of the state exposed to the threat of cholera. It was the crossing point between the eastern part, bordering on Russia and Poland, and the western provinces of the Prussian state with its "navigable streams, and river networks consisting of the Warta, Oder, Spree and Neisse rivers, intersected by the *Friedrich-Wilhelm-Kanal*. It was also an important marketplace that sponsored three major "fairs" because it was located on water and land routes that saw "lively and continuous commercial traffic in all directions." If cholera continued to follow past precedent along the rivers, the local administrative districts feared cholera would hit them especially hard.[103]

In addition, the Frankfurt Fair or "Martini Messe" that lasted for three weeks and was scheduled to begin on November 1 (an annual event) was one of the most important trade fairs in Brandenburg Province and contributed immensely to the income of the district and the state by receiving "extensive payments for its barge traffic."[104]

In addition to the Fair's financial importance to the state, the consequences of not holding the Fair had implications for the economic stability of Berlin and the surrounding area. It was reported that there had been much concern earlier about whether Frankfurt's trade fair should be discouraged because in Berlin alone "60,000 people worked in some capacity for the fair and would be unemployed if the ... strict measures were put in place in Berlin and the Fair closed."[105]

The concern with the unemployed as a result of the strict regulations and their effect on "trade and shops" thus leading to unemployment was not lost on the king or his officials. On August 31 for example, in advance of cholera, rising prices on food and commodities was being reported. It was expected that this could "produce the same problems as in Königsberg." This was undoubtedly a concern for the king and his officials. Shortly after the outbreak of cholera in Berlin he ordered a public works construction project in the Charité garden. Advertisements for the projects noted that they would be pay "customary wages" and the workers would be required to provide a certificate from the police that they were residents of the city and unemployed.[106]

Finally the cost of all these measures was weighing on the government. Earlier, the king had questioned Rust on the cost of all these measures. He wanted to know if it was all worth it. Although the government would not make the cost known, it was estimated that by July 26 the cost exceeded 50,000 million talers. The king himself had distributed 40,000 talers for the poor from his privy purse prior to the outbreak of the cholera. This amount did not include charitable funds raised within the city of Berlin to combat the cholera.[107]

The Royal Proclamation of September 6, 1831

For these reasons a change was needed to modify the strict measures. The turning point came with the Royal Cabinet Order of September 6, 1831, published in the formerly contagionist *Prussian State Gazette* on September 13.[108] The king after consulting with his cabinet and the Immediate Commission thanked the commission for all the work it had done. He then essentially repudiated the commission's handling of the entire affair and listed the major problems its policies had caused in Prussia. The same issue contained a notice by the commission, addressing the modification of the regulations required by the Royal Order. There was also another notice dated September 12, 1831, signed by Rust, offering employment to the Berlin unemployed in the construction of a building in the Charité hospital garden.[109]

The Proclamation issued under the auspices of the State Ministry and signed by the king specifically addressed; a change in quarantine and cordon policy, actions of the Immediate Commission, commerce and trade, the king's concern that the population not become violent, that the laws be enforced, and finally he called on the public to trust the government and doctors, and to follow their own consciences.

The Immediate Commission was not dissolved. It was expected to follow the king's "new revision of the regulations and instructions for April 5th and June 1st though modified several times in the past due to changed circumstances." It was not to "delay the changes and the relief" the king ordered.[110] The commission's policies had been under attack. The commercial interests were the most vocal, culminating in the Frankfurt merchant's complaints as well as concerns expressed on September 2 by Berlin officials. However, the uprising in Königsberg and other examples of unrest in the quarantined areas as well as the opinions of high government officials, forced the king and his advisors to re-assess the government position. The king did not decide to reverse the policy of the commission lightly. Rust was appointed to the commission because of his position and reputation as one of the leading medical experts in the state. His reputation was under assault. Rust also had an unyielding belief in his position on contagion.[111] Members of the medical administration viewed the change in policy as a political not a medical decision and done for the "sake of public opinion." The decision was made over the objections of Prussia's leading medical experts, Rust and the "Scientific Deputation."[112] His dissatisfaction with the decision was well known, one newspaper went so far as to report that "Rust has resigned his post as President." The report of his resignation was later proven untrue.[113]

Nevertheless, according to the *Augsburger Allgemeine Zeitung* the proclamation made a "favorable impression." It was also reported that "the words of the king on September 6, 1831, proclaimed by the State Ministry, had an electric effect" on the public.[114] This was an extraordinary announcement because it did not originate with any of the official medical or sanitary authorities (as had the regulations issued previously) but came from the State Ministry and the king, who evidently supported this change in policy by putting his name to the proclamation. He was directly mentioned by the Immediate Commission in their announcement that appeared right below the proclamation on the front page of the *Prussian State Gazette* on September 13, 1831. The king's Proclamation began:

> The most watchful care, the most unremitting efforts have failed to arrest the progress of the asiatick [sic] cholera has not withstanding the strongest measures of prevention this disease has forced itself across my Frontiers, into my Kingdom. In all those places, however where the orders given have been punctually executed, the dutiful exertions of the authorities; as it is by praiseworthy efforts of experienced Doctors, have succeeded in diminishing the violence of the pestilence and in confining the victims to a number small in proportion with that of those who have fallen a sacrifice to it in other countries.[115]

The king admitted cholera had spread into Prussian territory and the strict measures of the Immediate Commission, although not entirely successful, had succeeded in diminishing the impact of the disease. Secondly, the cholera's impact had not been as severe as in other countries. At the time there was some controversy over the phrase "In all those places, however, where the orders given have been punctually executed...." Chad wrote this referred to Schön and implied "censure upon this Governour [sic], whose disregard of his instructions has been the general subject of conversation here." Officially he had "not ... heard that this passage was intended to convey this meaning."[116] This was true. Privately the king did not criticize Schön for those actions but only for visiting cholera victims.[117] The rest of the document essentially repudiated the earlier regulations that Schön had opposed. As for the "efforts of the experienced Doctors ... "there was no direct evidence that they had "diminished the violence of the epidemic" as the means and methods for treating cholera were hotly disputed and the situation in Danzig and other areas had contributed to fairly high mortality rates.[118] The Royal Proclamation continued:

> ...as however during the prevalence of the malady upon our soil, experience and practical observations have enlightened the administration, I have caused all the regulations which have been published on this subject to be submitted to an examination and revision grounded upon change of circumstances, upon the present knowledge acquired by the treatment of disease that severe measures of separation effected by means of military lines on the frontiers of the Kingdom and the interior have already materially injured the industry and commerce of the inhabitants, and a continuation of them for a longer period would endanger the comforts and wellbeing of many families, and be more hurtful to the country than the disease itself, and the measures cannot be continued in their former degree, as the approaching autumn renders it impractical to preserve them without exposing the health of the troops by a continuation of this harassing service.[119]

Medical opinion continued to be divided on all aspects of the epidemic. The official medical organs, as well as administrative medical officials, continued to be contagionists.

However, the king was concerned about the adverse effects on the economy and industry of Prussia if the old policy continued. He ordered that all the previous regulations examined and revised in light of "changed circumstances." He was referring to scathing criticism by practicing physicians and Berlin city officials, the military costs and lack of public support. Most critically "the military lines ... have already materially injured the industry and commerce of the inhabitants" The king was incurring inordinate expenses to support these troops. He had come around to the opinion, expressed earlier in Königsberg (only this time it was applied to the entire country) that the continuation of these measures would "be more hurtful to the country than the disease itself."[120]

In addition to the economic impact of the military lines the precarious situation of the health of the military needed to be considered too. Dr. Becker wrote specifically about this issue and its importance to the meaning of the proclamation. Even with "our numerous and well-disciplined army, even with the assistance of the local militia, proved altogether insufficient for that purpose; and it was melancholy to observe, that the very troops of the sanitary line quartered in unhealthy situations, at the approach of the inclement season, suffered severely, not only from occasional cases of cholera ... but still more from endemic fevers of the country."[121]

Ambassador Chad was not so sanguine, writing that the "breaking up of the sanitary lines formed in the northern parts of the Kingdom; enable the government to move the troops there employed to the line of the Elbe. The ... cessation of hostilities in Poland, now therefore render available the greater part of the force in question."[122]

Based on the words in the proclamation distinct military pressure was being applied. With the conclusion of the hostilities in Poland it was critical that the western borders of the Kingdom be strengthened. This was not only to hinder the spread of cholera (as this was the reason for moving the troops). Also, there was the concern the army should remain healthy and be capable of protecting the western border from a French threat.

At the same time, the king and his councilors repudiated the Immediate Commission's entire medical policy. All its measures were re-examined and modified to limit some of the criticism (and not establish another unyielding policy). The king permitted local authority over quarantine measures. (Local control had been requested by the sanitary commissions and city officials). This was an important recommendation of the anticontagionists. The king underscored the change in policy:

> I have therefore with especial reference to the military lines, to the local populations of those provinces districts, and isolate places this till now, by regulations of the police escaped the malady, and also by shortening of the time of the quarantine decreed the institution of a Direct [Immediate] Commission with the further orders to publish immediately the subsequent alterations necessary to the decrees and directions already issued; and as this committee on a former occasion by most anxious precautions performed their troublesome office of averting and opposing the sickness to my complete satisfaction, it will now not neglect any experience which can contribute to alleviate the measures which have been adopted.[123]

The king for political reasons supported the past actions of the commission in the proclamation, the complete lifting of military lines along the northern border and in the interior where the cholera already had broken out was a reversal of past regulations. The commission lifted the military lines in East Prussia and in the interior. Nevertheless, a military line was continued in provinces still free of the disease. A cordon was imposed on the Elbe from Muhlenberg to Schnachenberg to protect western Germany. Cordons were established on September 14 on the Spree to the Neisse and on the frontiers of the Kingdom of Saxony. A military line was continued from Cüstrin to Ratibor primarily because the government district of Breslau had not witnessed an outbreak of the cholera by September 14. Cholera finally appeared in Breslau on September 23. The order stated that in all other places in the interior of Prussia, the quarantine was to be lifted and all persons allowed to "depart freely." Quarantines limited to five days would only be enforced for travelers and on merchandise from infected areas. Importantly, local authorities were able to determine points of entry and if desired establish quarantine regulations. The order allowed the free navigation of all rivers where the disease had already broken out (except those designated above). The provincial presidents were authorized to carry out these new regulations.[124]

Districts and even communes were now able to decide whether they would enforce quarantine procedures. Dr. Becker, a physician, in Berlin approved of this arrangement and called it a system of seclusion. He noted that this plan was "adopted throughout Prussia; the government having taken away all barriers to communication throughout the country, it having left to the option of all communes and districts to protect themselves by such measures as are compatible with the interests of the country at large."[125]

Administratively, reliance on local authorities to resolve problems in Prussia was not without precedent. Becker wrote, "It must be remembered that in "despotic" Prussia the business of the *Gemeinden* (parishes), and of the *Landkreise* (counties), is managed by a magistracy elected by the inhabitants, at the head of which are placed Burgomasters and *Landrathe* (district administrators) who are also chosen by their fellow citizens and approved by the king."[126] For example, the Prussian government took a similar tactic in regard to the *Städtordnung* of the same year (1831). Politically the king and his advisors thought it prudent to allow the cities of Prussia to exercise a local option as to whether the cities of Prussia should or should not accept the new ordinance. The grave situation presented by the cholera, local uprisings and general discontent combined with the merchant and industrialist opposition rekindled memories of the "July Revolution." A similar solution (local control of sanitary policy) was consistent with current administrative policy. Since neither the contagionist nor non-contagionist position was proven, the government was in a position to offer a compromise solution not based on medical evidence, but on what made political and economic sense for the security of the government and the economy of Prussia. The result was that on September 6, the king by issuing the Royal Cabinet Order to reverse the Immediate Commission's centralized policy was done to avoid massive opposition and allow local initiatives to predominate. This served two purposes, there was no central authority for the people to oppose (Becker explains the tactic very well) and costs could be minimized and absorbed locally.[127]

The solution was a success for the Prussian government. Looking at the government districts which had their first outbreak of the cholera after September 15, the percentage of cities and towns infected within the government districts was as follows: Potsdam (2.5 percent), Frankfurt (1.9 percent), Breslau (2.4 percent), Madgeburg (1.6 percent) and Cöslin

(1.6 percent). Compare these ratios to the initial outbreaks during May, July, and August in Danzig (11.3 percent), Königsberg (6.3 percent), Bromberg (13.7 percent) and Marienwerder (10.1 percent).

The number of sick per 1000 for the same government districts after September 15 was as follows: Potsdam (3.38) Frankfurt (3.08), Breslau (1.75), Madgeburg (1.69) and Cöslin (.33). Again compare these figures to the initial outbreaks during May, July and August in Danzig (15.81), Königsberg (14.56), Bromberg (23.32) and Marienwerder (19.53).[128]

Rescinding the military lines and easing the strict regulations regarding house quarantine and travel had come at a fortunate time for the Prussian government. The later cholera outbreaks were less deadly and limited geographically to smaller areas. In the government district of Breslau, and specifically in the city of Breslau, cholera struck after September 15, 1831, where it had its last major impact during this first epidemic in Prussia. It traveled along the Oder River breaking out in the city of Breslau on September 23 and lasted until January 2, 1832. The number of sick per 1000 were (15.42). Compare this figure to the initial outbreaks in Danzig (20.63) and Konigsberg (35.06) in May and July respectively.[129]

Again if we look at the figures for the entire government district of Breslau we find the impact of cholera considerably milder and less deadly than the initial visitations in Prussia. In Breslau, the city administration was probably better prepared to deal with the cholera, having learned from the experiences of other Prussian cities, and it was not restricted by the harsh orders of the Immediate Commission. The city instituted strict "administrative and hygienic measures." They attributed the "limiting of the progress of the sickness and hastening its termination" to these measures.[130] As Becker noted, local officials were authorized to decide on local public health policies. Breslau had opted for strictly enforcing the cleansing and quarantining of the homes of the sick. Meanwhile charitable committees had been organized in all sections of the city to care for the sick, and food was provided for those who needed it. Curiously, from the anticontagionist viewpoint, communications with the surrounding villages and suburbs of Breslau had remained open. For the seven weeks of the epidemic "3 to 4 thousand peasants" entered Breslau each day and returned to their homes. Extraordinary to one observer was the fact that only a small number of villages had cholera cases and for a greater number of villages there was no outbreak. To an anticontagionist this was proof that the cholera was not contagious but the product of local conditions.[131]

The remainder of the Proclamation of September 6, 1831, was an attempt to address the fears the government had toward the public and avoid an uprising in Berlin. First, the king had to modify a quarantine policy which was causing enormous problems for him and his ministers. Secondly, he had to defend the past actions of the Immediate Commission. Although the plans to modify the quarantine policy came from outside the Immediate Commission, the king continued to depend on it to carry out his orders. He had to maintain its credibility, because it represented the interests of the Prussian medical establishment and any major public disagreement would have demonstrated to the public an unhealthy divisiveness in the government at a time when overall public anxiety was at its highest. The government could not afford this with an epidemic ready to burst forth in Berlin.

In order to demonstrate that the government was committed to providing increased medical assistance the king stipulated:

The result of these orders however will only answer expectations if the inhabitants of separate dwellings animated by public spirit, unite in endeavoring to prevent the spreading of the malady among their fellow citizens, and to afford timely assistance to those attacked I have to that effect ordered the establishment of institutions, private nurses in each establishment and the immediate publication of rules respecting their regulations and duties.[132]

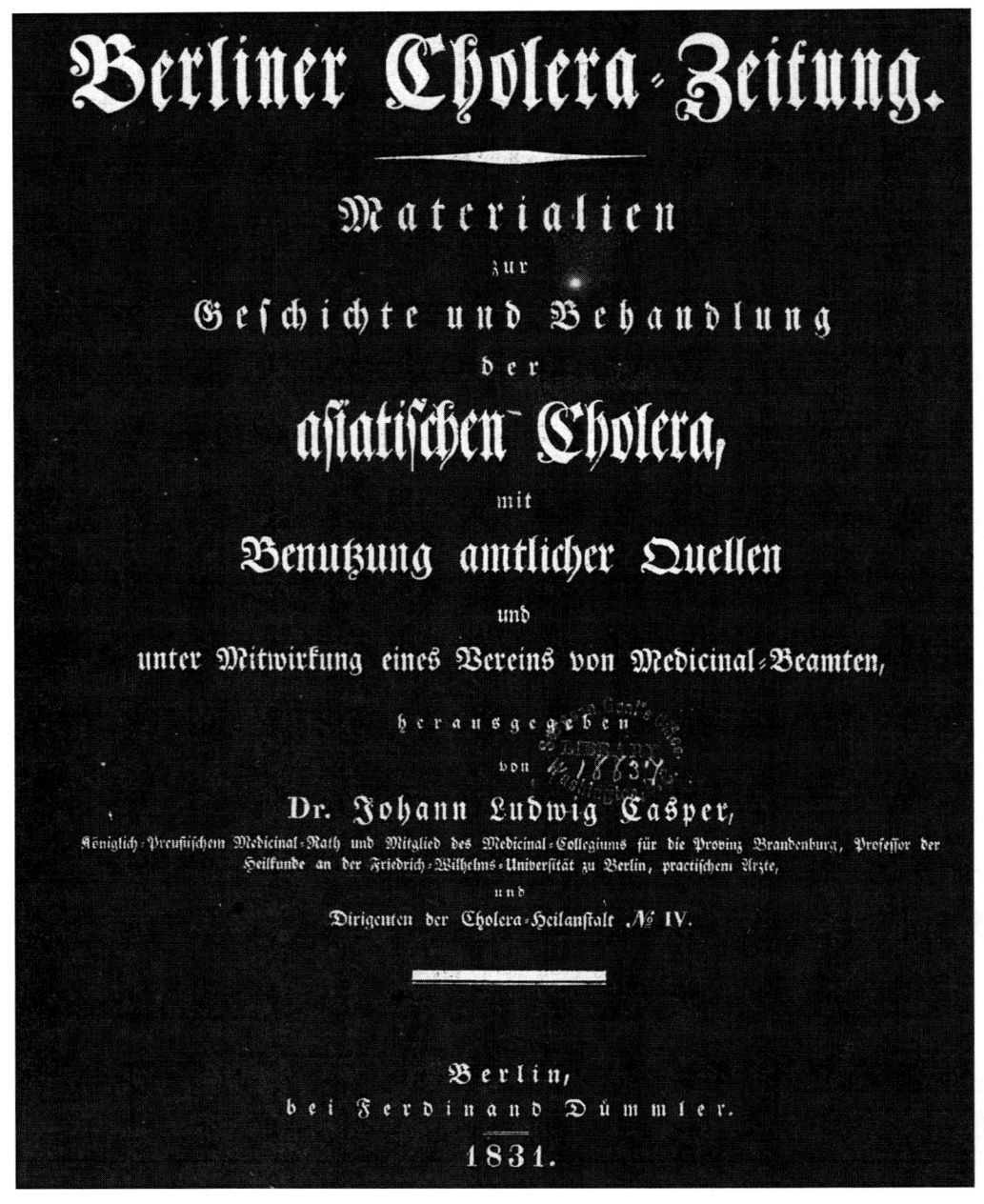

"Berliner Cholera Zeitung." The primary organ for communicating with the public during the cholera epidemic in Berlin in 1831 was the Berliner Cholera Zeitung. It was published in Berlin from September 24, 1831 to December 27, 1831, three times per week for a total of 36 issues (Author's collection).

The special mention of the cholera hospitals was necessary to allay the distrust which all classes had toward public hospitals. One writer in the *Berliner Cholera Zeitung* wrote that the population had a low opinion of the "hospitals" of the time and "more than one prejudice must be overcome in many classes, at the same time the natural connection to the family is understandable but the aversion to the hospitals is not a trifling matter."[133] Dr. Becker wrote, "prejudice against hospitals is greater in this country than in Great Britain" and that even after the establishment of excellent hospitals "a large proportion of cholera patients, even of the lowest classes has remained at home in all Prussian towns where the disease has prevailed."[134] In order to counteract this prejudice, between September 6 and early October the king ordered the establishment of six cholera hospitals in Berlin. Some of hospitals were opened for public inspection. For example, in hospital number IV (*Heilenanstalt*), visitors commented on the appearance and the attentiveness of the surroundings and the staff.[135] The idea of "allowing the public and particularly the lower classes, to visit the hospitals intended for the cholera patients," was to acquaint them with the "arrangements of such institutions" so they would "gain confidence in them."[136]

In Berlin, commune leaders, city councilors and administrative officials were all given credit for the excellent conditions in the hospitals. Specific regulations were also enacted in early September in which the Head doctors were ordered to ensure "that the sick were treated with consideration and gentleness ... unfriendly and inhumane treatment was to be avoided."[137] As an incentive to follow these regulations, nurses and other attendants were rewarded with additional wages of one to five talers and were publically commended for showing consideration toward cholera victims in their care.[138]

The king's proclamation, called on God to help him and his people through the coming trial. The king did not, however, intend to leave the consequences of the epidemic in God's hands nor did he view the epidemic as a punishment from God. The king ordered an active medical response to mitigate the ravages of the cholera. The king was prepared to offer employment to the poor through a limited public works project, because he feared the potential for popular unrest in Berlin. The king wrote:

> General attention should be universally given to funding employment and occupation for the laboring classes, and that the burden of supporting the poor should be rendered lighter to the parishes and the poor on their part must neglect nothing in order to further the welfare of their fellow citizens and maintain the general peace and quiet.[139]

Providing some means of employment resulted from the consequences and presumed manner in which the disease spread. Chad wrote the "indirect consequences of the prevalence of the cholera upon the lower classes are such as cannot fail to produce discontent."[140] He described the impact of the sickness on the different levels of the population:

> Many persons are entirely deprived of employment, as whilst the pestilence lasts, there is a general disinclination to admit unless in cases of absolute necessity workman of any sort into private houses. The effect upon the industrious poor in a populous Town is greater that at first sight it would appear to be. Amongst the sufferers are all those persons, who are interested in the sale of fish, fruit, vegetables-articles of food which are thought unwholesome. Poultry has also been added to this list.... The trade of shopkeepers is also generally very much diminished during the prevalence of the cholera, as the fear of buying infected goods prevents all purchases which are not absolutely necessary.[141]

Chad closed his letter: "If the determination of the Government to insulate all those houses in which the Cholera shows [*sic*] itself, has not been relinquished, the consequences would probably have been disastrous."[142]

On September 17 Rust advertised in the newspapers that all: "...necessitous persons would find work at the hospital of La Charité, where extensive building was in progress. The number of people that applied in their expectation of obtaining employment; and above one hundred of them proceeded in a body yesterday to the Palace at Charlottenburg and asked to see the King."[143]

Chad reported that an *aide-de-camp* was sent out to meet the crowd. The king gave orders to give the demonstrators either "bread or work."[144] The demonstrators were not "satisfied" and assembled the following morning. They "gathered at the castle gate which caused a stir in the castle." The king requested they submit their request in writing and permitted six of the men into a room where their complaints were heard. The king made a small gift of money to the men as they were "very poor people and some family men" the men went "quietly back to Berlin." The next day police officials commanded the six men who had signed the petition appear before them. Instead the 100 who had been there on the previous day appeared. They were told that they would have a guarantee of work by the following week.[145] Chad explained to Palmerston that the incident had caused no "sensation" in Berlin. Further the king had in fact previously distributed prior to the outbreak of the cholera "40,000 talers from his privy purse to be spent employing the Poor."[146]

The situation in Berlin could have become even more explosive than Königsberg. The king and his advisors were ready to use every means at their disposal to maintain order over the lower classes. The king was prepared to initiate a "public works" project, although it is evident that it was limited in conception and scope. Chad as earlier noted was convinced that if these measures had not been reversed the consequences would have been disastrous.[147]

The proclamation emphasized that the government was aware of the potential for disorder:

> I hope that the blamable disorders which at some places occurred on the breaking out of the cholera, proceeding generally from an absurd error, will nowhere be repeated and that all prudent and well minded persons will readily assist their superiors in the maintenance of public order and respect of Laws. Every resistance against superior arrangements, every attempt to create disturbances must give way to condign punishments of the partakers and exciters; if as I confidently trust, the measure introduced attest to all classes and conditions of my people that the administration, equally free from a destructive security and an overanxious fear, has had recourse to all known means at its disposal for suppressing the malady and at the same time has with the most candid earnestness occupied itself to prevent and lessen the evils attending it.[148]

The proclamation referred to disturbances in Königsberg, Memel and Stettin, but as official documents show, the disturbances were not limited to the larger cities.[149] Ironically, fear of the unknown and the acute anxiety was focused on those chiefly responsible for helping the sick: the government and its agents, physicians. The king attempted to point out the absurdity that physicians were in a conspiracy with the government against the infected. Official documents and personal writings continued to confirm the widespread belief in this conspiracy.

After the outbreak of cholera in a town following its appearance in Königsberg, one official wrote, the lower classes believe the "sickness was being used as a pretext to get rid of a part of the poor inhabitants, by the administration of a medicinal poison."[150] Initially, both protestant and catholic clergy spoke out against these "absurd ideas." As a result even they came under suspicion that they were in league with the doctors. Further, it was charged that government officials arranged the means of the poisoning with the doctors and for each "individual poisoning" the doctor was "honored by the state with 4 florins."[151] This created "a great bitterness in the lower classes, not only against the doctors but also against the upper classes in general."[152] These absurd ideas were not only common in the large cities when the cholera broke out "but also in the smaller towns, in local provinces and produced many disorders."[153]

Dr. Lorinser wrote in his autobiography the "poor believed doctors created cholera to earn money and to diminish the great number of the poor."[154] In Upper Silesia, as well as in other areas, the people were of the opinion that the wells had been poisoned.[155]

The pressures on the king and his advisors constituted a serious threat to the peace and stability of the Kingdom. Normally the king's intervention in State matters was limited. In this crisis the king took actions which were normally left to the bureaucratic apparatus of the state, in this case the medical experts. Naturally the rumors circulating in Berlin caused anxiety at court. The king's councilors and city officials advised him against instituting the Immediate Commission's severe contagionist policy. There is little doubt the king was involved in the major policy decisions concerning cholera and is illustrated from his initial appointment of the commission to the Cabinet Order of September 6. The subsequent royal proclamation was issued by the king without the agreement of the commission. The reason for this was the emergency situation created by the cholera as well as the revolutionary situation in Poland. One additional factor which may have motivated the king to act confidently in this matter was the support available from the military, various ministers and other high officials in his government.[156]

It could be argued from this document that the king reverted to an earlier, more conservative role as a "sacred and omnipotent figure" of the past "who resolves all pending conflicts" rather than to his contemporary and weaker role as the first servant in a bureaucratic state. For example, one historian has looked at the "social protest" of the construction workers in Berlin during the cholera epidemic and seen it as part of a pre-industrial early nineteenth century "conservative social protest." The king was viewed by the lower classes as an "integrative father figure" who knew what was best for the children of his country." His actions toward the workers confirmed the "status quo of the God given power of the monarchy." This "social conservatism" is clearly articulated in the proclamation because it is the king who is directly "resolving social tensions and rising conflicts in his Kingdom." He was the "protector of the land from foreign conquest or *sickness*" and was defending his people from destitution." With these words he attempted to remedy the "sudden unemployment and famine brought about by the trade barriers resulting from the cholera." From the context of the proclamation it appears in the king' hands "run together the threads of the economic, political and cultural processes."[157]

The king and his military officials had practical matters to consider as well. They were anxious about Prussia's ability to fight a foreign war. This was a holdover from the revolutionary days of July 1830, which cast events in 1831 in a different light. The tension and distrust of the government was recognized at the highest levels by the officials (as the public made abundantly clear in its reaction to the initial regulations of April 5 and June 1 imposed by the Immediate Commission). As a consequence, military officials were anxious as to whether Prussia was capable of waging a war if necessary against a liberal or national revolutionary movement. The Berlin cabinet wanted to avoid war. General Rochow wrote, "We have no constitution, we have a militia system which is much worse and it is not designed for a European power." As a result "we can only lead the nation in a war of opinion!"[158] A once strong Prussia that "had guaranteed peace in middle Europe was now weak."[159]

As one commentator at the time wrote, there were three intertwined phenomena seen as an expression of the 1830–31 period and recognized by Prussian authorities. All three manifested themselves in a variety of ways in the Prussian government's actions during this period and its response to cholera. They include "the enthusiasm for Poland; the idolatry of Napoleon ... and the fear of cholera."[160]

The support for Poland and the Polish insurrection in Germany was evident in the enthusiasm for the Poles especially among the youth and women in the German States. For many the Polish heroes were "fighting in a just cause." Included with this was the idolization of Napoleon. This was especially true among the Poles as well as many Germans. There had grown up a brisk trade in paintings, busts and statuettes in Poland of the image of Napoleon. These were produced in the German States also, and at a not "inconsiderable profit." Finally, there was the fear of cholera, a fear that seemed to inordinately affect men and higher officials than women.[161]

However, during the epidemic, the Prussian authorities relied on their medical authorities to plan a response to the cholera with the military lines on the borders and in the interior. It was not until the disease erupted in Berlin that the king and his councilors began to publically question the Immediate Commission and reverse its policy. This was not related to any change in the status of the Polish revolt but the practical experience of officials in Berlin, who now recognized the impracticality and exorbitant costs of quarantine and military cordons. Even the impact on trade and commerce placed Prussia in a weak position versus the potential of a French invasion. The social disruption could lead to a popular uprising in Berlin. They had been shocked by the uprisings in Europe in 1830, especially the July days in France. Prussian officials realized the powerful combination of the nostalgia for Napoleon, the enthusiasm for the Polish insurrection and cholera anxiety could act as a powder keg that could lead to instability and even popular uprisings. Although the non-medical Prussian officials feared cholera, they undoubtedly feared a popular uprising more and were willing to support the king in taking responsibility for mitigating at least one of the contributing factors to public unrest.

10

Berlin Organizes to Combat Cholera

There seems to be little doubt that when cholera finally arrived in Berlin the city administration and the Prussian government had learned a hard lesson from the previous strict sanitary policy. Officials in Berlin were prepared to mitigate the impact of the disease and take positive action to prevent many of the secondary effects. The king of Prussia advocated a series of positive measures that he wanted introduced and warned there would be consequences for those who acted against the interests of the state.

The first cases of cholera in Berlin began on the boats along the Spree and in the streets adjacent to the navigable part of the river. Nine of the first one hundred cases occurred on ships or barges and all were fatal.[1] Because the disease spread to the streets and alleys near the river, the disease was attributed to miasma. Those not near the river felt safe. By October 1, 1831, there were seventy-three cholera patients; most of the victims were near the water.[2]

At first the disease was slow to extend throughout the city and into the more highly populated parts of Berlin. Cases appeared on small nearby streets and alleys further from the river "occupied by the lowest orders."[3] On September 3, 1831, Carl Müller at 8 Kaiserstrasse (in the eastern suburbs) died. Although he did not live near the river, he worked in the mint near where cholera had broken out. Between September 3 and 22, five other cases occurred in different houses on the same street.[4]

Another case, also removed from the river area, occurred on September 3 in a large workhouse, containing about "700 inhabitants of the lowest classes," who found employment there. During the month of September, 57 cholera cases occurred in this workhouse. In a nearby building with 550 inhabitants there were 36 victims. Unfortunately, the first case was not reported until September 8, five days after the disease first appeared in the workhouse (not an uncommon occurrence). The disease spread to the central part of Berlin in the northern and eastern suburbs inhabited primarily by laborers. Once it reached these "districts it moved with as great an intensity" as it had in the streets and alleys along the river.[5]

In the 58th district, primarily inhabited by laborers and far from the Spree River, a local doctor, Dr. Oppert saw his first case on September 10th (by this time cholera had been in Berlin for twelve days). His patient died on September 14, 1831, "on that day his landlord, who had shaved him during his illness and a woman who lived next door to him were taken ill and died." Three days later a fourth person was attacked and died in the same house. Shortly afterward cholera spread to "seven houses on the same street."[6]

Of particular concern to the city officials in Berlin was the 59th district. This included five six story tenements built to hold thousands of people and considered the first tenements built in Berlin.[7] At the beginning of the 1830's approximately 2,300 people lived in the five building complex. They were the "most wretched part of the population ... [and] ... lived, crowded together in a deplorable manner, sometimes several families to a room." These tenements were "commonly called Family houses, originally built by an avaricious speculator" and "universally considered as our greatest nuisance."[8]

The buildings commonly known as the Wülcknitzschen (as they were referred to in contemporary accounts named after the original builder) or Family houses, located at no. 92, 92a, 92b, 93 and 94 Gartenstrasse, were built in 1821 by Baron von Wülcknitz, a local speculator. The tenements quickly became the residence of day laborers, weavers and poorer artisans. The buildings were originally planned with a garden in the courtyard. Over time the courtyard had become a swamp with run off from the septic system. In addition, "the privy in the courtyard had 98 seats for 1,450 people in 1831." The rooms "served as work areas, sleeping quarters and kitchens with "eight to ten persons per room."[9]

The living conditions in the tenement complex had concerned the authorities when cholera first threatened the capital. Trying to take advantage of the situation a new landlord Herrn Wieseke, in June 1831, made a list of tenants who were in arrears on their rent. He sent this list to the Magistrate along with a proposal to clean and fumigate the rooms. He would also permit a small building at 93 Gartenstrasse to be used as a lazaret. In return, he demanded the rents be covered by public means when the families returned after disinfection. If the Magistrate did not accept his proposal, he threatened to begin evicting his tenants. He warned he would "hold back their furniture, tools and looms." Not content to deal with the Magistrate alone, he also requested an interest free loan of 15,000 talers from the state authorities. He said if he was given this loan he would not have to evict the tenants from his buildings. He reasoned this sum would be sufficient to protect his investment in the case of a cholera outbreak. The head of the poor commission was alarmed. Wieseke's request was not honored. On July 27, 1831, he obtained a court order to begin the evictions.[10]

The police arrived to begin the eviction. Immediately a "large crowd gathered, insulted the officers, was generally insolent and challenged them." Thirty soldiers from the artillery barracks and police on horseback soon arrived. The police report blamed the event on the "lack of employment and low factory wages," although there were probably no factory workers living there. The police also reported there was also "talk of rebellion."[11] The real cause of the unrest was the combination of the planned evictions and anxiety over cholera. The actions by the authorities would lead to a loss of income and deprive them of bread. The police reported "they cried out, they could respect no law and that they would die anyway because it is hunger that causes cholera."[12]

The poor law commission began payments to stop the evictions and peace returned to the Wülcknitzschen tenements. However, on August 17, 1831, the poor relief administration decided to stop the outstanding rent payments and see if cholera would break out in the tenements.

The cholera first showed itself in the 59th district where the tenement buildings were located. It did not occur initially in the Family houses. On September 3, the first victim in the 59th district was a weaver named Joseph Müller. On September 10, the second victim was a working woman named Poschinsky. She was found behind a fence on Gartenstrasse near the tenements. The third victim, another woman, was found on September 12.[13] The expectation, attributed to miasma, was the overcrowded tenements in the 59th district would soon suffer from cholera. Because these tenements were far from the river there were also some who thought they might escape cholera. The Wülcknitzschen tenements remained free of cholera for three weeks. However, on September 21, the first case occurred at No. 94 Gartenstrasse. The victim, the son of a weaver, died followed by a sibling and an infant all in the same family.[14]

Of the Wülcknitzschen tenements the one at 92 Gartenstrasse had the highest morbidity rate. It peaked at 7 to 8 cases per day by the middle of October. The *Berliner Cholera Zeitung* reported 88 cases for 92 Gartenstrasse (it did not distinguish between a, b, and c) from September to the end of November.[15] Out of a total of 1,447 inhabitants, 112 individuals became sick in these tenements during the epidemic.[16] On September 19, the two story building at No. 93 Gartenstrasse was converted into a forty bed sanatorium (this had been part of an original proposal by Wieseke back in January).[17]

Nevertheless, the number of cases in these tenements was considered relatively small considering their living conditions. This was ascribed to the actions of Dr. Thummell, who "caused patients to be removed, as soon as notice was given, to an appropriate hospital."[18]

Once cholera broke out the pending evictions were postponed. By the middle of November with cholera in decline, additional tenants were now forced to vacate their rooms. The deal that Wieseke had tried to make with the Ministry of the Interior was rejected on December 27, 1831. Realizing a loss, he mortgaged the property and like his predecessor Baron von Wülcknitz took the money and fled to Paris.[19]

Other districts in Berlin remained remarkably free of cholera. According to Dr. Becker on one of the streets, Wilhelmstrasse inhabited by "very poor weavers, whose dwellings can by no means be regarded as healthy; still they have not suffered from cholera." He attributed this to their "secluded mode of life." They did not "mix with the inhabitants of the infected districts." There were some individual cases of cholera even in the better districts. These occurred primarily among the poor residing there. The cause was easily traced to "communications which the patients had with the infected districts." Dr. Becker was a member of the 13th district protection commission that contained 5,000 inhabitants (his district was located in the best part of town). From September 4 to November 4 only six cases occurred in private homes and an additional five cases "among the attendants of an institution founded for the relief of the patients of this district."[20]

In Berlin, by the end of October, 1,912 individuals were sick and of this number 1,057 died and 588 recovered. In November, the epidemic became less violent. For example during the week of October 16–22 the number of sick was 282 and dead 171. Approximately one month later November 13–19 the number of sick per week declined to 66 with 31 deaths.[21]

The Berlin Commune "Protection Commissions" and Their Activities During the Epidemic

In some respects Berlin was fortunate because the central authorities had early recognized that due to the political and economic situation in Berlin many of the strict measures ordered for other large cities and regional districts would not prove suitable for Berlin. As we have seen, besides the practical aspects of restricting access to a large city like Berlin that would lead to social and economic disruption, there was an almost ideological belief that "in large cities under the influence of the commercial interest, which, in consequence of the restrictive regulations, everyone looks with horror upon the doctrine of contagion" and its consequences to trade and commerce.[22]

The reality was, of course, that there was a commercial class with a horror of restrictive quarantine measures, doctors who were opponents of contagion, and the lower classes who saw themselves as victims of overzealous regulations that restricted their ability to earn a living. The result was many of these regulations were ignored because they were seen as more damaging than cholera.

With the changes in the strict policy Berlin was better organized and equipped to respond to the effects of cholera and the local resistance to government measures. The attempt to show that the city government was trying to be helpful and respond compassionately to this crisis was evident from the words and actions described in the *Berliner Cholera Zeitung* as well actions by the king and higher authorities.

The first example can be demonstrated in the organizations to combat cholera, specifically the sixty-one protection commissions ordered in each Berlin commune. As noted previously, the Chief Sanitary Committee of Berlin was responsible for these sixty-one commissions. This organization was directly responsible for dealing with the poor on a daily basis. These commissions "appointed men who were to be had at a moment's notice, and whose business it is to attend the patients, as well as prevent the intrusion of strangers."[23]

Besides the commissions, in each commune there were several doctors and surgeons responsible for observing the sanitary conditions of the people in their districts. They attended to the sick and most importantly were required to make known to the commission the number of sick they treated.[24]

Each member of a protection commission had special duties to fulfill. The doctors had to present themselves twice daily to the commission office and remain an hour or more. The commission office was located in a local hospital or sanatorium established for cholera sick. The doctors had to identify the houses they had visited in the district and report ill patients or those who had consulted them. The Police Commissioner was charged with overseeing the measures adopted by the Chief Sanitary Committee. He had the right to admit a foreigner living in the district at the time to the local hospital. Other members of the commission distributed any funds received, they regulated all administrative affairs and one member remained permanently at the office to deliver aid. The commissions had to report each day to the Chief Sanitary Committee, the number of sick, dead and recovered in their district. All citizens were required to make known to the commissions the existence of persons ill from cholera. If the sick person lived in a house the commission member had to determine if the victim could be treated at home or had to be sent to a hospital. In the first case, the patient was allowed to choose a doctor that "suits him." The commission member was only responsible for the immediate relief of the patient, and this might include making provisions for a steam bath, or obtaining therapeutic supplies for treating the patient. Commission members were responsible for quarantining houses. They could order anyone who had contact with a patient isolated for five days and order guards to prevent communication with anyone else. If the patient required transport to a hospital the commission member was responsible for bringing in porters to carry the patient to the hospital.[25]

Besides the regulations necessary to combat cholera, the Chief Sanitary Committee was also concerned with a number of non-regulatory activities. This can be seen in a notice published in the government newspaper for the benefit of the Berlin public. It was a justification of what was necessary to maintain public health. The public was ordered not to hide cholera cases because this inhibited "rapid and efficient service to patients." The public was not to impede the transportation of the sick to a cholera hospital. In addition, the public was told the regulations imposed had been proven by experience to be effective. Also regarding the cost, "temporary monetary sacrifices" had to be made now, so that others do not have to make more "painful sacrifices" later. Finally, "the poorer residents can relax in their afflictions" knowing that "paternal care" was assured by the local authorities. The notice also attempted to assure the working poor that "the country has begun to control unemployment and the lack of food through a comprehensive building ... [program] ... and further aid is graciously promised." Arnim, who signed the notice, concluded it with an optimistic exhortation "So let us with courage, with faith in God ... and perseverance in this combat serve as an example to our fellow citizens."[26]

According to Arnim and the other members of the Chief Sanitary Committee, a primary responsibility of the commissions was to demonstrate to the public they were trying to help the sick and the healthy. The novelty of the illness combined with the variety of opinions about the cause of the disease and how to prevent it caused great anxiety. Ironically, according to one doctor "It is well known that in Berlin, the class of society which entertained the most exaggerated fear of cholera, remained almost entirely free from the disease" while it suffered from what "I have formerly adverted under the name *anxietas cholerica*." In Berlin, any remedy for cholera advertised in the newspapers was "found and bought in all the shops the next day."[27]

As a result of this great anxiety, city authorities especially in the first days of the epidemic directed "in personal meetings with the heads of the commissions" they attend to what they perceived as a general carelessness of control everywhere. For example, there remained the need to identify houses where the disease had broken out with warning signs, replacing military postings in front of houses with civilian guards, and transporting the sick and dead. These were to be approached in the usual manner. Quarantine was also reduced to five days.[28]

There was still "much prejudice" in the lower classes that needed to be overcome. Many sick perished because they would rather stay with their families, and had a "natural aversion to the public hospitals." In order to counteract this fear the Chief Sanitary Committee published a notice stating that some classes were of the opinion that a patient sick with

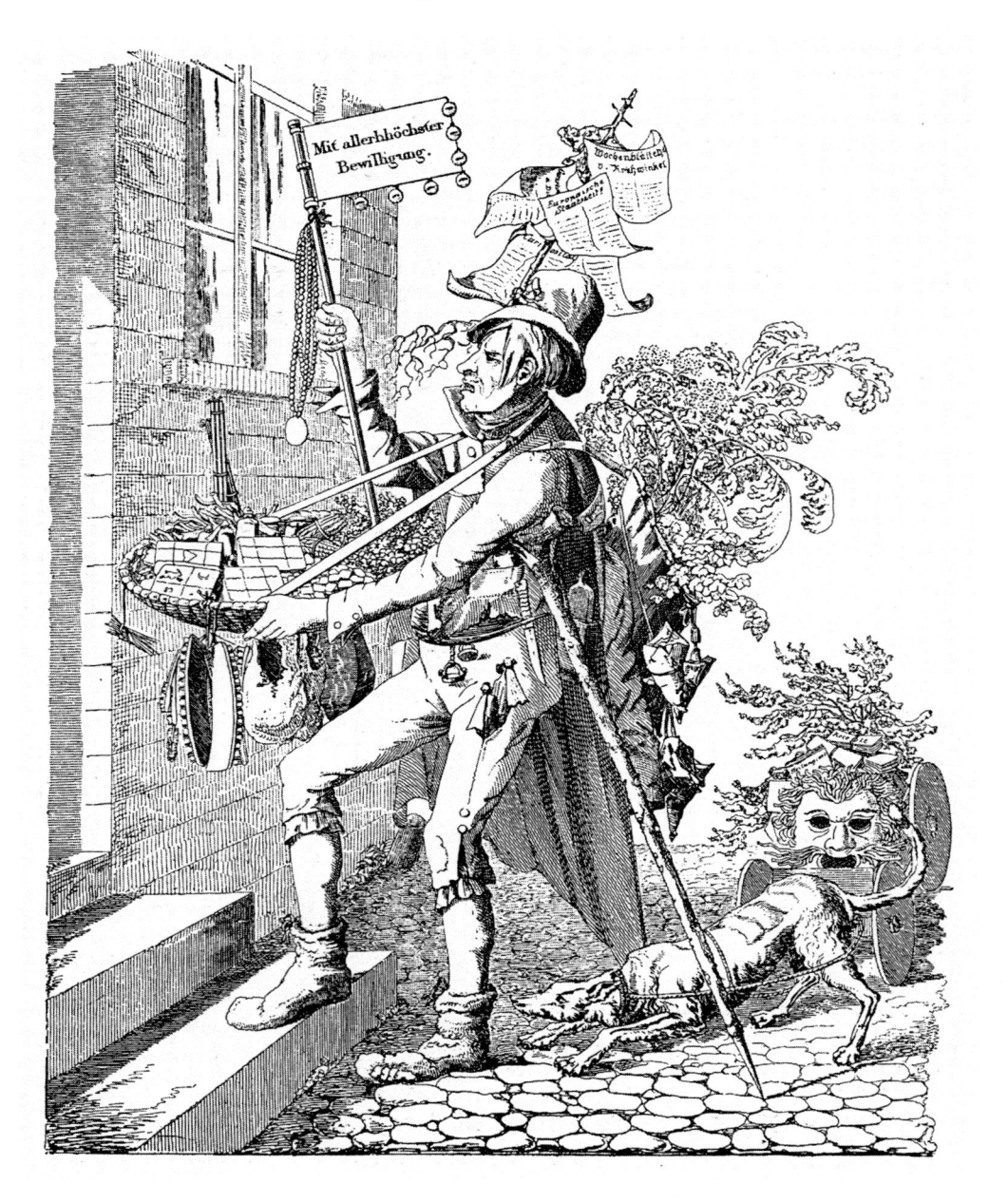

A German caricature of a peddler selling cholera nostrums door to door. Eugen Holländer, *Die Karikatur und Satire in der Medizin: mediko-kunsthistorische Studie*, 2nd ed., Stuttgart, 1921, p. 178.

cholera was to be forced to go to a local cholera hospital. It was noted that no such regulation was decreed. That the regulations published by the Chief Sanitary Committee on August 23, expressly stated that the patient could remain in his home if he could be treated and cared for properly. The local commune or district hospital was there to help out if the patient lacked adequate assistance. Those treated in the public hospitals had a better chance of recovery than those treated in "private dwellings" and that this could be confirmed.[29]

It was also the job of the individual deputies and doctors of the commission to control this prejudice as well as prevent the concealment of cholera cases and deaths from the authorities. In addition, guards and servants were required for the "rescue and recovery of the poorer classes of cholera patients." Those who performed their duties well were rewarded with one to five talers and their names were made public.[30]

The impact of government regulations on the poorer classes was of special concern. A scarcity of the necessities of life would result if external traffic with Berlin was prevented. The idea of a quarantine of Berlin had for a long time been given up (although there was occasional discussion about whether it might have to be imposed i.e., Arnim). All barriers that threatened trade were as much as possible eliminated. Even, special arrangements were made with the factory owners so that in spite of the "unfavorable conditions" they could maintain production in the midst of the epidemic. The factory owners "in securing their interests" and naturally cautious about their workers, "each morning obtained a health certificate from the commission whether cholera had occurred in the dwellings of their workers." According to this report, "With this the working class acquired a secure income." In addition "His Majesty the King had graciously here, as in other places ravaged by cholera ordered several buildings to be at once built, including the proposed enlargement to the Charité hospital with the aim of bringing the promised urgent need to the poor. Also, the immigration of foreign workers and craftsmen into the city looking for work was prohibited for the duration of the present conditions."[31]

In Berlin, as in other large cities there were a great number of unemployed. Many found employment in what we might call the "cholera industry." This included nurses, porters, watchmen, messengers, disinfecting services and other employment in the new district sanatoriums and hospitals.[32]

When the administrative authorities had their first conference with the heads of the commissions, concerning the larger issues of patient care and acquiring the trust of the poor, they also confronted practical issues. These included the establishment of private hospitals in their districts, securing charitable support from well-off residents, and hiring servants, porters and guards at wages between ten and fifteen talers per month. Additionally they acquired supplies that included baskets (for transporting sick patients), woolen blankets, warming devices, first aid kits and disinfection devices.[33]

The commissions were supported by a host of charitable contributions to assist with the cholera sick and unemployment. These included collections by the local commission by means of monthly subscriptions from its wealthier citizens. Even the arts community organized large kitchens in different sections of Berlin that served between "4000 and 5000 free portions of soup" daily. Other associations provided clothing and took care of children who lost both their parents to cholera.[34]

The Establishment of Cholera Hospitals in Berlin

The general hospital in Berlin was the Charité. According to Dr. Becker when there were "occasional cases of cholera in the wards" of this hospital these cases were immediately moved to one of the official cholera hospitals established by the Chief Sanitary Committee. Because some of the mentally ill who were generally separated from the general population were occasionally seized with cholera, this was seen as evidence that cholera was not contagious. Dr. Becker pointed out that anyone who was familiar with the operation of the hospital would know that there was constant communication between the medical and other staff members as well as "the lunatics who are occasionally employed in menial service."[35]

As a result of the orders of the Chief Sanitary Committee, five large cholera hospitals were established in Berlin. Three were situated in various sections of the city and one was placed in the center. The first hospital was opened on September 6.[36] The chief administrators of these hospitals were the physicians who became experts on the treatment of the cholera in Prussia and led the medical treatment response to cholera in Berlin. These physicians supervised and reported on the efficacy of the treatments administered to the sick in their care.

The five cholera hospitals were official receiving stations. The sick were selected by the local commissions and sent to one of the five hospitals. As noted above, initially there was great hostility among the population toward hospitals, and alleviating this fear was the aim of official government policy.

Cholera hospitals were regulated by the Chief Sanitary Committee of Berlin. There were instructions for the maintenance of sanitary and dietary measures, financial records and medical reports. Each monthly report documented the number of cholera cases admitted to the hospitals, attempted therapies, the course of the sickness for each patient and a report on all autopsies which were performed under the supervision of the chief physician.[37]

In addition the commissions also established private sanatoriums with 6–12 beds in their respective districts that provided the advantage of proximity to the victims. These were usually established with donated funds from wealthy inhabitants within the district. If the local officials could not raise sufficient funds the Chief Sanitary Committee made up the difference. Also, all the citizens in each district had the right to be treated in these local sanatoriums.[38]

After establishing the local sanatoriums, the commissions quickly hired nurses, servants and porters for a monthly wage between 10–15 talers. They also acquired baskets for transporting the sick, woolen blankets, warming apparatuses and some had pharmacists available to provide medicines and most had physician assistants.[39]

The primary treatment centers for cholera were the larger cholera hospitals established by the Chief Sanitary Committee, These cholera hospitals were initially founded to sequester the sick. Most therapies did little good for the patients and the medical officials were the first to admit (at least in their reports) that at first "everything did not go well." One visiting doctor noted that when hospital I was established "a private house was hired" and the hospital "lacked everything that is said that an orderly hospital should have ... it was crowded with cholera patients" and because of that "implementing sanitary measures was not possible ... nor the disinfection of cholera patients." The physician "made the same observations in the other hospitals."[40]

One problem noted immediately was the number of attendants and other medical personnel who became sick. In hospital II for example, of the ten male and female attendants and three medical assistants, six attendants and two assistants got cholera within three weeks. It appears that all recovered. In hospital I within four days of the hospital opening two assistants of the head doctor became ill. Both later recovered. One was given an emetic and recovered the other it was found necessary to "bleed" (a common medical procedure at this time). This did not appear to work and he was given an emetic and finally recovered. Next, two nurses both contracted cholera and one later died. Soon after, two men employed in carrying patients and dead bodies became sick. One recovered and one died. Finally, a washerwoman, a male attendant and the hospital superintendent became ill a second time and after treatment recovered. In general, employees connected with "hospital service" at hospital I (about 35 out of 70–80) "occasionally complained of "diarrhea, vomiting and drawing pains in their extremities" and were treated with a "good diet" and other "simple remedies" all eventually recovered.[41]

The death rates in the five cholera hospitals averaged over 60 percent. The total number of patients brought to these hospitals was 926 of which 351 recovered and 575 died.[42] Eck wrote, that as the epidemic progressed the "public began to trust ... [cholera hospitals] ... as the best place for both medical and dietetic care."[43] It is more likely that as the epidemic continued the severity of the cases diminished and the recovery rates of patients increased.

It should also be noted that there was concern in Berlin among contagionist doctors due to the inordinate amount of "transmission of cholera by hospital attendants, and by the porters and servants of cholera committees in Berlin." The medical men "observe some caution" in communication with "other persons ... predisposed to the deleterious action of the contagion." They recommended that "other persons employed in cholera hospitals, or in attending cholera patients in town, all the servants of cholera committees should be under some control."[44]

Another matter of concern was allowing the visiting of friends and relatives of cholera patients into the public hospitals. Although considered, necessary and unintentionally cruel not to allow visits, it appeared to be "prudent" if one could not altogether forbid visitors, then at least to "reduce to the least possible extent the visits of strangers to the hospitals."[45]

As for medicines, it was reported that, "at no small cost" for the remote parts of the city, three drug dispensing institutions were established by the authorities, each with an apothecary sign, and these were managed by experienced persons. Also, a place for free disinfection was included in a private sanatorium, with a pharmacy included that dispensed drugs free of charge. These benefits were not restricted to any one group of individuals.[46]

During the epidemic in Berlin, public health officials stationed in the cholera hospitals also reported on the experimental therapies they undertook and the results. Because these physicians were able to officially study a large number of cases they recommended that other practicing physicians use the recommendations of the "Report of the Directors of Cholera Hospitals." The doctors were satisfied with their reported "results" and saw them as the basis for the "future therapy" for cholera.[47] The physicians did not conceal their attempts at experimental therapies and many communicated them publically in articles in the *Berliner Cholera Zeitung*.[48]

Experimentation on patients did not end with their deaths. Numerous autopsies were performed by Dr. Romberg and Dr. Phoebus, Prosecutor of the Charité hospital.[49] "From the beginning to the end of the epidemic in Berlin in all cholera hospitals, ... autopsies were performed on cholera victims." Romberg reported on the results of over 200 autopsies in cholera hospital I and Dr. Phoebus performed over 65 himself, some in private homes while others were performed in cholera hospital II.[50] Many of the autopsy reports were merely descriptive and suggest an attempt at a nosological analysis of the disease in keeping with comparable activity in the other European capitals. In a broad sense cholera emerged as an opportunity for Prussian doctors to practice clinical pathology on a greater scale than previously possible. As Virchow later noted, Prussian doctors never had the selection of bodies that would typically be found in Paris, Vienna or London even during normal times. The "paucity of larger hospitals in the German states and the difficulty of carrying out autopsies limited our countrymen's opportunities in precisely the two practices most important to the exact practice of pathological development."[51] For Dr. Virchow this explained why clinical pathology made rapid progress in France and England "where there were larger and more numerous hospitals than in Germany."[52] Virchow later suggested that there had been some earlier progress in clinical anatomy in the Prosectorship at the Charité under Phoebus (the first Prosector). Phoebus wrote "many doctors were present at my ... [cholera] autopsies."[53] But as Virchow later concluded "the great stimulus brought about by the occurrence of the first ... [cholera] ... epidemic had no lasting effect, and young medical men who wanted instruction found themselves obliged to go to Vienna, in order to draw on the rich resources of the schools there."[54]

The Prussian medical administration not only established hospitals for sequestering the cholera sick and applying experimental therapies, they also communicated the results of their therapies and medical advice to the public through the contagionist *Berliner Cholera Zeitung*.[55] The most important information was the official lists of the sick and deceased. The editors believed that this information was not without "scientific interest concerning the relation of those being overtaken by cholera, its course and cause."[56] The list was published using only official reports and generally ran 14 days behind.[57]

Two major issues that faced the Berlin authorities was forcing patients to go cholera hospitals and quarantining private dwellings after the initial report that the inhabitant was ill. The first issue was resolved by the Chief Sanitary Committee on September 12, 1831, when the committee issued a new order stating that cholera sick could remain in their dwellings "cared for and treated there, and not be forced to go to a cholera hospital." On the second issue the quarantining of houses or dwellings in which cholera occurred. If the patient was removed to a hospital, recovered or died, the authorities followed current regulations. By September 12, 1831, house quarantine had been reduced to five days.[58]

It had been up to the local commissions to appoint men to make sure that the sick did not have contact with other patients. Interestingly enough, on September 29, 1831, Dr. Albert Sachs, the editor of an anti-contagionist journal, "invited the heads of the commissions to give their opinion" in relation to the "still existing quarantine regulations." The editors were "most pleased with the results" and summarized them for their readers on October 31, 1831. The questions were answered by the heads of fifty-nine of the sixty-one

"Beilage zur Berliner Cholera Zeitung." (Supplement to the Cholera Newspaper). The supplement provided a list of the names of the sick, the number, the name, age, occupation, residence and whether they recovered, died or continued sick. This supplement was the first one published in the Berliner Cholera Zeitung and is dated Saturday, September 24, 1831. Note it has been labeled disinfected (Author's collection).

commissions for their districts. One district had no cases of cholera and did not reply; seven district heads maintained quarantine was useful and believed the disease was contagious. Fifty-one district heads were against quarantine regulations and wanted them repealed or at least further modified.[59]

The first question asked was if the quarantine of the homes achieved its purpose of isolating the substance of the disease to lessen if possible the transmission of the disease to others? The answers covered the logistics of quarantine including the time the doctors and attendants arrived to regulate the area. They concluded that too many people had come and gone to make this an effective procedure. Also, the doctors and attendants did not stay but left the patients. The guards could not be counted on as they came from the lower classes and needed to be paid. Good people did not come because they did not want to be quarantined for five days. Finally the issue of greatest concern to the district heads was that the "quarantine for the length of the disease" was too expensive.

The second question posed was: did the house and apartment quarantine harm patients? A summary of the responses included the following: the fear of quarantine had terrible results because people hid the sick and when aid came it was generally too late and they died; others fled the sick because they did not want to be locked up for five days; nurses were quarantined for five days, reducing the number of skilled care givers; other compassionate individuals who did not fear contagion knew if they assisted the sick, they might be imprisoned with them or with a dead body; and in the end, because of these quarantine measures the sick had only a paid guard to depend on. Finally, for the patient the regulations surrounding quarantine confirmed he was suffering from "a dangerous sickness" and this intensified an atmosphere of "terror and fear" that affected the patient "up until his last moments."[60]

The last question was whether "quarantine regulations were injurious to the healthy subjects and relatives of the sufferers?" The responses indicated regulations were injurious. The journal editors wrote, "These are the stated reasons why the commissions concluded the current quarantine regulations could not be considered appropriate" and that in fact it seems when "arrangements were made according to the regulations, in most cases they were rarely carried out in as severe a manner as prescribed."[61]

These answers confirmed Dr. Becker's observations that members of the commissions generally agreed that due to the great number of people involved it was impossible to watch and control these patients. It was also too expensive. This policy "created a loud expression of public opinion against the system."[62]

The five day house quarantine was eventually given up as "extremely irksome and useless." One solution for the removal of quarantine, according to Dr. Becker was the person exposed to contagion was taken "to other buildings established for that purpose, internal quarantine." Thus "placing these persons out of the sphere of the continued action of the effluvia, of providing for their wants where it was necessary, of constantly observing their state of health, and having immediately recourse to the proper treatment when symptoms of the disease showed themselves, and at the same time of preventing their communication with other persons, and the risk of infection through their medium." This would put them in an environment that would help them "to restore the body and mind in a healthy airy building where their wants are kindly attended to."[63]

There were at least twenty cases in Berlin where persons placed in quarantine had by the third or fourth day been attacked by cholera? For him there was "no doubt that their chances of recovery were rendered much more favorable by their having been under strict medical observation and by the necessary measures for their cure being immediately resorted to."[64]

The modification of the official government policy was a practical approach to moderating government sanitary policy at the beginning of the cholera epidemic in Berlin. It was accomplished by the king and his officials without regard to a resolution of the medical conflict between "contagionists" and "anticontagionists" or "miasmists." It was based on the observation of the continual failure of quarantine for cholera. Other factors were the exorbitant cost to the state, the negative impact on trade and the potential for popular unrest unless the situation was mitigated. As for physicians in Berlin, whether contagionists or miasmists, in practical terms they continued to treat their patients accordingly. What was required next was a solution to bridge this gulf and serve as a foundation for a future policy that would meet the needs of the Prussian medical community, while satisfying the economic needs of the Prussian government with its emphasis on free trade and support of *laissez-faire*. The attempt at finding a third solution bridging the gulf between these two ideological viewpoints based on experience learned from the first cholera epidemic in Prussia, are discussed in the following chapter.

11

The Medical Legacy of the Cholera Epidemic of 1831

Following the end of the cholera epidemic in January 1832, it was evident that the Prussian government needed to develop a comprehensive policy to deal with cholera and other contagious diseases.[1] Prussia had no previous contagious diseases laws, except for the earlier plague legislation of 1709. Any future policy would need to serve as a foundation for legislation and for the practical medical administrative measures required to deal with epidemics. Because of the experience gained from the partially discredited absolutist approach, it became apparent that cholera did not seem as contagious nor did it spread like plague. As a result of these developments, the disease was viewed as a lower category contagion, while plague continued to be viewed as highly contagious and was not included in the new regulations. The government wanted to bring uniformity and better control to sanitary legislation concerning contagious diseases.

Immediately following the dissolution of the Immediate Commission on January 19, 1832, the king assigned General Thile the task of developing general regulations and procedures to be followed for all contagious diseases. The end result was the Prussian Contagious Diseases Law of August 8, 1835. The following concerns the development of the law and its importance for future sanitary legislation in Prussia. It arose directly out of the Prussian experience with the cholera epidemic in 1831.

Contagionists, Miasmists and the Government's Intermediate Position

The success of implementing less restrictive and more beneficial measures among Prussia's chief non-medical bureaucrats, officials and the monarch may have been a political success by September 6, 1831, but the contagionist view continued to dominate the Prussian medical administration as well as the official *Berliner Cholera Zeitung*.

With the cholera outbreak in Prussia, Berlin had become the focus for foreign observers. Soon these foreign and local physicians became embroiled in the controversy over contagion. This was to be expected. Berlin was a "hothouse" environment, especially for Prussian physicians because the majority of the state and private physicians lived and

11. The Medical Legacy of the Cholera Epidemic of 1831

practiced in Berlin.² The contagion controversy was so contentious that Ambassador Chad reported to the British Foreign Office:

> We have a Congress of Doctors here from different parts of the World, they quarrel from morning to night, and split into contagionists and anti-contagionists, Partisans of Mercury, and the Partisans of the anti-spasmodics.... I do not see that either side has the advantage as to successful practice."³

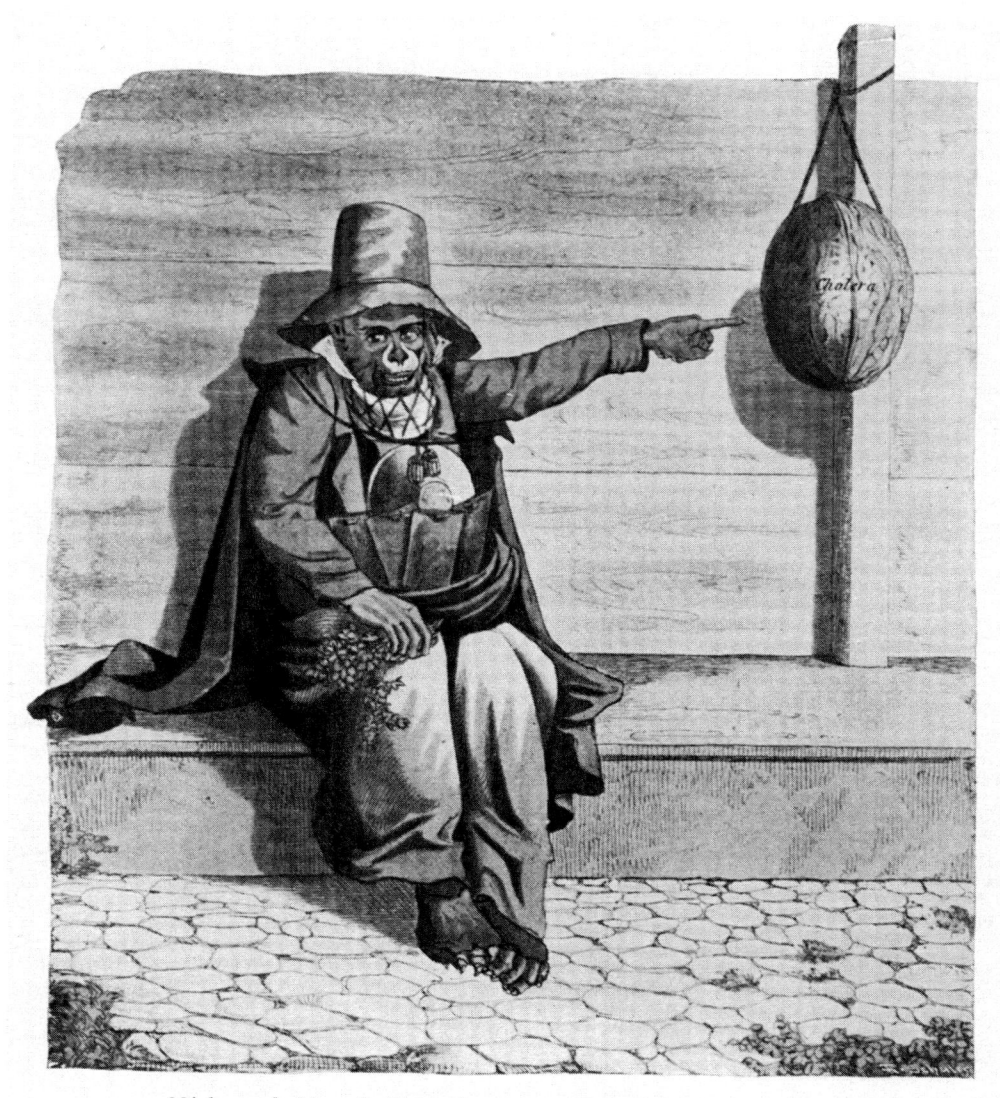

Mich nach Vorschrift zu bepacken, unterließ ich nie,
Doch das Nüßchen dort zu knacken, heißt die Frage — wie?

"Der Präservativ Mann Gegen die Cholera." German print, early 1830s. Caricature of a monkey seated on a bench and pointing to a walnut shell, labeled cholera. He has a metal plate on his stomach and is holding herbs. The bottom line concludes, the question of cholera is a "hard nut to crack." Reproduced from Eugen Holländer, *Die Karikatur und Satire in der Medizin: mediko-kunsthistorische Studie*, Stuttgart, 1905, p. 100.

In this "hothouse" environment it was only natural that some doctors whether government employees or especially physicians in private practice would try to make their names known by contesting theories about this new disease. This would be a natural choice in a society that had recently loosened the traditional social structures that had limited upward mobility for middle class professionals like physicians. These men saw an opportunity using cholera to enhance their own status and profession by writing treatises and performing experiments to prove their theories, cure their patients, and gain official and public recognition.[4]

This was especially true in Prussia. The majority of physicians were state employees and in order to enhance prestige in state service the physician had to find an opportunity to be noticed, unless they had been appointed because of social connections. Otherwise the chance of rapid advancement was limited. This helps to explain why provincial doctors and younger doctors took the opportunity with the outbreak of the cholera to write treatises in support of the "liberal" or anti-contagionist position. For example, the treatise by the state district physician Dr. Barchewitz, or the important writings of the various doctors in the Medical Association in Königsberg. In Berlin there were those like Dr. Albert Sachs in private practice, who championed anti-contagion and edited *Tagebuch über das Verhalten der bösartigen Cholera in Berlin*. Of course for state employed physicians, taking a position contrary to official policy came at a cost, as we will see later, Dr. Carl Lorinser found this out.[5]

Some of the younger anti-contagionist doctors were even willing to experiment on themselves to prove their own theories. Dr. Becker described a notorious experiment at the time. "Dr. Calow one of the loudest adversaries of contagion" and three doctors assisted in a "dissection" in Berlin on September 5, 1831, and "not satisfied with the information derived from their senses ... thought it proper to ascertain the properties of the blood and the contents of the intestines by tasting the fluids."[6] Shortly after this incident Dr. Sachs, published an account of the death of Dr. Calow, in support of a "fellow brother," who was attempting to resolve this "contentious question." The "deceased friend" after attending to the sick (there is no mention of the dissection or his tasting of the contents of a deceased person's intestinal fluids) became sick himself after exposure in the apartment of a former cholera patient. He later passed away on the evening of September 7. Later other family members in the same building died. Their deaths were attributed "to the cholera developing in multiple family members ... under the influence of a musty, damp, unhealthy home" and a "mephitic atmosphere."[7]

For anti-contagionists, cholera was not introduced into a place but was created from an unhealthy environment. The person became sick by their own inappropriate behavior comparable to any natural occurrence that caused sickness. An example was an individual who not taking proper precautions in a thunderstorm was struck by lightning. By appropriate behavior (proper diet, clean, open and sunny environment) or "common sense" cholera could be avoided. The moral argument was neatly summed up by Dr. Baer in Königsberg, "He who gets the cholera has only himself to blame" and it was no wonder, that the lower classes who suffered from "a lack of character and moral turpitude" were the most common victims, the latter was one area where both "camps seemed to find common agreement."[8]

The doctors in the *Cholera Zeitung* (Königsberg) argued cholera was a naturally occurring event and that it was humanly impossible to prevent outbreaks of disease. In order to "secure protection against the cholera infected atmosphere ... the heavens would have to be shut off from the earth ... because the air which we cannot do without is filled with poison and contagion." State officials saw that the goal of the "miasmists" was to free themselves from the "constraints" of State interference by arguing "preventing an epidemic was not the business of the state" and that it was "important to withdraw the states' influence on the medical system" concerning infectious diseases.[9]

Meanwhile, following the death of Dr. Calow, an unsigned letter was later published in England describing the events that led up to the cause of his death from cholera. The letter was undoubtedly written by Dr. Becker. It contradicted the "mephitic atmosphere" as the only cause of his death and concluded Dr. Calow, who "denied the contagious nature of the cholera, and who, in order to establish his opinion had made some very disgusting experiments upon his own person, caught the malady, and died of it yesterday, after a few hours' illness."[10]

The conflict continued in multiple publications and letters between opposing camps. With many opinions communicated abroad. Throughout the debate the Prussian medical administration under Rust's leadership remained committed to contagion and quarantine based on past experience. They also considered themselves responsible for the health and welfare of the general population of Prussia. This notion was later powerfully summed up by Rust, who wrote that the anti-contagionists wanted to "remove all protective sanitary regulations. I would regard this as a crime against humanity."[11]

The turning point in the medical argument in Prussia concerning the debate between the two extreme positions was an article that appeared in the strictly contagionist *Prussian State Gazette*. Dr. Hufeland, physician to the king, published a short article on September 11, 1831. He attempted to find a middle ground between the two opposing views entitled "A Word to My fellow Citizens Concerning the Contagiousness of the Cholera and the Best Means of Protection." It began:

> You argue about the question: Is cholera contagious or not? The answer is simple, like the colds one gets in the spring it is a result of "a peculiar corruption of the air." Once human beings become sick it evolves to a higher level and can be "communicated to someone else." This "requires a special susceptibility in humans and this thank God is very rare" as shown by those working in the medical institutions who rarely become sick. It is in our power to prevent "this susceptibility to the disease" by avoiding the cold and not indulging in a poor diet. To avoid getting the body cold one should wear a woolen sash around the waist (a common recommendation at this time) and to avoid cold feet wear woolen socks. For your diet, moderation in food and beverages, avoid fresh fruits, raw milk and an excess of alcoholic beverages. Finally a "firm faith in God with whose help anything can be overcome in times of danger.[12]

The anti-contagionist *Cholera Zeitung* (Königsberg) noted for the first time the *Prussian State Gazette* could "resist the truth no longer" and had begun to change from an organ of pure contagionism by publishing Hufeland's article. However, the *Cholera Zeitung* could not completely agree with Hufeland's thesis. It argued that for "nearly half a century.... [He] ... sought to take an intermediary position in all physician medical disputes and this did not lead to the happiest or most successful conclusion." He had been less "successful in mediating on two occasions when called upon on animal magnetism and homeopathy." The former was subject to "serious deceptions and errors." The latter something less than

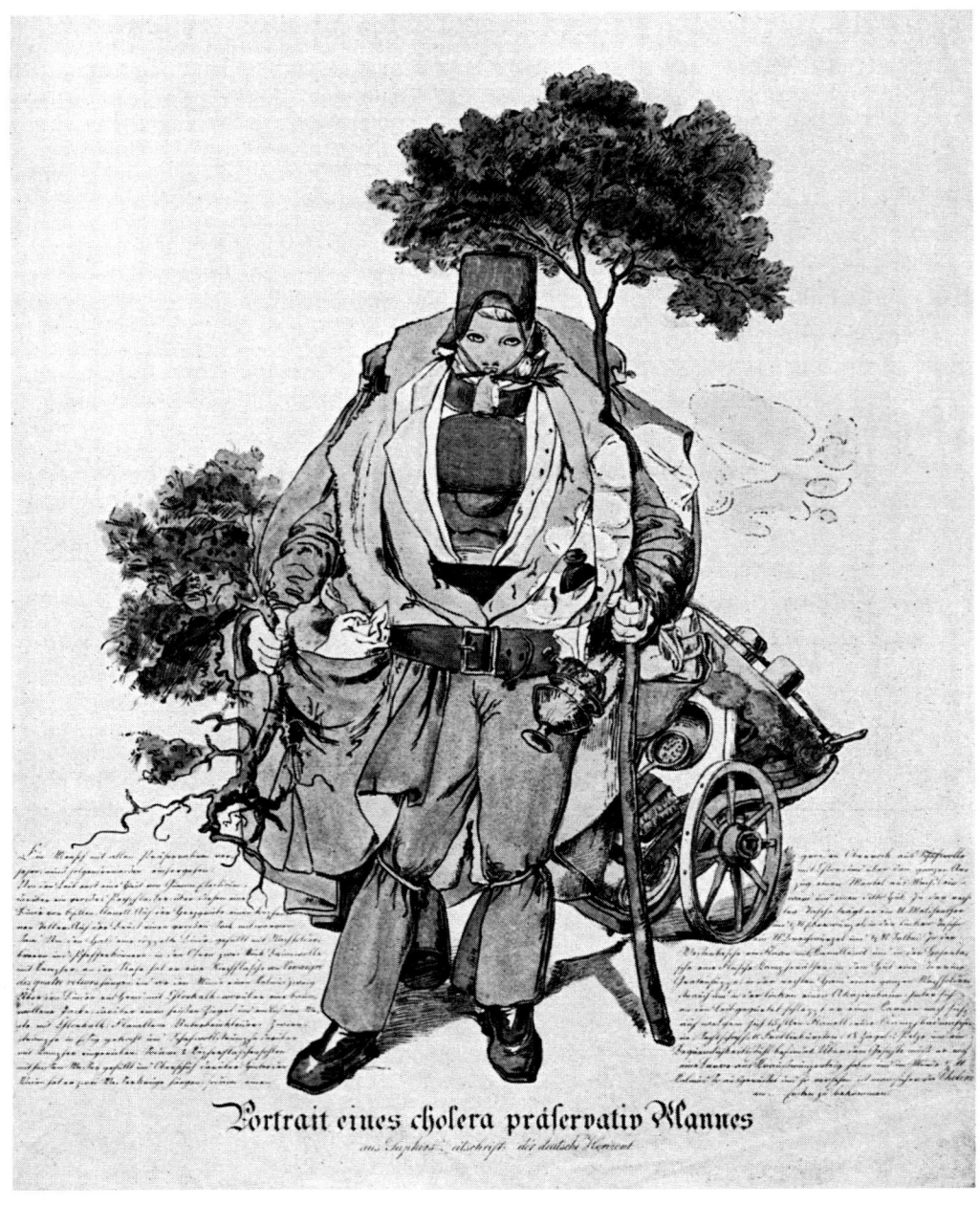

"Portrait eines cholera präservativ Mannes." A figure dressed in a cholera safety suit. German etching after Joseph Petzl, 1832. According to Eugen Holländer, one of the most popular and copied prints of the time. The caption begins "A man who wants to be immune to the contagion of cholera must be dressed according to the following description. First the chest must be fully wrapped with elastic gum; on the overcoat we apply a large patch of pitch, covered with a strip of flannel six yards in length. On the pit of the stomach is placed a copper plate. The chest is covered with a bag of warm sand. Around the neck a double bandage filled with peppercorns and juniper; in the ears two pieces of cotton sealed with camphor and on the nose a bottle of vinegar; and a cigar in the mouth...." Reproduced from Eugen Holländer, *Die Karikatur und Satire in der Medizin: mediko-kunsthistorische Studie*, 2nd ed., Stuttgart, 1921, pp. 180–181, 187.

"absolute rejection." It was pointed out that the recent "question of the contagiousness of cholera argued with great animation among physicians ... is too important to science and urgent for the state."[13] Hufeland was criticized for not previously expressing his views except "in several ... scholarly treatises" in an attempt to mediate between the two positions. Hufeland had criticized physicians in both camps in a previous article in August. He wrote that it was a wonder to him that one found doctors disputing the subject on the contagious nature of the cholera because it was a long established fact that "a disease can come from the atmosphere and also be generated by contagion, for example the common cold."[14] His greatest sin was combining both positions. The newspaper criticized him for allowing contagionists and non-contagionists to appeal to him as an authority. If the matter were not so important this would not be such a great issue, but the conflict strikes at the very "marrow of the state." However, his article concluded that the decision has already been made that the disease is contagious, but no more than a cold or the ague. The author noted that in all other respects, he agreed with Hufeland's admonitions "to avoid the cold, be moderate in the diet and to trust in God's providence and aid."[15]

The Lifting of the Quarantine

As noted earlier, the king's anxiety concerning the strict sanitary policy surfaced in early July 1831, during a dinner with Rust when he complained about the severity of the cholera measures. The economic and social constraints of the stringent policy as well as the contentious medical debates in Berlin only increased the feeling of anxiety and panic in the city. Both camps were determined to prevail and to influence officials as well as the king. Certainly the king was eyeing the potential of unrest having read the reports of earlier experiences in Danzig and Königsberg and the more recent events in Memel and Stettin. Earlier he introduced a series of measures to provide employment to counteract the effects of the strict quarantine regulations that had contributed to the unrest. In addition, his officials were warily observing the rising cost of the price of a bushel of rye, a grain staple more critical than wheat for the lower classes in Berlin and Potsdam. The price of a bushel of rye had been steadily rising and by September was 13 percent higher than its price in July. Even by lifting the internal quarantines in early October the price increased over 22 percent by November. The on-going escalating price of rye can also be attributed to the residual effects of the restraint in trade due to earlier quarantine restrictions, hoarding and lack of help at harvest time especially in the east.[16]

In order to reverse the government's sanitary policy, the king and his non-medical officials required the medical expertise and reputation of Hufeland, who had worked out this intermediary position. Hufeland's theory would not require the government to continue to take such a strict position and it could defend reversing the absolutist public health measures advocated by Rust and the Immediate Commission. The reversal of the latter could be accomplished if enough doubt could be raised and justification found for supporting a more moderate policy. In order to make the latter palatable to the public and other officials the new measures had to be presented in broader terms understandable to the public. This was still necessary because the government had invested in innumerable official notices on quarantine, personal responsibility and the dire consequences for those who transgressed these measures. This included long term imprisonment and even execution.[17]

What was required was a common sense explanation understandable to the lay person of Hufeland's theory that would permit a reasonable accommodation by the government with trade and still allow the government to maintain control over sanitary policy. The arguments required to support this more moderate policy came from Dr. Carl Lorinser, a young provincial physician, whose three part article on anti-contagionism became a *cause celebre* when it was published in the *Prussian State Gazette*.

Doctor Lorinser originally submitted his article to the *Jahrbücher für wissenschaftliche Kritik* and claimed he did not know how or why his article suddenly appeared in the *Prussian State Gazette*.[18] Undoubtedly, the king and his advisors had been looking for a clear statement of a less extreme "anti-contagionist" position, and Lorinser's article met the requirement, making a practical case for non-contagion modeled on Hufeland's intermediate position. It was considered suitable for a wider audience and published in *Prussian State Gazette*, giving it the official imprimatur of the Prussian government. Lorinser's motivation was to demonstrate "that the pestilential cholera disease could not be fought with quarantines." His article was not originally written as part of a "rarefied medical controversy" but written in words and concepts that could be understood by non-physicians. His "common sense" way of laying out the facts showed why the cholera was not contagious. This was exactly what the king and his advisors required to gain the additional support of the general public for modifying current policy in opposition to their own medical administration and Immediate Commission.[19] The solution soon appeared in an article submitted to the liberal opinion journal *Jahrbücher für wissenschaftliche Kritik* by Dr. Lorinser. Not so strangely, Dr. Hufeland served as the medical editor for this publication.

Dr. Lorinser was a physician from the administrative district of Oppeln in Silesia. When cholera broke out he was forced to implement strict cholera regulations in his district even though he personally claimed to have opposed them. He traveled to areas where the disease had broken out and observed patients in the lazarets. He said he had to impose policies that he thought were ineffective. Traveling throughout the different districts where cholera was present he found himself suffering from occasional "heavy sweating" and an unusually "susceptible nervous system that manifested itself in his stomach." He attributed this to "epidemic influence," a moderately warm atmosphere, combined with humidity, and still air with noxious exhalations from the soil or as a "miasmist" physician at the time would say, an environment suitable for contracting a contagious disease.[20]

However, the "epidemic influence" and queasy stomach was not his most unsettling experience; it was the "angry mob" he and a fellow physician confronted near the city of Ratibor:

> When I returned after the outbreak of cholera in Ratibor … [Upper Silesia] … with the Ostrog district physician, where I had visited the sick, we were greeted at the bridge which was closed to ordinary traffic, by a threatening mob shouting and exclaiming: Here come the torturers! Into the water with them! The mob began throwing stones … were it not for the two gendarmes accompanying us for our protection we would not have reached the bridge in time nor gotten to the other side.

After this experience, Lorinser returned home and soon became involved in an administrative controversy which he considered "his greatest triumph."[21]

Lorinser was a member of the, *Die Societät für wissenschaftliche Kritik* (Society for Scientific Criticism) since its founding in Berlin. He was asked to review three books for the society about cholera in its publication the *Jahrbücher für wissenschaftliche Kritik* a publication founded to "discuss the great questions of the day." He wanted to bring his ideas before men of science and submitted his manuscript to the latter publication at the end of September. He was "astonished" to find his essays published on the 4, 5, and 6 of October 1831, in the *Prussian State Gazette* instead of the *Jahrbücher für wissenschaftliche Kritik*. With the exception of Hufeland's earlier article, it "so far had been the most zealous supporter of contagionism and persistently justified all government measures!"[22]

Lorinser believed his article convinced the government to lift the military cordon on the Elbe and the Oder in early October, eliminate cordons along the internal provincial borders and terminate the internal quarantine stations.[23] However, based on his article Lorinser was not just bringing "his ideas before men of science" but was highly critical of the government's policies and of the officials implementing these policies. He used his article as a vehicle to call into question the underlying rationale for the government's policy as well as the integrity of the doctors and officials responsible for preventing the cholera. Although Lorinser did not seem to recognize the antagonistic thrust of his article toward these officials, in his autobiography written well after the incidents he describes, it helps to explain his treatment by government officials in subsequent years.

His article was ostensibly a review of three books. He chose the books under discussion because with the invasion of cholera much strife had been created in Prussia. These authors discussed their experiences in different lands, India, Russia and Poland with a greater impartiality than was "the case of most others writers on cholera."[24]

He proceeded with a general discussion of how some diseases spread differently than others. He noted that it was difficult to determine whether the cholera is contagious (contagious defined here means the seeds of the disease reproduce in an individual and spread from one individual to another with the assistance of a suitable atmosphere, the earth or a combination of the two). Trying to determine how diseases spread was compared to "looking for a snake in the grass while it twisted and turned about." He discussed the atmospheric and telluric theory as a source of the contagion and argued not all sicknesses are unconditionally contagious. He used smallpox and scarlet fever as examples "because not all men get the sickness," (some diseases are simple infections and are transmitted from individual to individual and are not contagious because the atmosphere is not suitable to spread the contagion). He then discussed plague and Rinderpest (cattle plague) to show how isolation prevents these diseases from spreading. He gave the example of Austria and its military lines, cordons and quarantines that had prevented the plague from entering Austria from neighboring Turkey over the past 70 years. He wrote that cholera is different than plague and, even though Austria imposed strict plague measures to prevent the cholera, it continued to spread from Austria breaking through "line after line" until it crossed into Hungary. He concluded "cholera spreads differently than a purely contagious disease."[25]

Lorinser pointed out that most contagious diseases have one property "in that it affects the individual, usually only once in a lifetime and gives the individual the ability not to contract the same disease again." But an individual can be "infected repeatedly by the cholera." Further, in the case of contagion, those close to the sick become ill themselves, "but with cholera those close to the sick or caring for a patient generally remain free of the cholera, including those who handle cholera corpses." In addition, goods do not seem to transmit the disease and even when the "sick touch their belongings it seems to be harmless."[26]

Cholera did not appear to spread like most contagious diseases. He speculated that cholera was spread through the atmosphere or by "epidemic influence." The intensity of the disease in an individual was an effect of "need, poor diet, dampness and the cold weather" and not purely contagion. He added that it was "strange that officials, who treat the disease like the plague, warn that poor diet and the cold are also causes of the disease." To illustrate his point he described two Polish corps following the battle of Iganie in April 1831. The first marched through the marshes and the cold weather and contracted cholera. The second group "camped on higher ground where there was no shortage of food or good water and remained free of the disease."[27]

He provided historical background for a variety of diseases that had become epidemic at one time or another in Europe, especially in Germany that acted like cholera He was especially taken with malaria (like Hufeland), he saw it as a similar "atmospheric disease" and favorably compared the autopsy results that doctors found between cholera and malaria.[28] He later concluded that if one considers the cholera spreading as a result of favorable atmospheric conditions combined with the seeds or germs of the contagion like other "atmospheric diseases" then there is "little that can be done" and "there can be no protection by cordons and quarantines."[29]

Next, he criticized doctors and officials who readily accepted foreign opinions on the cause and spread of cholera, especially those who accepted the opinion from St. Petersburg that the cholera was "like plague and contagious." Scarcely had this opinion been formulated, when "hundreds of pamphlets and booklets" appeared by defenders of contagion. Many of these men he argued were "worthy men" and persisted in the dispute seeing it as a "duty." For others it seemed to be the "safest course" and those who would not see the disease as contagious were accused of being "blind" and of engaging in criminal behavior.[30]

Under these circumstances, with the physicians in disagreement, the government had "no choice but to impose ... stringent measures for the protection of the people." He added that "scarcely had it been decided that the cholera was to be treated like plague" when it became "sanctioned" by government officials "with the certainty of truth."[31]

Lorinser saved his most damning criticism for government officials who embraced the views of the contagionists before anyone had experience with the disease. He wrote, the "great masses" of the people "actually held no opinion" until the public authorities committed themselves to the principles of contagion, acceding to it rather than "examining" it further. Some officials were being overly "cautious," while others were simply "selfish and by flattery hoped to bring some advantage to themselves." Quoting the playwright Schiller, he wrote that these officials had "sold their vote for bread and boots," and it was no longer in doubt whose opinion these so called "neutral groups had embraced."

Cholera's Wahlverwandtschaft

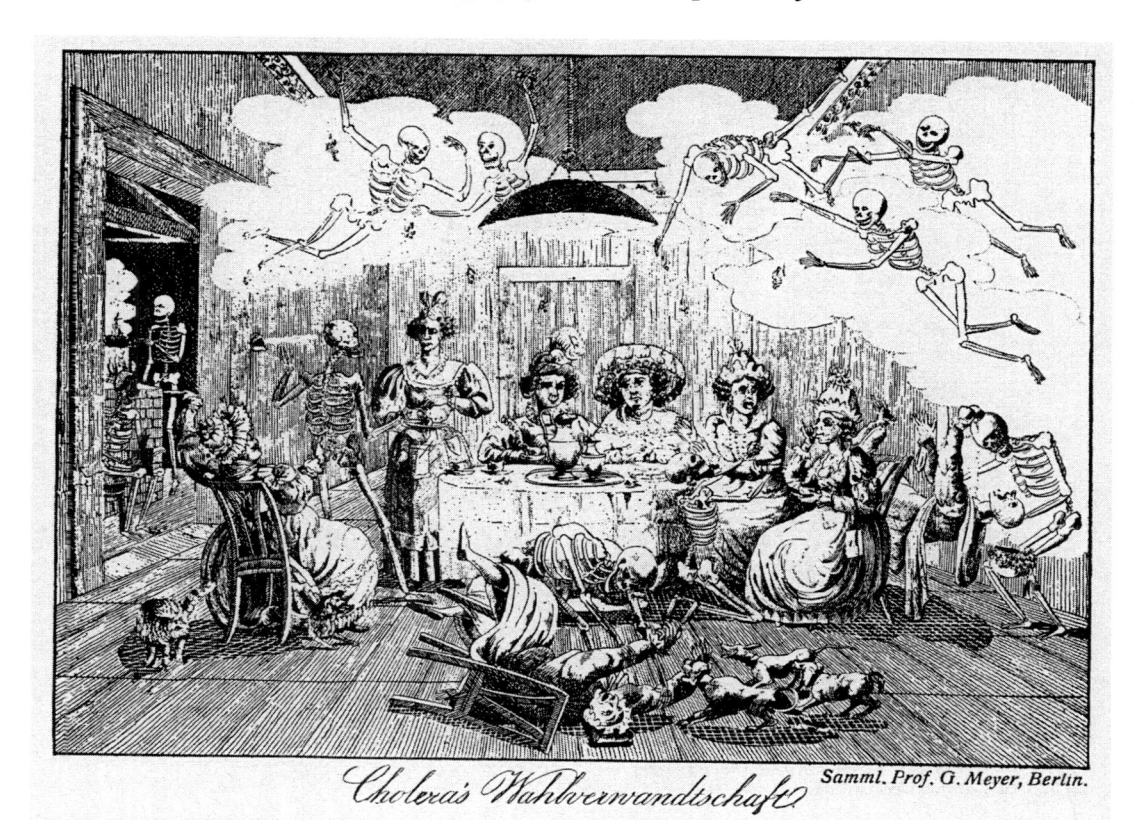

"Cholera's Wahlverwandschaft" (Cholera's Electric Affinities). Berlin. An early caricature of the medical theory that "cholera had a certain elective affinity between its nature and the peculiarity of an individual. Because of this special relationship cholera only affects that individual and no other." *Cholera Orientalis*, Heft 1, (1832), 178. The image shows cholera attacking specific individuals at a party and seemingly leaving others alone. In general the poor were thought to be the most susceptible to cholera. Reproduced from Eugen Holländer, *Die Karikatur und Satire in der Medizin: mediko-kunsthistorische Studie*, Stuttgart, 1921, 184.

The state authorities now spoke with "unanimity" and "authority" giving basis to the opinion that cholera was contagious. However, most of them had "not yet seen the cholera, whereas the majority of physicians in the areas affected by the disease had gradually come to the opposite conclusion." Accordingly, there was "no basis for the proof" that cholera was contagious. As for further proof, we only need to look at what was "prophesied to us from Russia, that Germany would be spared the epidemic if its government recognized ... [cholera was] ... contagious and the eastern border ... closed by cordons and quarantine."[32] Later when cholera "with inexorable progress had reached our gates many hoped that the leading states of Germany would stop the evil measures and decide on a safer course concerning the contagion." Finally after nearly half of Prussia and two-thirds of Austria was covered by the disease, he wrote:

> The great experiment which the governments were compelled to undertake has failed in the main, the sequestering of the sick from the healthy is not useful, nor can the spread of the disease be inhibited by cordons or quarantine stations. The moment has come when this must stop....

> The coercion and misery generated by the plague policy is felt everywhere and even more deeply and more painfully than the disease itself. For the great cost and losses which were sacrificed in vain to the supposed plague we have gained nothing but experience and this remains a precious legacy to posterity.[33]

Lorinser concluded he had previously studied plague and observed cholera patients. The "course of cholera and the way it spread was very different from plague," and if his recommendations had been followed in the first place "the results of this great experiment would have been "happier and we would have seen fewer victims."[34] Finally he recommended:

> We should accept the disease without fear and care for the needs of poor people, isolate the sick in their homes in case of possible infection, give attention to the most careful cleansing and improvement of their diet, as is done for ordinary infectious diseases and abandon the routine methods of treatments introduced by the English and followed by us with submissive acceptance while we improve our own treatments.

He finished the review writing, "I have spoken and saved my soul."[35]

The Controversy Over the Lorinser Article and the Repeal of State Quarantine Regulations

To Lorinser the destructive effects of the cordon were "generally visible" to the public. The hatred toward cordons and quarantine was "astonishing." In Berlin there "ruled the vilest atmosphere against its author, protector of this torture..." Dr. Rust. This attitude toward Rust existed not only among the public but also among other doctors and "in the highest circles" of the government.[36] Under these circumstances, he believed that his "frank review" was "received with the greatest jubilation by the majority" and greeted by the "blind contagionist with scorn."[37]

Lorinser wrote, he was never able to discover "how the article was so quickly published in the *State Gazette* which thereby allowed the king to dissolve the cordons and Kontumazen." However, as noted previously, there is little doubt that the king was aware of its imminent publication and that it was probably his personal physician, Dr. Hufeland who advised him and the editor of the *Prussian State Gazette* to publish Lorinser's three part article.

The *Prussian State Gazette* was the organ of the Prussian government and rarely published articles which "would stir a thinking individual to support the state." However, two articles were published in 1831, about foreign policy, that were applauded by liberals throughout Germany. These were published in error because the editor could not read the king's corrections. It appears to have been standard practice for the king to be aware of what was published in the *Prussian State Gazette*. In another example, he ordered his Foreign Minister, Bernstorff, to order a retraction of something published in the paper.

The three part article authored by Lorinser was completely contrary to what had previously been official policy. The king had to have been aware of its content and would have approved of it before publication. He may even have ordered its speedy publication. If the article had not been approved by the king he could have ordered an immediate retraction (as he had done in the past and besides the entire article was stretched out over three issues).

As further proof of the role the king played in this matter, one only has to look at what occurred in September 1830, when the poet and government official Karl Simrock wrote a poem praising the French Revolution. The king "impressed on the censors that in the future they exercise more rigorous control over the newspapers," and on his own issued a cabinet order dismissing Simrock from his office.[38]

Nevertheless, the publication of his article was highly controversial. Lorinser compared it to "lightning setting a rotten building aflame" and wrote "nearly all the public papers took part in the controversy and several ... printed the entire essay. In magazines and special booklets, authors spoke out on their different opinions and the dispute was soon so unpleasant that I did not want to read any more about it." He claimed that he refused to participate in the debate "further" because he "had achieved his goal to quiet the contagionists."[39]

Meanwhile Rust prepared an essay published in the *Prussian State Gazette* on October 12, 1831. It followed Hufeland's and Lorinser's essays. It was entitled, *A Word of Appreciation for the Protective Measures against Cholera*. He defended the blockades and other barriers recommended by the Immediate Commission. He wrote that as the medical community became more familiar with the disease the Immediate Commission began "altering the measures" called for in the original regulations. This resulted in the modified regulations of August 22, 1831, and September 12, 1831, especially the "abolition of the military cordon of infected towns and regions." Nevertheless, he continued to argue the original measures were correct at the time, his cause was not lost and people were "freed of the disadvantages of strict barriers" and "the anxiety of the repeal of all security measures." He finally gave thanks to the king for his "paternal care" and in "whose wisdom was found the correct middle ground between two opposing extremes."[40]

Politically the absolutist cause had been lost. Beginning early in October the government supported a more moderate anti-contagionist position and ordered specific military cordons lifted. Meanwhile, even though Rust and the medical administration had lost out to other government officials on their absolutist policy it did not mean that the battle within the medical community was over. Rust continued with his stubborn adherence to contagionism. Observing that the "disease" travels with war and having realized the danger to Prussia with "two warring peoples" on the Prussian border, he believed the measures he had introduced actually prevented cholera from spreading further into Prussia. Rust invoked Austria's defense against plague as a model for his medical policy and reasoned that "Austria prevented the plague for 100 years by using a sanitary cordon." Rust was convinced that if the cholera had come overland through Turkey that the Austrian sanitary cordon which had protected Austria from plague would have prevented cholera from entering Europe. He based this on the belief the public truly feared the plague and supported regulations to prevent its spread. He reasoned they would have done the same for cholera. Rust and his followers were simply not willing to overturn a body of medical knowledge they relied on because the government had taken a contrary position.[41]

A year later Rust wrote more truthfully about his real feelings about the king's actions. He said the king had acted outside his jurisdiction.[42] Rust's attack fell within the ethos of the modern Prussian bureaucrat that included holding "in check any possible capriciousness of a monarch within the quasi-legal system of specialized bureaucratic knowledge." The program to combat the cholera originated from a "consensus of officials," the only true source of legislation in a monarchical state. As part of a "deputation of learned physicians and scientists ... whose findings should be acknowledged as correct," he argued, in a "monarchical State" this manner of developing administrative policy serves as "the basis for legislation." Otherwise there only exists the "free play of arbitrary actions and despotism."[43]

These were strong words to have written nearly a year after the event, and indicated the extent of the feeling the king had stirred up in his leading medical expert. Rust continued to insist that he had acted on the basis of the support of medical experts, and that the original cholera "regulations" were appropriate. For Rust, it was not a question of supporting one opinion over another but that the king should support his medical experts and not give in to uninformed public opinion.[44] He had the support of Altenstein, who complained to the king that anti-contagionists like Sachs in their publications were "impertinent" and "scoffed at the Ministry of Justice's legal regulations." In his view "it is dangerous to permit private opinion to influence regulations made by the state."[45]

Lorinser attempted to avoid the subsequent medical debate because as an employee of the Prussian State his chief supervisor in the medical section was Rust. Nevertheless, as a result of his essays he emerged at least publically as the chief enemy of the contagionists.[46] Dr. Horn, a medical councilor, and member of the Scientific Deputation for Medical Matters, and a contagionist, later replied extensively to Lorinser's criticism of the quarantine and isolation policy. Dr. Horn wrote that Lorinser supported the erroneous anti-contagion position "most ingeniously." He stirred "debate among young doctors and excited non-doctors alike, raising serious doubts and magnifying the difficulties for the opposed administrative arrangements."[47]

Lorinser's arguments and understanding of the cholera were originally derived from the reports of the Indian doctors (English) as reported in the *Hamburger Magazin* where "foreign medical literature was published."[48] Because his essays were not written originally for the medical community, but for a political publication with "liberal sympathies," he argued more by example and experience why cordons and quarantines were ineffective. He wrote, "unlike other contagious diseases, cholera moved easily through the cordons" and the "exertions of the administrative officials against the private interests of so many thousands ... must be viewed with the cordons as a great and lasting hindrance." This for many readers appeared demonstrably true.[49]

Dr. Horn replied that the cordons had initially worked to impede the cholera but the area to be covered was too large and the resources limited. The Polish-Russian war stimulated an "increase in neighboring trade." The cordon failed because, "War, disbelief ... [in the contagious nature of the cholera as a consequence of the protests of local doctors] ... trade interests, corruption and smuggling ... were in most places insurmountable obstacles" to an effective program.[50]

Further, there was no sense in comparing the cordons for the plague in Austria with the cordons established for cholera in Prussia. Quarantines and cordons between Turkey and Austria were successful, because the borders were easily patrolled, there was no doubt about the contagious nature of the plague, people believed in the integrity of the system and the population realized the consequences if quarantine broke down.[51]

Lorinser had countered that the cholera did not behave like a regular contagious disease. There was no direct proof that a person that was sick with the cholera communicated it directly to another person. Isolation of an individual did not guarantee the disease would not break out sporadically in a community. The medical community was "confused" about the nature of the disease and had not yet experienced it.[52]

Lorinser's conclusions suited the king and the commercial interests who were applying pressure to his government. In reply to Lorinser's argument that this "great experiment was unnecessary and ... had failed," it could no longer be "concealed that the course of the sickness cannot be prevented through cordons or through quarantine stations."[53] Horn answered the first was partly true. Not because of atmospheric conditions (miasmic) nor because the sickness was like influenza and thus rendering a cordon useless, but because of the "enormous extent and spread of the disease on the boundaries of the neighboring lands." Additional reasons included smuggling and other schemes to prevent the proper implementation of the regulations. Probably the most serious charge by Horn, concerning Lorinser's advocacy, was the "popular beliefs of the non-contagiousness of cholera" that undermined the "strenuous efforts of the authorities" to establish and maintain an effective and suitable quarantine policy.[54]

In spite of the popular support for Lorinser's views on cholera, he was viewed with disfavor by his superiors, President Rust and Minister Altenstein. He believed this was a result not only of his article but because of his great success in communicating his views outside the Ministry. He wrote, the only reason they tolerated him was because both had to take public opinion into account. Both tried to "take steps" against him and he was aware of the "scorn and resentment" directed towards him.[55]

In March 1832, Lorinser believed his official position was threatened. All prospects of promotion or salary increase had vanished. He traveled to Berlin to meet with Rust and Altenstein to resolve his differences with them. Lorinser considered Rust his greatest adversary and believed he had wounded his vanity. "He possessed an extraordinary talent ... and most feared his great influence." By now Rust's "rage had subsided and he found himself deserted by the public and abandoned by most of his colleagues." Even Alexander Humboldt, "one of the most intelligent men in Berlin had declared himself against his views." The next morning Rust met with Lorinser. He "marveled at the seeming naturalness and ease ... [he] ... was received." Then "a very quiet conversation" followed about the issue at hand but with no success, "each retained his own opinion." Rust spoke extensively about the "tribulations and persecutions he endured. He expressed his astonishment that I, as a government Medical councilor declared myself publicly against the prescribed regulations." An hour later Lorinser left convinced such "conciliatory and moderate behavior" by Rust was deliberate and was done less out of benevolence, but rather from other considerations.[56]

The next morning Lorinser met with Altenstein, who as he suspected would be "ungracious and serious" and would speak to him in a way that Rust intentionally avoided. According to Altenstein, "My essay, he said, was indeed written properly, the problem lay in the fact that it was a violation of my official duty, because I protested against the measures of the government and published these contradictions in a newspaper."[57] Moreover, he said, he "should not believe that the lifting of the cordons ... had occurred as a direct result of his essays," that there were "earlier deliberations" which questioned the efficacy of the cordon and the quarantine facilities."[58]

Altenstein paced back and forth and puffed on his pipe. He continued to berate Lorinser, who listened patiently. Altenstein became quieter and removed the pipe from his mouth. He invited Lorinser to sit at his side on the sofa. Lorinser began defending himself and explained that all his official acts had been in keeping with the law. He was asked "exclusively for an academic paper" and did not intend it to be transferred to the state newspaper, this happened without his knowledge ... and he could not change the ideas he had expressed." The last, produced a striking change in the mood of the minister. It seemed as though he calmed himself down, "and steered the conversation to other subjects. At the end of the long audience, he showed himself fully reconciled, gave me a friendly handshake and invited me to visit him whenever I returned to Berlin."[59]

Lorinser was surprised by the turn of events, and later found out that he was received in such a civil manner because public opinion was generally in his favor and two respected physicians, Dr. Hufeland and Army Staff Doctor and Privy Chief Medical Councilor (and member of the Immediate Commission), Dr. Weibel had "declared ... [his] ... valuable essays had come at the right time." In addition his article inspired the same sentiments in Dr. Bittner, physician to the General Staff and "in many other higher officials."[60]

Lorinser's timely writings and common sense arguments gave the king additional support to cancel the cordons. However, at this time already two-thirds of Austria and most of the Prussian provinces had been infected.[61] In his order cancelling the military cordons on October 9, 1831, the king justified it by noting that now that the cholera had broken out in Madgeburg, and Breslau, and thus has also crossed the Elbe, all military cordons, as well as water and land quarantine stations were to be eliminated on the Oder, Neisse, Spree and Elbe. The same orders were given for all internal waterways. There was to be free movement between provinces, however, prudent measures like health passes for travelers would be maintained.[62]

For the government this order came at a critical moment. With "the restrictive measures off, the panic in Berlin subsided." Not surprisingly, when the order was given to repeal the military cordons Berlin was increasingly under attack from cholera and it appeared to the officials that the only way to avoid "unrest as a result of the restrictive measures imposed by the "Immediate Commission" (with Danzig and Konigsberg as examples) was to demonstrate the easing of these regulations by lifting the internal quarantines. One official went so far as to admit that the Berlin situation was actually worse than official reports. The reports did not "contain all the cholera cases because many are in private houses, kept secret and not announced to the police." Based on the reports from other cities the evidence for the need to lift the internal quarantine can be shown by the increasing number of reported deaths from cholera in the *Berliner Cholera Zeitung*. During the three weeks from September 4, 1831, to September 27, 1831, initially there were 373 cholera deaths and then from September 28, 1831, to October 15, 1831, cholera deaths increased by forty percent to 513 in Berlin. It was during this height of the epidemic in Berlin that discussions were held to modify the strict cholera regulations.[63]

The Conclusion of the Epidemic in Prussia

Lorinser's article in the *Prussian State Gazette* marked a "turning point" for official government policy. With the repeal of the internal provincial and waterway barriers it seemed a follow-up response was required to clarify a number of other issues raised in the Cabinet Order on October 16.[64] This included the need to continue to disinfect goods, letters, and money. The mayor of Berlin sent a special petition to the Immediate Commission asking it to modify quarantine regulations on individual houses and apartments. The mayor also asked that it provide further instructions on the disinfection of dwellings, and the effects of the cholera sick, dead and recovered. According to Thile, Hufeland's pronouncements on contagion and a petition by the local magistrate were the significant reasons for revisiting this cabinet order.[65]

A special session of the commission was convened to consider these issues on October 17, 1831. It included members of the commission, specialists from the technical section of the medical administration and three independent doctors. The questions posed by Rust concerned the elimination of quarantine and quarantine stations on the border, and whether to disinfect goods, money and letters. For the doctors the larger question was the "pestilential" nature of the cholera, and whether it had been correct to cancel the cholera measures previously ordered by the commission.[66]

General Thile wrote to the king to inform him on October 25, of the results and took this as an opportunity to criticize Hufeland for being out of touch with previously ordered measures. Hufeland had not attended the special session and in his place he submitted a report. He agreed with the majority of the findings of the commission and added further recommendations. General Thile took exception to two recommendations. The first that "oil cloth clothing ... [worn by physicians and other persons to protect themselves] ... only prolonged the illness." Thile complained that Hufeland was "wrong" not to make his opinion known earlier. Secondly, he recommended the "forcible removal and transporting of the sick" to hospitals should cease. The General pointed out these measures had already been stopped and were made public on September 11. On September 12, the Chief Sanitary Health Commission in Berlin also published a notice in the *Prussian State Gazette* that read "each cholera patient could remain in his home, be treated and cared for."[67] If the patient did not have the means to care for himself he could be brought to a cholera hospital. The notice concluded by assuring everyone that "the recovery rate in the hospitals was better than in a private home."[68]

As for other issues, these included supplying a "warming apparatus" for the baskets used to carry the cholera sick to the hospitals during cold weather, removing restrictions on funerals and cemeteries, and easing of travel regulations. The disinfection of dwellings was turned over to the local sanitary committee under the authority of the provincial presidents.[69]

On October 30, 1831, the *Prussian State Gazette* contained the following regulations issued by the Immediate Commission: (1) the disinfection of goods etc., was not required because "experience and general evidence show there was no demonstrable evidence of the transmission of the disease" by these articles; (2) the effects and dwellings of cholera patients require disinfection and purification; (3) goods transported over water where cholera exists need to be disinfected; (4) a number of requirements for ships and their crews was listed; (5) cholera patients are to be watched over in their homes, their needs attended to including disinfection under the authority of local sanitary commissions; (6) travelers require current health passes; (7) travelers had to report to local officials when staying overnight and have their health passes authorized; (8) referred to specific paragraphs regarding the duties of officials etc., published in the public notice of August 22, 1831, and (9) referenced additional provisions given earlier on October 16, 1831.[70]

The commission also lifted the ban on the important Frankfurt on the Oder "Messe" or Fair. It ordered the fair be held in the "ordinary way." However, because of the prevailing conditions there were stipulations enumerated by the Interior Department. Travelers to the fair were to follow the main routes and report to the police in the major cities along the routes. They had to have health certificates with the health conditions from their home districts written on the certificates. As long as the paperwork was in proper order they had to be allowed to pass. Foreigners wanting to attend the fair needed to produce a passport showing health conditions from their place of origin and if cleared "admitted unhindered." Without proper paperwork travelers were required to undergo a five day quarantine which they would have to pay for themselves[71]

Even more importantly and to show the good intentions of the king and his government, the king pardoned anyone who violated the law to prevent cholera enacted on June 15, 1831. It was a harsh law that contained seventeen paragraphs listing various transgressions that ranged from passing through quarantine lines, trading in forbidden areas, and confronting guards at quarantine stations. Penalties ranged from ten years in prison to the death penalty.[72] A November 22, 1831, cabinet order was decreed that pardoned anyone who had "violated" the June 15, 1831, law. Local police authorities were still responsible for "the investigation and determination of punishments for any infractions of purely sanitary regulations relating to cholera."[73]

The lifting of the quarantines in early October was probably the most significant direct action taken. It acted as a prominent public pronouncement that the government was moving in a more realistic direction. Lorinser had provided the public face and support for the removal of the quarantine lines. Hufeland the intermediate solution that bridged the criticism of both camps at least in the view of the government. Hufeland wrote in December 1831:

> To me it is, in fact, inconceivable, how among physicians there can be any dispute on this point, or how they should, as in some instances, have been divided into two parties, contagionists and anti-contagionists, standing in hostile opposition to each other. Is it not a long-recognized truth, that a disease may originate from epidemic influences and there develop a contagion, and that the same disease may at the same time be produced by the atmosphere, and by a contagion?[74]

The intermediate position Hufeland advocated later influenced Prussia's comprehensive *Measures against the Spread of Contagious Diseases Act*. However, in October 1831, the Prussian government was concerned with the importation of cholera from abroad. It ordered "quarantine against foreign countries in Silesia, in East and West Prussia and in Posen remain in force."[75] In addition, the measures of October 30, 1831, still contained fairly strict regulations concerning travelers. They required health passes and the disinfection of goods from abroad from known cholera districts. Local officials were ordered to keep a close watch on the cholera sick and ensure that their household goods and dwellings were properly disinfected.

From then on the Immediate Commission found itself discussing more mundane matters, disinfection, sanitary measures for the sick, travel regulations and procedures for handling mail.[76] The sweeping powers the commission had enjoyed prior to September 6, 1831, were reduced to less important decisions. These were now being decided at the local level. Rust later wrote the situation was probably worse because:

> in recent times in public papers, published articles and judgments about cholera and statutory police measures against infectious diseases, everyone it seems is smarter than a whole College of the most experienced and respected doctors ... and no one feels called upon to obey the lawful regulations.[77]

Nevertheless on December 22, 1831, while discussing regulations concerning travelers, seemingly the last refuge of the previous strict policy, a question concerning the quarantine regulations in Prussia was raised once again. However, members of the commission "differed on their opinion" about quarantine. Finally, one commission member maintained that further "regulations against the cholera were not necessary, that the relief in having lifted them was great, inasmuch that the commission had received complaints from all sides concerning the continuation of the general regulations."[78]

The minutes of that meeting show that support for lifting the regulations had originated in the "Ministry of Trade, the king and among other doctors."[79] Rust stubbornly insisted that the original policy had been successful. He saw the reason the disease had not spread further or been as severe as in other countries was because of the early actions of the Immediate Commission. He refused to yield on his position. He requested that the Immediate Commission hear a motion and vote on whether the "cholera regulations should be re-imposed." He insisted that members of the "Scientific Deputation were in the majority for continuing ... [Cholera] ... regulations."[80]

On February 9, 1832, the Berlin Health Committee made it known that Berlin was free of the cholera. Berlin was the last major city in Prussia to enjoy this relief. Danzig had been free of cholera since October 25 1831, Posen since November 28 1831, Königsberg and Breslau since the beginning of January 1832.[81]

The Medical Administrative Legacy of the Epidemic

Fortunately for the government and people of Prussia the number of cholera cases declined by the end of October. It is difficult to determine the exact reason why cholera abated in Prussia in the late fall of 1831. Certainly the application of basic hygienic standards and the sequestering of the sick limited the opportunity for cholera to spread further. Perhaps as Becker noted, those areas that exercised direct control over their own public health regulations were able to prevent or limit the entry of the cholera into their communities. The winding down and subsequent end of the rebellion in Poland in September also eliminated large troop movements on the Prussian border (which would have been a source of re-infection). There was less movement on the roads as workers returned to their farms to help get in the crops for winter. Finally, as the cold weather settled in, the opportunity for cholera to spread was hindered by winter shipping, which slowed down or ceased on the frozen rivers. By January 1832, cholera stopped being a major public health issue in Prussia. The number of new cases declined to zero. On January 30, 1832, the Immediate Commission was disbanded, but not before it was asked to write new cholera recommendations that were subsequently incorporated into a cabinet order in early February.

The Cabinet Order of February 5, 1832

The seriousness which the government originally supported the Immediate Commission was demonstrated in the cabinet order of June 15, 1831, which authorized the "death penalty" for a serious transgression of the quarantine.[82] With the cabinet order of September 6, 1831, and Hufeland's and Lorinser's subsequent articles in the *Prussian State Gazette*, the official Prussian medical establishment saw its strict quarantine policy dismantled. Although Prussian non- medical officials were able to modify the contagionist policy, they did not convince the Prussian medical establishment, under Rust and his superior Altenstein to adopt their anti-contagionist views. Rust continued to insist on the contagion theory of cholera even writing to Alexander Humboldt that there are those who "want to go further into this and remove all protective sanitary policy measures.... I concede as long as I have an influence on this, it will never be done with my consent."[83]

For Rust it was not just a policy issue. After all he had made many enemies with his stubborn insistence on the contagiousness of the cholera and this had taken a direct toll on him. He wrote to Altenstein in December 1832 asking for additional compensation:

> No other activity has acted to simultaneously destroy my mental and physical existence as the [Immediate] ... Commission on Cholera Affairs. It affected my health, popularity, and my existence as a practical physician, in short everything that is dear to me ... and worthy of sacrifice, without even the sight of God and the world entitling me recognition, let alone any compensation for such a well-known victim ... [for doing] ... my part on behalf of the state.[84]

Even with his commitment to contagion and reputation Rust assisted in writing the cholera legislation of February 5, 1832 (dated January 31, 1832, the last meeting of the commission). He later played an important role on the newly appointed commission that led to the Contagious Diseases Law of August 8, 1835. This was demonstrated by the special thanks and gift he received from the king for his service.[85]

Notwithstanding Rust's unrelenting contagionism, the legacy of the Prussian cholera epidemic and the conflict between the contagionists and anti-contagionists led to more moderate and acceptable regulations for the commercial interests and to the public at large in Prussia. This was immediately shown in the cholera legislation contained in the cabinet order of February 5, 1832. It was one of the first laws enacted in Prussia concerning a contagious disease (excluding plague) and can be attributed directly to the cholera epidemic. The introduction stated, this "Cabinet Order is partly a repeal and partly expanded instructions on the regulations that had been initiated prior to and at the outbreak of the sickness."

The commission was ordered to write the new regulations "apart from the opposing views of the doctors at this time" and the "inexplicable nature of the sickness."[86]

The cabinet order explained the "nature of the cholera, its cause, appearance and its manner of spreading had still not been satisfactorily investigated."[87] The end result of these regulations was that cholera was contagious but neither cordons nor a general quarantine was required. It was a cautious document that recommended quarantining a patient's house or isolating the patient, but only if he lived in a rural area where it would present "few difficulties."[88] In other circumstances a room or part of a house could be isolated.[89] For inland shipping, it was up to the discretion of the provincial president of the province or the local police officer to determine whether a ship should be put under observation (limited to five days). The observation of a sea going ship from an infected country coming into Prussia was limited to five days.[90] These regulations demonstrated a pragmatism which could only have been learned from experiencing the epidemic itself. This practicality was continued beyond the hysteria of the epidemic. The commission looked at prior regulations concerning Danzig as an example of the damage a strict contagionist policy could do. Without a sense of what occurred previously, later regulations may seem to be strictly contagionist, but it is clear that the Prussian medical administration had made great concessions over its initial response.

An additional development that arose from the recommendations during the epidemic itself was the establishment of "Schutz" or "Revier" commissions. The new instructions recommended the appointment of special commissions during a cholera epidemic. They had been popular and effective during the epidemic. Their members had to include "at least a doctor or surgeon, a police or commune official as well as townspeople elected by members of the commune." The local "Schutz" commission was independent of the sanitary commission. The commissions were an attempt on the part of the government to allow local control in what was considered a potentially volatile situation. During the epidemic, the provincial presidents and other officials at the local level had been given more responsibility in determining the community's response to the cholera epidemic. The new legislation continued this effort.[91]

The Contagious Diseases Law in Prussia and the Ministries in Conflict

In order to avoid another catastrophe, like the one Prussia had experienced, the government stated the justification for the legislation. "It was only by the occurrence of cholera that people became aware of the necessity of sweeping legislation, to order and enforce in this connection, sanitary police regulations for contagious diseases." Therefore Prussia required specific laws regarding "contagious diseases." Up to this time there were no legal requirements dealing with epidemic disease (excluding plague and the cholera cabinet order just mentioned).[92]

As a result of the need for legislation, following the dissolution of the Immediate Commission the king asked Thile to head a new commission to develop regulations and procedures for contagious diseases. The king requested the new commission be composed of former members of the commission. The reason the king relied on the former members of the commission to craft what would later become the Contagious Disease Law of 1835 was due to the on-going internal conflict between Ministry of the Interior (especially the police section under von Brenn) and the Ministry of Religion, Education and Medical Affairs under Altenstein.[93]

As we saw earlier the conflict intensified during the months leading up to the cholera outbreak. Von Brenn believed the Police Section of the ministry alone should have jurisdiction for ordering the measures to prevent cholera. In November 1830, the two ministers openly disagreed over which ministry had the authority to impose preventative measures. Altenstein justified his ministry's jurisdiction (the educational and research division) because of conflicting opinions over the treatment and prevention of cholera.[94]

At the end of the cholera epidemic and with the disbanding of the Immediate Commission, jurisdictional conflict between the two ministries returned now that the emergency was over. Von Brenn argued that the Interior Ministry of Police should be responsible for the administration of cholera regulations. Altenstein countered that his Ministry should participate in this matter because the "nature of the disease had not been sufficiently investigated to establish valid standards for administration, the scientific interests of the Ministry required it and it was still necessary to obtain a more precise knowledge of the progress of the spread and the nature of the disease."[95]

Von Brenn wrote to Altenstein on April 30, 1832, that it made sense that the Interior Ministry of Police have jurisdiction over medical matters because it had to balance trade, transportation and the public life of the state in the applying sanitary regulations. Altenstein's ministry was responsible for the "administration of the poor, sick and communal matters." Because this was "an inseparable relationship" the Ministry's Medical Affairs Department should be united with provincial officials and police and should be subordinated to the Ministry of the Interior.[96]

Altenstein replied on October 3, 1832, he recognized the current separation of the medical administration from the medical police led to "attendant evils." This could only be prevented be joining the two under "one hand." Here was an example of Altenstein's "humanist" philosophy being brought to bear on this practical matter. For him the benefits of "education" and "research" as the basis for progress were more important than a strictly technical approach. If the medical department of his ministry was subordinated to the Ministry of the Interior "scientific progress" would devolve to a "formal handling of existing regulations" while scientific progress would be "unnecessarily curtailed."[97]

Altenstein desired the two medical sections be reunited under the Ministry of Education, Religion and Medical Affairs. The conflict between the two ministries dragged on despite the repeated suggestions of the Minister of the Interior and the "stubborn silence of Altenstein." Finally, von Brenn forwarded a proposal to the State Ministry on April 19, 1833, requesting that it re-open the investigation of the 1824 State Budget Commission's decision that led to the original separation of the unified medical administration. He requested the technical and scientific sections be re-united and made subordinate to the Ministry of the Interior.[98]

The State Ministry postponed a vote on von Brenn's request. The overlapping areas of jurisdiction continued between the two Ministries. The two separate medical administrations were not united until twenty-five years after the original decision that separated them. In June 1849 both were assigned to the Ministry of Education, Religion and Medical Affairs following a report from the State Ministry that reversed the original 1824 decision.[99]

The Origin of the Prussian Contagious Diseases Law of August 8, 1835

Knowing about the ongoing conflict between the two ministers following the end of the cholera outbreak the king asked General Thile to head up an expert commission to write new regulations the government deemed necessary concerning contagious diseases as a result of its experience during the recent cholera epidemic. The king required the commission to write these regulations with the concurrence of the two ministries this also contributed to "delaying the work of the commission."[100]

Though the members of the commission were former members of the Immediate Commission it seems a majority were willing to mitigate the danger of the cholera and include it with less contagious diseases and sanction the modified cholera regulations ordered in the latter part of the epidemic. Dr. Rust was singled out for "special merit" in the development of the regulations concerning the procedures for handling contagious diseases. The king "expressed his greatest satisfaction with Rust" in the cabinet order of November 8, 1835." However, as Thile explained in a letter to the king, and showing the influence of Rust and his like-minded colleagues, the contagious diseases law of 1835 did not include what was believed at the time to be the two most highly contagious and dangerous diseases, plague and yellow fever.[101]

On the above matter, the origin of the work of the commission included less serious contagious diseases (cholera had come to be included here as well) and the regulations included diseases that pass from animals to humans as well. The commission's work was divided into three parts: regulations for the sanitary police; disinfection procedures; and instructions on the nature and treatment of contagious diseases. This latter part was intended "to be given to the medical commissions for the guidance of the public at the outbreak of a contagious epidemic, or in cases of necessity with the most appropriate instruction in the manner of assistance to be immediately provided."[102]

According to Thile the document was an "important supplement to the regulations, and fills a gap in the previous instructions on the procedure for contagious diseases, that the commission was obligated to retain it" and although originally extensive because of the issues it addressed, it had to be made concise:

> Plague and yellow fever, as I said, are not in the regulations but have been taken into account. The Commission was prompted by this for the following reasons: the existing measures for the prevention of plague in the countries which are compelled to enact those measures due to their

location, like Russia, Austria, etc., are made as soon as the plague in the neighboring country appears. They consist of an absolute barrier of the land on the borders and combine military cordons with the strictest application of quarantine stations and a quarantine of the land and sea. At the outbreak of the disease within the country a military containment system is initiated and thus a complete isolation of the places overrun by plague.[103]

Given the recent experience with cholera, Thile, as well as other members of the commission realized this approach had failed with cholera and probably would not be entirely successful with plague on the Prussian frontiers. It appears from the document that there was some attempt to develop regulations but in answer to this there was the following explanation:

If the Royal Commission appointed by Your Majesty would now have to design plague regulations, as they did in fact attempt to carry out the necessary preparatory work, it soon became convinced, by its own lack of experience with this disease that the only model they had were the previous procedures in place that had worked for the past 100 years in the states mentioned.[104]

The document concluded that the specific experience of the cholera in 1831 and 1832 had convinced the officials this type of "sanitary legislation was incompatible" with contemporary life. "All the circumstances of such a populated and busy country like ours, how little our vast land borders could be hermetically sealed, as it is, and how inadequate would be our means," it would be inappropriate to retain them. However, the contagionists on the commission were willing to accept modified regulations for cholera that resulted in the new contagious diseases act but could not agree on plague.[105]

Thile recommended that a new commission be assigned to Vienna and Marseille for several years to prepare new plague regulations.[106] As for yellow fever, the commission accepted the judgment of one physician who argued that in a northern climate, although yellow fever "could get here, it could not spread the way it does in the hot southern countries and would thus cease to be such a dangerous contagious disease" i.e., the Prussian climate was not conducive to the "epidemic influence" or "atmospheric" requirements to create the conditions for a yellow fever epidemic.[107]

On August 8, 1835 Prussia enacted a new and comprehensive law, *The Measures Against the Spread of Contagious Diseases*. This was the first general regulation for "the most common contagious diseases." It included cholera, typhus, smallpox and dysentery along with a number of less deadly diseases. As a result of one lesson learned in the cholera epidemic, it specifically stated that in order to prevent the spread of contagious diseases, education about these diseases and the cooperation of the public was necessary.[108] Many of the original recommendations of the Immediate Commission based on the experience with cholera found in the cabinet order of February 5, 1832, were incorporated into the legislation of August 8, 1835.[109]

The recommendations included the "Protection" commissions, local control, limited quarantine for cholera patients, health passes for travelers, measures for inland shipping and for ships arriving from suspected cholera ports. The regulations were similar to the regulations enacted toward the end of the cholera epidemic in Prussia. The Cabinet Order of August 8, 1835, replaced all previous instructions and cabinet orders for cholera.[110]

The Prussian experience with the cholera in 1831 had shown the government that no group in Prussia was satisfied with the earlier "contagionist policy." The upper classes had complained about these policies, and even the highly placed Foreign Minister Bernstorff's wife complained about cholera regulations, writing, "the people murmured, the higher estates grumbled, and what of the government? It produced general confusion during these days with all its previous excesses."[111]

A coherent approach to contagious diseases was developed directly from the experience with the cholera epidemic in 1831. The commission was able to develop a category of less formidable contagious diseases that now included cholera. It developed regulations that minimized the impact of these diseases on the general public and commercial classes. These diseases were considered less contagious than plague. The commission could not recommend these less stringent regulations for plague until further study, thus the recommendation to send a commission to Vienna and Marseille (a French port that had experienced the plague as late as 1720).[112]

The policies and instructions that were found to have worked during the cholera epidemic were later incorporated into the new regulations which emerged in the Cabinet Order of August 8, 1835.[113] There was without a doubt, a direct connection between the early response to the epidemic in Prussia and subsequent modifications of cholera regulations over the course of the epidemic. This had a direct impact on the enactment of this first of its kind legislation in Prussia. In addition, the latter order resulted from a compromise that was not issued by fiat from above by the medical administration of Prussia, but was the result of direct experience acquired by the government in 1831.[114]

Undoubtedly the resulting conflict over which medical department was to be responsible for cholera policy in the future contributed to the tension between the two ministries and weighed on the government and the king's inability to resolve the on-going conflict between the two ministries. This made it impossible to assign responsibility to either Ministry to write the regulations for the Contagious Diseases Law. Just as the king relied on a special commission to prevent the cholera he now turned to the former members of the Immediate Commission to write the new contagious diseases regulations. He appointed them under the leadership of General Thile to a new commission with this responsibility. The commission did have to obtain the agreement of both Ministries to complete its task and this as noted earlier contributed to the time involved from the appointment of the commission to its final enactment into law in August 1835.

However, the primacy of former members of the commission serving on the new commission contributed to the Contagious Diseases Law of August 8, 1835, being more of a compromise than what might have emerged from a united medical administration either under the ministry of the Interior or the Ministry of Religion, Educational and Medical Affairs. After all, Rust continued to represent the medical establishment in Prussia and the establishment continued to support the contagionist position even in opposition to the king and public opinion.[115]

For the king and his officials there could be no return to what had been perceived by liberals as a misguided "reactionary medical policy." It was now replaced by a more enlightened policy guided by practical considerations even though the more extreme critics continued to speak out against all restrictive measures. Over time "the anti-contagionists, miasmists and localists of every stripe found their ranks swelling, and theirs was often considered the dominant opinion." The contagionists were on the defensive and found themselves moderating their position "while advocating measures that caused as little offense as possible or replacing them with other measures, sequestering the ill in a less drastic manner."[116]

The Contagious Diseases Law in Prussia although not a full retreat from contagion allowed for a latitude and flexibility and was suitable for the new demands of a rising social and economic middle class in Prussia without imposing excessive burdens on the lower classes and trade that the initial regulations had imposed at the outbreak of the epidemic.[117] The Cabinet Order of August 8, 1835, emerged as a working compromise and a future plan in which three major groups obtained benefits they required, the king and his advisors could continue to rule without fear of unrest in the event of a similar outbreak of cholera or other contagious diseases, the liberal economic interests and the lower classes obtained a maximum of freedom of trade and movement without subjecting themselves to a too restrictive policy and the rest of the population was prevented from unlimited exposure to epidemic diseases.

In some sense this Contagious Diseases Law could be said to be the final legacy of the career of Dr. Hufeland who spent much of his professional life attempting to reconcile opposing points of view in a variety of controversies. The Contagious Diseases Law remained on the books as the only infectious diseases law until it was superseded in Germany by the Contagious Diseases Law of 1905.[118]

12

Prussia, Cholera and the Polish Refugee Crisis

In the middle of July 1831, on the eve of the cholera epidemic in Königsberg and its later spread to Berlin in September, two events occurred that placed Prussia in an awkward domestic and international position and led to later repercussions that affected Prussia's standing with Russia. They also generated intense criticism from the western powers of France and England and the Polish emigré exiles in the west. The first was the defection of General Gielgud's Polish army corps into Prussian territory on July 13, 1831. The second event followed the storming of Warsaw and its fall on September 6, 1831. The subsequent mass exodus of civilians and government officials sought and received refuge in Prussia. The exodus culminated in the later defection to Prussia of the main Polish army under General Rybinski on October 5, 1831.

Prussia was not prepared for all these refugees. Once it accepted the refugees Prussia had to find some way to absorb them. At the time of Gielgud's defection in July, because of the impending epidemic in Prussia as well as the known cholera in the Polish army, Prussia had to implement quarantine restrictions to prevent cholera from spreading further among its own population. Prussian officials were aware that in other countries the worst outbreaks of this "dreaded disease" occurred when civilians came into contact with the military.

This chapter addresses the cholera arrangements made by Prussia on behalf of the refugees, the impact of these arrangements on the refugees, the population and the government, and the Prussian attempt to resolve the refugee problem following the resolution of the quarantine policy. It concludes with a brief discussion of the final disposition of the refugee problem and its effect on Prussia's international reputation.

It is clear that strict cholera measures implemented in Prussia in July, at the time of General Gielgud's defection, and the orders to quarantine the Polish army units were not imposed to impede the Polish war effort. They were part of a domestically focused sanitary policy orchestrated by the Prussian government under the auspices of the Immediate Commission. There was an actual fear of cholera because it was an unknown disease. Prussian doctors had limited or no experience with the disease. By early July, cholera had only broken out in isolated areas in Prussia, except for the significant outbreak in Danzig in late May. The king and the Prussian military (the latter acting under the orders of the Immediate

Commission) realized measures were needed immediately to prevent a wide spread epidemic. The borders were secured by the Prussian military, a cordon was in effect to protect the small towns on the border districts as well as the city of Königsberg (nevertheless, an outbreak occurred on July 23, 1831, a few days after Gielgud's defection). The cities, towns and even government districts attempted to do everything in their power to prevent a cholera outbreak. For example, when the cholera broke out in Riga in May 1831, there was a sudden intense fear of cholera in the district of Stralsund in New Pomerania (a Prussian Province). "A coast guard was immediately arranged to prevent any clandestine landing of ships, and [the local authorities] began to quarantine all incoming ships. The fear was so great that even after September when the King cancelled the cordons Stralsund was permitted to protect itself against cholera at its own expense.[1]

Prior discussion over Prussia's treatment and holding of the Poles that defected with Gielgud to Prussia is based on a lack of acknowledging the on-going evolving internal medical policy in Prussia during the months that the Polish military refugees were held in the quarantine camps at Packmohnen and Schernen. It was during this time that the government's strict policy *vis a vis* the public and the strict measures advocated by the Immediate Commission were under scrutiny and later modified by the king's proclamation on September 6, 1831, as ineffective, costly and more harmful to the economy and his people than the sickness itself.[2]

Gielgud's Defection and the Establishment of Quarantine Camps in East Prussia

There had been serious disagreement between Prussia and Russia over the constant demands from the Russian government to stop the rebels who fled into Prussian territory and return them to Russia. Czar Nicolas insisted at least the main leaders of the insurgents and members of the Polish government whose names were on a provisional list given to the Prussian government, be returned to Russia if they sought refuge in Prussia. The emperor had written to his Vice Chancellor, Count Karl Nesselrode on March 9, 1831, he had learned "with deep sorrow that individuals guilty of high treason against him and all crimes that rebellion brings in its train ... had found refuge under the protection of Prussian laws and a false principle of humanity had provided them the means to carry out elsewhere their resentments and their plans of vengeance and subversion."[3]

However, on this particular issue the Prussian government refused to relent. It had previously communicated to the Russian government on December 9, 1830, it had decided it would not deliver to Russia any Poles who "found refuge in its territory." This response was necessary due to "the feelings which prevailed among the people of the Kingdom of Prussia."[4]

On July 12, 1831, on the Prussian border near Schnaugsten, a local staff officer and a *Landrat,* learned that General Gielgud and General Chłapowski had announced their intention to seek protection in Prussia. The *Landrat* rushed to the border to make the necessary arrangements. That same evening both generals moved their remaining troops, totaling 2,500 men, into Prussian territory.

The plan to cross into Prussia was based on the fact that the Prussian king had issued an order February 11, 1831, permitting the "two warring parties if they crossed into Prussian territory a slow return to their homeland." The Polish generals were aware on April 10, 1831, that Russian Colonel Bartolomo had taken advantage of this order and crossed into Prussian territory after being pursued by insurgents from Samogitia on the Prussian-Lithuanian border. He was allowed to rest in Memel and return with his men to Kurland by sea. The Polish generals expected to be treated in the same way, and thus returned swiftly to Poland to continue the fight against the Russians.[5]

General Chłapowski asked if the same order applied to Poland (even though Prussia did not recognize the Polish government). Due to the conditions on the border the Polish generals were in no position to negotiate further. The Polish soldiers were given refuge. Later, on August 22, 1831, after undergoing quarantine in Prussia (see below), General Chłapowski sent a message to the Prussian king asking if he and his men could return to Poland. The king did not reply until September 5, 1831. He clarified his original order of February 11, 1831, and wrote "he only had in mind a small number of men seeking shelter in Prussia but it could not be applied to a large number of troops."[6]

In addition conditions concerning cholera had changed since April 10, 1831, when General Bartolomo was allowed to return to Kurland. In late May, cholera broke out in Danzig, meanwhile the Russian transport ships arrived in Danzig harbor. The merchants in Königsberg continued to complain about the recent incident of landing supplies for the Russian army in Prussian territory and secondly about the Russian transport ships still in Danzig harbor. In addition, new strict regulations were imposed with severe punishments in Prussia on June 15, 1831, for transgressing cholera regulations. The measures were "considered necessary because of the cholera outbreak in the bordering foreign lands, and to ensure compliance with official measures. A strong and swift punishment" was ordered for those who violated the regulations.[7]

In order to answer these complaints on June 18, 1831, Schön ordered a double cordon on the Polish and Russian borders. The dual cordon included military and the local militia men to better protect against unauthorized border crossings. As for the ships in Danzig harbor, "because they had already arrived, the ships and cargo were to be subject to a strict quarantine" and the "crew isolated from the ships" so that "no substance can spread the disease." Schön attempted to answer these complaints, which continued and culminated in the Königsberg merchant's petition to the king at the beginning of July. However, the Polish army defection under the two Polish generals, was unexpected and an order of magnitude beyond Prussian expectations. When combined with the public fear of armies on the march spreading cholera, the Polish military defection required a public response from the Prussian government.[8]

On the afternoon of July 13, the Polish troops of Generals Rohland and Szymanowski approached the same place where Gielgud and Chłapowski had crossed into Prussia. With the arrival of additional troops, and not seeing any Russian troops pursuing them, the soldiers became "restless."[9] When General Rohland's men learned what General Gielgud and

General Chłapowski had done, the "news was like a thunderbolt." They did not want to abandon the national forces to Prussia but wanted to save them for one last battle." The soldiers saw their Polish brethren surrounded by Prussian guards. To avoid this "terrible example" they wanted to move along the Prussian frontier and escape back to Warsaw.[10]

At this time, General Gielgud was surrounded by several officers on horseback. He was speaking to the Prussian Landrat. Captain Skalski of the 7th Regiment, a Polish officer, galloped forward, took a pistol from his holster and shot General Gielgud through the chest, whereupon he fell from his horse dead. The assassin fled without having been detected. According to one eyewitness, the assassin was one of General Rohland's officers, who performed this act "out of a fanatical love of his country" He justified the act by Gielgud's "incompetence" and therefore "could not be blamed for treason."[11]

The troops, now full of martial spirit, resolved not to follow in Gielgud's footsteps. Under their two generals they marched along the Prussian border pursued by Cossack patrols and regular Russian troops. Many of the soldiers tried to care for the sick and wounded. Some had to be left behind. But they were running low on ammunition and general supplies. The soldiers became demoralized. Other soldiers were recent Lithuanian insurgents who were untrained. If Lithuanian insurgents surrendered to the Russians they believed they would be sent to Siberia. The choices were either to take the battle to the enemy, surrender to the enemy or seek refuge in Prussia. As a last resort they decided to do like Gielgud and Chłapowski, retreat into Prussia, and lay down their weapons with the hope that at least they were "dealing with a civilized nation." They hoped "after some time, to serve the fatherland once more."[12]

Generals Rohland and Szymanowski met with General Krafft and agreed to the same terms as the other two generals. The most important condition was "they turn over their weapons and war materials." If they agreed, the generals and their troops would be "assured protection" and they could stay on in the Prussian territories.[13]

There were additional conditions for sanctuary after their arms were laid down. The Polish general could maintain command of his troops but they had to voluntarily give up their weapons, artillery and some horses. Officers could retain their swords, non-commissioned officers and soldiers their knapsacks. Officers and men were separated from each other, with only one squadron officer to maintain the discipline of the troops. For the sake of sanitation, all Polish officers and men were required to submit to twenty-day quarantine immediately. They were to be divided into several divisions for this purpose and would be placed under a military guard during the quarantine period. Huts for the Polish troops, straw as well as fuel would be provided. Polish troops would receive rations comparable to the portions Prussian soldiers received. Once Polish troops entered quarantine, "Prussian sentinels and patrols must be obeyed, otherwise force of arms would be employed in the strictest manner." Any contact with guards was to be avoided. The Polish generals' planned for themselves and their troops to be held in a twenty-day quarantine, would not leave without orders of the king of Prussia. Prisoners from the Imperial Russian army were to be freed immediately and permitted to return to Russian territory, if they wished.[14]

The most important condition was the laying down of weapons. Of the seven additional conditions, at least three related to the quarantining of the Polish soldiers. These pre-conditions were not as the *Warsaw Gazette* wrote at the end of August, implemented "under the pretense of cholera" but were part of an on-going attempt to prevent cholera from spreading into Prussia. The strict measures in the two quarantine camps that were shortly established were comparable to the same measures applied to the civilian population in Prussia in mid–July when the defection occurred. This is demonstrated in the Prussian government's measures to prevent the cholera and the previously referred to *Law for the Punishment of those Offenses which Relate to the Violation of the Regulations Adopted for the Prevention of Cholera on June 15, 1831*. The punishment for the transgression of these regulations included imprisonment and if warranted the death sentence.[15]

In addition, accepting Polish military refugees, who most likely had been exposed to cholera, was of concern back in Berlin. Friedrich Ancillon, Director of the Political Section of the Ministry for Foreign Affairs under Count Bernstorff informed the English ambassador in Berlin, Chad, that Polish officers would be sent to the city of Memel and regular soldiers would be disarmed and placed in villages along the frontier. Chad reported there was "great apprehension ... that the cholera will by this means be propagated and many exclaim against the injustice of subjecting these villages to the dangers of Infection, and those that complain add that the cholera was introduced into Hungary by the ... [Polish] ... soldiers of General Dwernicki's Corps." As Dankbahr wrote, "perhaps this was not entirely without reason" as the "two warring armies were then regarded as the carrier and distributor of the dreaded disease."[16]

The fear of infection by the Poles was so great that individual local authorities were granted the power to blockade themselves against the cholera (as noted earlier in the example of Straslund). Some communities took extreme measures to prevent contact with Polish soldiers. The city of Tilsit was expected to be the primary supply depot and hospital facility for the quarantine camp at Packmohnen. The city refused in the strongest terms, until August 8, to accept wounded officers from Packmohnen. Tilsit also refused to accept sick Prussian soldiers from Packmohnen even after the Commandant ordered them to be moved to Tilsit for better care. The city attempted to prevent all relations with Packmohnen, even though in mid–July the army had made plans to make the city a main source of the camp's food, other supplies and maintenance.[17]

Eventually, this public relations nightmare required a public notice on the "health" of the Polish quarantine camps. A notice was published in the Königsberg Official Gazette on August 14, 1831, and August 18, 1831. It was reported that the quarantine camps, Packmohnen (14 miles from Tilsit) and Schernen (4.6 miles from Prökols had "no suspicious health circumstances."[18]

The second question to be settled was whether the Prussian government would allow the Polish refugees to remain in Prussia. Almost immediately after the Polish generals and their men defected to Prussia, a Russian General named Kreje, began negotiations and demanded the release of the Polish refugees. However, as one Polish officer's bitterly recounted, the reason why the Poles were not delivered to the Russians was because the "Prussians were not able in the eyes of Europe to violate the law of nations even though in their hearts they would like to have done so."[19]

That the refugees or at least their leaders would be assured sanctuary in Prussia was still not certain. Russia was applying pressure to deliver the generals and some of the leaders of the insurrection to Russia. On July 13, 1831, the day of the defection, Vice Chancellor Nesselrode in Russia wrote a confidential dispatch to Baron von Maltitz, who was appointed *chargé d'affaires* at the Berlin court in the summer of 1831 following the death of Count Alopeus. Nicholas requested the Prussian government extradite generals Chłapowski, Gielgud, and Rohland as well as several other leaders of the insurrection.[20]

On July 22, 1831, Chad wrote, that he was informed that three Russian generals had approached the "Prussian authorities to deliver up to Russia the Polish prisoners who have taken refuge on the Prussian frontier." He expressed his concern to the Prussian Minister of Foreign Affairs, Count Bernstorff "that the request not be granted." Bernstorff carefully avoided committing himself by stating that he was "respecting the manner in which the King may think proper to decide upon this question." Chad concluded, "I feel it in my own mind that there is no probability that the Prisoners will be delivered to Russia."[21]

Baron von Maltitz delivered his note to Minister Ancillon on August 6, 1831, "demanding the release of [Generals] Szymanowski, Roland and other Polish and Lithuanian insurgents, as well as arms, rolling stock, horses and artillery."[22] Nevertheless, even with all the protests the king had already made his decision on July 14, 1831, when General Krafft offered the Polish generals a signed document proffering them "protection and residence" on behalf of the king in the Prussian territories if they laid down their arms and underwent quarantine.[23]

Although not prepared for such a major defection General Krafft began making immediate arrangements for the quarantine of the Polish troops. General Chłapowski and his troops were sent to two camps, a small one for officers called Aszecken and nearby a larger camp at Schernen for non-commissioned officers and soldiers near the Minge River. The two camps were in the Memel district. There 249 officers and 2,361 non-commissioned officers and soldiers quarantined in the two camps. Generals Rohland and Szymowski and their men were quarantined at Packmohnen near the city of Tilsit. This camp contained 359 officers and 3,904 non-commissioned officers and soldiers. General Krafft had to find accommodations and supplies for over 611 officers and 6,265 non-commissioned officers and soldiers almost immediately.[24] This total did not include non-military servants, officer's wives, and the wives of fallen officers from the last battle. In addition, accommodations had to be found for camp followers and laundresses who also had to be quarantined.[25]

Information concerning conditions in the quarantine camps, especially Packmohnen, is of interest because it addresses the Prussian attempt to prevent the cholera from spreading throughout Prussia and the treatment Polish refugees received during their quarantine in Prussia. From the Polish perspective, the treatment the refugees received during the time spent in Packmohnen can be best expressed in the well-known Polish proverb when commenting on living conditions "as poorly as in Packmohnen"[26]

The Prussian military was not prepared for the influx of this many refugees and the order to quarantine them. The Polish soldiers were inspected for any illness especially cholera, the sick and wounded were separated and cared for immediately. The king ordered a special allowance of provisions for the Polish troops, equivalent to the same rations as the Prussian soldiers. The arrangements were made under the most "strenuous conditions possible." The Prussian officers planned to provide provisions for the camps at Schernen and Packmohnen with stores of food warehoused near the two camps. The supplies for Schernen were to be obtained from Memel and for Packmohnen from Tilsit. However these provisions were not available until shortly after the troops reached the quarantine camps.[27]

The Polish officer, Konstanty Gaszyński, wrote an account of his journey from the Prussian border to Packmohnen and of his stay in the camp. Following the signing of the agreement between General Krafft and General Szymanowski, the general returned to his troops and communicated to them the terms of the agreement. At seven that morning, the men began to walk into Prussian territory. The officers were permitted to keep their swords. The troops had to surrender their weapons at the border. The men proceeded along a narrow path surrounded on both sides by Prussian guards who stood approximately five paces between them while local villagers reluctantly eyed the passing soldiers.

After spending the night nearby, the next morning they continued their march to the camp. They marched for an hour and stopped for an hour. There was no shelter, the heat was unbearable and there was no water available. After another hour they continued their journey and soon the town of Laugallen appeared before them. The soldiers could not go into Laugallen but instead they entered a yard with "double the number of guards on both foot and horseback. According to his account the soldiers requested something to drink from the Prussian officers. The Prussian guards did not have rations for them. The soldiers were forced to purchase food and drink from the locals."[28]

The food that was available included milk, bread with butter and water. The soldiers began to feel better but complained with no future wages or salaries where would the money come from to pay for food later. As it was, they had to pay dearly for the bread and water they received. Fear of cholera made the people suspicious of the soldiers. They refused to give the soldiers the food directly. Also some felt the Polish money was infected and so "some of the money went unclaimed."[29]

The soldiers slept on the ground in the hot sun. They waited for food and straw to be distributed as promised by Prussian General Major von Stülpenagel, chief commander of Packmohnen and Schernen. Meanwhile, the soldier's horses were becoming weak as a result of the scorching sun. That evening, the soldiers were informed that they would be taken to a healthier location and supplied with water, food and straw as well as a finished barracks for the officers and soldiers.[30]

In the official report for the Prussian government undertaken by a Captain Dankbahr he explained that there was an inevitable delay in laying out the camps and their locations because the king had to take "partly into consideration the disinfection and quarantine of the Polish troops, and partly where they should be quartered later." In the first case, the health of the soldiers had to be investigated to determine if they were completely free of cholera. They were placed in the camps because the plan was to move non-commissioned officers and soldiers once they had completed quarantine, north to Samland in East Prussia between the Baltic Sea, the Lagoon and the Pregel River. The officers were to be quartered in Königsberg and in the towns south of the city. However, before they could be released from the camps the soldiers had to be certified free of cholera before they could leave the camps and be distributed among the population.[31]

The next morning supplies arrived as promised and the men received "bread, meat and vodka." They marched between their Prussian guards who had arranged themselves in a fencelike formation for approximately 4.6 miles along the road to the camp at Packmohnen. Packmohnen, was "excessively humid and near a lake devoid of any greenery, cold with only a small cottage that housed the two generals and their staffs."[32] The other officers and soldiers were given straw and a few sticks and sent into a barracks. The camp was divided into two parts closely guarded by Prussian soldiers on foot and horseback. Also, stationed on the other side of the lake were armed Prussian soldiers standing five paces apart. They "could not have been more closely guarded if they had been "prisoners of the Russians."[33]

Because cholera was considered contagious at the time it explains why the Polish soldiers were interned in quarantine camps with unusually strict controls (based on regulations issued by the Immediate Commission on April 5, 1831, and June 1, 1831). Further, it explains why they were treated more like "prisoners" than refugees seeking asylum and why they were threatened with severe punishments if they tried to escape from the camps. According to the regulations of June 15, 1831, those who tried to evade quarantine (this included the Prussian civilian population) and "evade the guards and patrols," after being warned by them, the guards could "use their weapons and without further consideration, shoot the transgressors."[34]

However, the Polish officers may not have known how strict the quarantine measures were for civilians in Prussia, or been aware of the palpable fear these soldiers created when they first entered Prussian territory as refugees. In April, when it appeared cholera would enter Warsaw, the original policy was to try to isolate Warsaw from the military on the orders of Governor Krukowieki. The attempt at a quarantine was seen as an "embarrassment" by the government and with the support of medical opinion (and the war conditions) the plans for the 'strict isolation of the sick" were reversed.[35] The Polish soldiers had no long-term experience with strict quarantine measures. Their government had not imposed quarantine but rejected it. They must have been puzzled by the officious way these regulations were carried out by their Prussian guards, including orders to shoot any transgressors.

Ironically, Polish newspapers in Warsaw published numerous articles on the Polish soldiers stay in Prussia. On July 21, 1831, one newspaper reported the soldiers were in a quarantine facility similar to the facilities on the border. It was reported as a fenced in area with three buildings. Each building staggered the inmates according to their time of arrival and if someone became ill they were taken to a military hospital. There were chambers for men and women. In addition there was a shed for fumigating their effects, adequate food and straw for sleeping on mats. However, in an excerpt in a letter from an officer being held in one of the camps published by the same newspaper on August 2, 1831, the reader was informed the soldiers had been "enclosed in a cholera camp and were under the open sky for 21 days."[36] The cholera camp for the Polish soldiers was not modeled on the standard quarantine facility but neither were the soldiers entirely under the open sky for the entire time of their internment (as huts and barracks were provided).

Nevertheless, the soldiers were strictly supervised and as Dankbahr explained, at the time of Gielgud's defection "the strict measures used to guard Gielgud's bivouacked Corps were dependent on the still prevailing view of the contagiousness of cholera" and "the state laws were strictly applied as were the official medical regulations." The fear of infection from the Poles produced an attempt in some communities to implement even stricter blockade measures against cholera than called for in official regulations. Localities were given permission by the Immediate Commission on August 1, 1831 "to isolate themselves from contaminated areas ... the inhabitants had to stand guard themselves and pay to move the post office to the outskirts of the town."[37]

The Polish Soldiers in Packmohnen

Between the accounts by Dankbahr and Gaszyński we can obtain a reasonably good description of the Prussian treatment of the soldiers in the camp at Packmohnen, the conditions of the soldiers in the camp, the later Polish resistance to their "captivity" and the reasons for the strong Prussian response, especially toward those attempting to escape.

From the beginning the king ordered that the Polish soldiers receive the same amount of food as the Prussian troops. The Commandant "made strenuous efforts to meet this requirement." The proximity of Memel and Tilsit to Schernen and Packmohnen where food storage warehouses were located made it easier to carry out these instructions.[38] The Prussian authorities maintained a daily grant for the Polish troops. Generals were allowed two talers, officers one taler, lower officers five silver groschen, non-commissioned officers and soldiers three silver groschen and six pfennigs. Clearly, General Stülpnagel believed some of this was too generous and said so, since "gentlemen officers have no need to pay for housing and food" that money should be "automatically deducted."[39] He also asked General Rohland if individual officers preferred "food rations in kind or money?" The officers preferred to purchase their own food.[40] As for the distribution of rations, the generals received 6 times the daily rations, the lieutenant colonels, majors and the Chief Medical Officer three times the daily allowance, the remaining officers one and a half to two times the daily allowance and the rest a single ration.[41]

The average number of food portions received daily for July 16, 1831, through July 31, 1831, for the Packmohnen camp (excluding the hospital) was 3,774 and the average daily food portions for the total period from July 16 to August 31, was 3,780. For the lazaret, the average number of food portions from July 16 to August 31, was 185. The latter was based on the number of sick with the peak period from July 23 through July 30, averaging 248 food portions.[42] Dankbahr reported that due to the adverse weather at the beginning of August the soldiers were granted extraordinary portions "as a preservative against cholera, especially soups."[43] We have evidence that an increase in rations did occur although the word extraordinary may be somewhat of an exaggeration. According to General Rohland's accounts, food portions from August 1, 1831, through August 7, 1831, averaged 3,865 per day an increase over the average daily portions of 3,780 for the overall period under discussion.[44]

In addition, the oldest General was also given 1,000 talers to "remedy the pressing needs" of his men. Packmohnen camp soldiers were undoubtedly "poorer" because many of the detainees were not Polish but Lithuanian partisans.[45] These men had not had the time to be either considered or promoted to the rank of officer. On average they received lower food portions and money grants. In an attempt to remedy the situation General Rohland ordered that some of his soldiers that suffered from low wages be promoted to officers. Rohland saw this as an effective way to maintain better discipline and raise the wages for some of his men so they would be qualified to receive higher daily payments of food and money. By August 26, 1831, the number of officers had increased from the 361 at the beginning of the internment to 421.[46]

Another factor contributing to the charge of low wages, especially for the lowest ranked soldiers, was a market established outside the camp at Packmohnen. It was set-up to "improve the food and supplies" by having them brought in from around the countryside. The market maintained the quarantine because it was specially surrounded by a military blockade in a fortified area with strict controls. Here the local inhabitants could sell and purchase goods from the soldiers.[47] Gaszyński reported the citizens of Tilsit did not miss the opportunity to sell their goods to the refugees at highly inflated prices. Each day "liquor merchants, tobacco sellers and purveyors of other goods that included butter and vegetables set themselves up in front of the camp in a place marked out by the authorities." The soldiers complained, however, that they had to pay dearly for this "Prussian hospitality." For example, a "bottle of wine that cost two francs in Tilsit" cost at least "seven francs" at the camp market. The prices of other goods and supplies were also inflated.[48]

The Poles complained bitterly they had to sell their precious horses in the most unfavorable manner to merchants who "mercilessly stripped them of their money" for oats and hay. "They had to sell their horses at half-price, the price the merchants set themselves."[49]

Nevertheless, the buyers were still cautious of disease in purchasing from the Poles. They received their money on "a long spoon and washed the money in vinegar." Another example of this caution was the visit of a cousin of one of the Polish officers from Tilsit. The visitor had to stand "twenty paces away while Prussian soldiers stood by with rifles and bayonets." The Polish officer was told that if he took "one step they would use their weapons." Another story concerned a tailor from Tilsit who looking to make a living got into the camp and was taking measurements of a few officers." He was caught and returned to the city where he was "placed in a separate room for a few days, bathed in vinegar, isolated, and set free"[50]

Gaszyński wrote, "despite all these ridiculous precautions against cholera our troops remained in the best of health while of the Prussians policing us, at least twenty of them passed away but not from a contagious disease" He attributed their lack of resistance to disease to the fact they had for too long become accustomed to comfort and a soft bed. When deprived of it for a few days they became weak."[51]

Traces of cholera in the Prussian troops first appeared in Scherzen and later in Packmohnen. Fortunately these remained limited to individual cases. According to the official report, the Polish troops were less subject to the cholera, "most likely because they had already experienced the disease, thus reducing their moral and physical susceptibility" to cholera.[52]

When the Gielgud Corps was placed in the quarantine camps, the prevailing view of cholera was that it was highly contagious and the public feared infection by the Poles. Individual communities were given the power with the consent of the authorities "to interdict themselves to a higher degree than the regularly prescribed measures" against cholera. The city of Tilsit, until August 8, wanted to forbid all relations with Packmohnen, even though it was expected to be the camp's primary source of supplies.[53] Tilsit's reaction was completely understandable as the government of Gumbinnen in early July had wisely advised that "a strict barrier was the best means of protection against the disease" and that "the outbreak has always been shown to be the consequence of a break in the [medical] quarantine" and most tellingly, through "secret communications with Russian and Polish subjects." In early August there were reports of a series of local cholera outbreaks that occurred August 2 through August 6. The government concluded the "reason for the spread of the disease was communication with these infected localities"[54] In the end only the strong intervention of Schön was able to avert a "growing embarrassment" for the government. The city of Tilsit was required to ease its restrictions and supply the camp at Packmohnen.[55]

On August 13, 1831, the Immediate Commission, perhaps to avoid such an embarrassment elsewhere, issued an order that "specified that the local regulations could not be more severe than those observed on the sanitary cordons." On August 28, 1831, additional regulations were issued stating that "major roads had to remain open, persons with valid identification, as well as military forces, had to be allowed passage through the quarantined localities."[56]

Description of Daily Life in Packmohnen

The Packmohnen camp was composed primarily of small huts where officers played cards, smoked pipes and talked with their colleagues. The soldiers, along with the Prussians and horses, bathed in the lake. The camp laundresses also washed clothing there. Meanwhile the soldiers used the lake water for cooking, cleaning and as a source of drinking water. (Ironically, Packmohnen had the better sanitary report of the two camps, with no cholera cases reported).[57] The soldiers cooked their food in clay pots. In the background one heard the "neighing of horses and the singing of songs about the nation and of their faith." Ever in the distance was the "grim silence of the Prussians standing guard. For the soldiers "life was monotonous" and for most of the time their lives were "inactive and dismal." The soldiers looked forward to the twentieth day when it was promised their "bondage would end."[58]

When the twentieth day came, the soldiers were informed by the camp commandant that they would not be returned immediately to Poland but would be quartered in the cities and villages in and around Königsberg. He informed them that before they could be released he needed to wait for an order from the king and there had been a delay in the arrival of the letter. They expected to remain only few more days in the camp.[59] According to Dankbahr, the delay was caused because the disinfection of the Poles had not been completed and the immediate location of where they would reside following their release was still under discussion.[60] Further evidence indicated that the refugees had not yet been officially certified as healthy, necessary in order to place the refugees in the apartments and houses in the villages and towns of East Prussia.[61]

However, before this occurred some of the refugees in Packmohnen attempted to take matters into their own hands and break free of the camp. Frustrated by this turn of events and stuck in quarantine with weather conditions deteriorating, they feared cholera might spread throughout the camp. The "rain and rough weather" lasted until mid–August.[62] As the rain fell the barracks and land began to flood, meanwhile, the "soldiers and officers were forced to occupy a small hill."[63]

In addition as General von Krafft noted on August 6, the Poles were saddled with a multitude of delusions including the rumor that "French ships would land in Memel harbor with weapons for the insurgents" or that the Poles had recently won glorious victories over the Russians."[64]

Desperate from despair, on the night of August 6, 150 soldiers, including Lithuanian insurgents and Lithuanian partisans who had been expelled from Samogitia on July 15, and quartered in Packmohnen under Rohland's command, attempted to break out from the camp.[65] The soldiers started to riot and break through the Prussian soldiers ringing the camp.[66] Naturally there was a great uproar and two squadrons of Prussian soldiers "stood ready for battle" against dozens of people armed only with "sticks and despair."[67] The Prussian soldiers fired their weapons. According to Gaszyński two Poles in "their barracks were wounded." The next morning the escaped soldiers were returned to the camp. However, other witnesses, including General Rohland, reported "the Prussians used their weapons and some on the Polish side were killed."[68] The Prussians worked through the night and the next morning positioned two Prussian guns across the lake.[69]

The camp commandant came to the Poles and asked if this was how they paid for the hospitality shown by the king. The Poles answered by making jokes. Someone "strung white handkerchiefs together as a sign of surrender." Another group of soldiers built a simple mound of earth works and added two small kegs of beer to resemble cannons to "show how absurd the two gun positions were in a camp of defenseless people." The jokes seemed to have been effective because the guns disappeared the next morning. However, the number of guards was doubled and the Prussian general met with General Rohland "to require that every regiment commander, give his assurance in writing of his subordinate's cooperation." Gaszyński reported, the declaration was given with the warning that the Prussian government keep its promise that "we linger no longer in quarantine." According to General Rohland, General Stülpnagel blamed the camp uprising on the Lithuanian partisans and threatened to remove 20 officers and 200 soldiers and turn them over to the Russians. As a result, Rohland agreed to maintain peace in the camp. This satisfied General Stülpnagel and he did not follow through on his threat.[70] To make the situation worse for the Poles, "every day came some news of the struggle in Poland and it was hard to remain idle while their countrymen were shedding their blood."[71]

The Poles tried to escape by bribing villagers to help them with clothing and guide them to the border. However, the frontier with Poland was completely guarded, "almost all the officers who tried to escape were caught." On July 20, General Rohland was informed by General Stülpnagel they had captured two officers who were "refugees from" from the camp at Schernen. However, some soldiers did escape including an officer who was helped by a Prussian and made it to Paris. Another escapee made it to Boston with the help of an American naval officer. The Lithuanian press reported some Poles had fled with the help of Lithuanian partisans. On August 28, 1831, the *Warsaw Gazette* reported 1,500 interned men had fled the camp. One eyewitness wrote this "number was exaggerated."[72]

When the soldiers were captured they were treated as criminals. According to Gaszyński, two officers were locked in a small fortress called Weichselmunde in a room containing two cholera corpses, they were told that until they gave their word of honor that they would not leave Prussia without the king's permission they would not be released from the room.[73] These men and others refused to sign the declaration. They realized they would not be able to leave Prussia until the end of the Polish campaign. The soldiers continued to hope that the king would free them from the quarantine camp. They remained in quarantine heavily guarded for over thirty days.[74]

The Quarantine Camp at Schernen

In his diary General Chłapowski, who commanded the troops at Schernen, refused to discuss his stay in the camp. However, there is some limited information from his diary concerning the quarantine camp at Schernen and from other sources although they are not as extensive as those for Packmohnen.

Dr. Flemig, regimental doctor of the first regiment of the Royal Dragoons, found himself on the border region near Memel as a result of the new sanitary cordon policy of May 18, 1831. He wrote on July 13, 1831, that some 3,000 men of the Gielgud-Chłapowski Corps sought royal protection and entered Prussia at the village of Schaugsten. They had been encamped for a few days on the left bank of the Minge River at Schernen some few miles northwest of Memel. The lay out of the Schernen camp and accommodations were similar to that of Packmohnen except rather than being situated on a lake the camp was on the left bank of the Minge River a non-navigable river with many shallow locations making it easy to cross. The camp was divided in two terrace shaped divisions and the space between them was a swampy area with a pedestrian bridge. Chłapowski wrote that the camp was "at least on a river with clear water and about three miles from Memel."[75]

The soldiers were settled in two quarantine camps. The smaller camp was called Azecken and was reserved for officers. The larger quarantine camp Schernen was for non-commissioned officers and enlisted men. Those soldiers in the Schernen quarantine camp were not as fortunate as those at Packmohnen or Aszecken concerning cholera.

The smaller camp Aszecken, housed 162 officers and 183 soldiers that served the officers. In Schernen there was one general, 98 officers, 221 non-commissioned officers and the remaining were enlisted men. The troops in Schernen were housed in straw huts in the camp, with a few Polish women functioning as domestics.[76] When Chłapowski's troops first defected, Dr. Kohler, who became the director of quarantine for the two camps, investigated the sanitary condition of the troops. He determined there were 308 wounded men and 20 who were sick, but none with cholera.[77]

By the time the two camps were established both contained infirmaries. The infirmary in the smaller camp contained 40 wounded and 7 sick, the larger camp infirmary contained 9 officers, 88 enlisted men and of these 46 were wounded and 51 sick. At this time "there was no sign of cholera."[78]

However, Dr. Flemig who was assigned to the Memel district and also to the quarantine camp noted on July 18, one soldier, an invalid, became sick. He was not familiar with cholera and so was extremely cautious in his diagnosis. He later wrote that "after every doubt had been eliminated [the victim] was found to suffer from the cholera." Flemig described this first victim who he found at the edge of the swamp behind "a makeshift straw shelter." The victim had "sunken eyes, a raspy cholera voice, wailing and flailing his limbs and with soiled clothing." The following morning "his corpse was found with his limbs distorted and his body dark blue." He concluded "cholera was ... in the Polish camp."[79]

The following morning another person was found dead with the same cholera characteristics. On July 19, five more men sickened from cholera. The prescribed quarantine measures were implemented in the camp as there was no doubt the cholera was spreading. Dr. Flemig left the camp to treat a sick Prussian royal dragoon with cholera symptoms who he found in a barn serving as a storehouse. He later attended to another dragoon who was diagnosed with cholera. He died on July 28. He also treated civilian cholera victims in Memel before he returned to the camp.[80]

Flemig returned to Schernen on July 28 and wrote a report noting that a number of royal Prussian troops (in their encampment) and Polish soldiers in the camp had become ill with cholera. The treatments employed were standard for the time and included bleeding, prescribing opium and making the patient sweat. He concluded this was about as much as could be done given the circumstances in the camp.[81]

Flemig reported that a short distance from the camp there were two small houses "about 100 steps from the river." He had the two houses designated "as cholera lazarets." The sick were immediately removed from the camp and placed in this "isolated area. The houses were small with only two rooms each, one room was a little more than five feet high the other a windowless room. Because of their size no more than five men could be placed in each house. The secondary rooms were used for supplies."[82] Due to the outbreaks in Schernen, Schön published an announcement on August 10 in the *Königsberg Amtsblatt* that the Prussian military had been "ordered to blockade" the camp.[83]

According to Dr. Flemig, the number of patients that contracted cholera in Schernen from July 28 to September 3, numbered 32. Of the 32 sick, 31 were cholera cases; of the total sick, 17 recovered and 15 died. Flemig concluded there were two factors that led to this high death rate: first this cholera was especially acute; and second, too much time passed before the victims were taken to the lazaret for treatment.[84] Not included in this number were two Prussian soldiers who contracted the cholera and were taken to Memel to be treated. Both subsequently died.[85]

Dr. Flemig observed the sanitary conditions in the Polish camp were better than in Memel; this was shown by the fact that the number of sick was considerably less in the camp than in Memel. He attributed the better conditions to the movement of fresh air in the camp as compared to many of the dwellings in Memel where the "trapped air in the homes was favorable to the distribution" of cholera. In addition, none of the medical personnel working in the lazarets became ill because most of their work was done in the "open air and all the requirements for the patients were kept outside."[86]

In general the camp at Schernen was "quieter" than Packmohnen. Some of this can be attributed to the Lithuanians (many were insurgents and not trained soldiers as noted previously) who were quartered at Packmohnen.[87] Oddly, Chłapowski had been so successful in Lithuania that it was said he raised new regiments as if he had a "magic wand." In recognition of his success the Polish government awarded him a Commander's Cross and made him Chief Commander of Lithuania.[88]

Unfortunately, two weeks later he entered Prussia and laid down his arms, resulting in a flurry of harsh criticism for his actions.[89] At the end of July, he received the order dated June 29, 1831, appointing him Commander of Lithuania. Along with the appointment came 100,000 złoty for "war needs." Even though there were complaints of conditions in Packmohnen where the majority of the Lithuanians where located, he did not want to distribute these funds on foreign soil and wished to return the money. His officers forced him to divide the funds among themselves. Later in 1833 all the monies were returned to the Bank of the Kingdom of Poland.[90]

Conditions in Schernen could not have been as trying as reported in Packmohnen if Chłapowski did not feel it necessary to distribute the funds he received specifically for the support of his troops. However, the Schernen camp had its share of unrest but not as a consequence of poor conditions or ill treatment.

The Decision to End the Quarantine for the Polish Soldiers

By early August an official decision had been made concerning the fate of the Polish soldiers. In order to move forward on the decision a public acknowledgement of the sanitary conditions in the camps was necessary. At the beginning of August, the camp Commandant, General Stülpnagel came to the Poles at Packmohnen to tell them "he had finally received the order from the king that the soldiers would be quartered in the small towns and villages in the Königsberg district. But he had to wait for a delegation of doctors, who had not yet "arrived to assess the health of the soldiers." According to General Krafft the order to inspect the health of the Polish troops was "in anticipation of the highest order of his Majesty the King, concerning the future destination of the Polish troops based on their continued shelter in the Prussian Royal territory, and the utmost rigor of their accrued time in quarantine."[91]

On August 11, 1831, government medical councilor, Dr. Albers and Dr. Linden a regimental doctor, inspected the officers and enlisted men at Packmohnen. They confirmed the soldiers had since July 15, 1831, been observed on a daily basis and at no time had there been a case of cholera, nor was there now any current suspicion of cholera. They declared the troops at Packmohnen "free of cholera ... their clothing and effects were completely clear of the sickness as well."[92]

According to General Krafft the two camps of Schernen and Aszecken were inspected on August 14, 1831, by a delegation that included the camp commandant Major Tiedwiss,

Regiment Doctor Flemig, Dr. Köhler, Captain Mack and Dr. Albers. The troops were declared cholera free. The inspectors noted that there were individuals in the infirmary wounded and sick. They appeared to be suffering from the intermittent fever and gastric disorders but with no suspicion of cholera. The inspectors concluded that it had been nineteen days since the last cholera case had occurred in the camps on July 26, 1831. They reported "the quarantine at the Schernen and Aszecken camps of the sequestered Polish troops can be lifted without concern. These troops can be declared completely healthy and above suspicion of cholera ... there is little danger from the Polish troops who may come in contact with our own population."[93]

At the time the Poles believed they had been held in the camps under quarantine by the Prussian government until the Russians had taken Warsaw. However, as Gaszyński observed they were always given the reason that they were guarded with such care because of the "fear of cholera." They were given to understand that, at least in that year, the Prussian cholera policy was "prudent." They were especially mindful that "in many places in Prussia and especially in the vicinity of Thorn and Königsberg, the disease had spread violently throughout the entire region and even in other cities."[94]

When the delegation arrived in Schernen on August 14, 1831, it was 19 days since the last cholera case in the camp. By the time the Poles were expected to be released from both camps, 20 days of quarantine would have elapsed since the last case in the camp. In retrospect this would have been in keeping with their original intent of keeping the Poles for 20 day quarantine or until they were sure they were free of the cholera.[95]

By this time the Prussian government had resolved the problem of what to do with the Polish soldiers. They were made to swear an oath in Packmohnen on September 4, 1831, that "during the duration of the present war between the Kingdom of Poland and his Majesty the Emperor of all the Russia's" they would not return home until given permission by the King of Prussia. The plan as reported by General Stülpnagel was to distribute the officers and men throughout the towns and cities of East Prussia. Those who refused to swear not leave Prussia without the permission of the king were imprisoned.[96]

In order for this plan to work, the public had to be assured that the refugees posed no immediate danger. By a detailed notice published in an official journal, the population was notified that all precautions had been observed, and that the soldiers had been held long enough to assure both the doctors (who had to truthfully attest there was no cholera) and the government that there was no chance that the soldiers would spread the disease further in Prussia.

On the day the medical delegation arrived in Packmohnen, the soldiers were ordered into the square. Dr. Albers and Dr. Linden walked between the rows of men declaring on a form that the men were healthy. The soldiers thought they were at the end of their captivity but were told they needed to remain in the camp to dispose of their quarters. Perhaps because there had been no cases of cholera or suspicious cases in Packmohnen since their arrival, the officers, were allowed to leave on horseback and even go into the city of Tilsit. According to Gaszyński, they could now "enjoy the beauty of nature" and, compared to what they had just been through, "the city of Tilsit, although small, seemed to us like Paris."[97]

Finally on September 8, 1831, the Poles in Packmohnen in their 53rd day of quarantine finally marched out of the camp and were quartered in the villages lying between the Pregel and the Friedrich-Grabe. However, according to Gaszyński, the conditions were still difficult. Officers attempting to travel in Königsberg, faced innumerable difficulties. They had to "beg General Stülpnagel in writing for permission to leave and to report afterward to all civil and military offices [this was not much different than the regular cholera travel restrictions at this time] after the expiration of the time period of a visit. If one suddenly changed travel plans he had to report to the police. They allowed only the sick and the wounded officers to live in Königsberg. Every few days, Prussian doctors would visit the latter to find out whether the patient was healed. Those that had recovered were forced to leave immediately to convalesce in the local garrison.[98]

The conclusion of the quarantine did not go as well at Schernen. The camp in general had been "quieter" than Packmohnen; however, the deteriorating weather conditions, the fact that many of the Poles felt they would never return to fight for the revolution and an "atmosphere in the camps ... of distrust and anxiety" all contributed to a mutiny on August 22, 1831. The mutiny occurred two days before the "health conditions" of the Poles in the two camps was published in the Königsberg *Amtsblatt*.[99]

As a result of the mutiny General Chłapowski, petitioned the king on August 25, 1831, after two and a half months of quarantine. His request was based on the king's order of February 11, 1831, that stated "fighting troops crossing the border will be permitted to return to their homeland." He wrote it was "no coincidence ... that the Russians retain their weapons ... [while] ... the Poles had to offer their arms at the border."

The king answered Chłapowski on September 5, 1831, but it was not communicated to Chłapowski by General Krafft until September 14, 1831. At this time, the General and his soldiers had already been in the quarantine camp for fifty-five days. They were released on September 8, 1831, and settled in the district of Fischhausen in East Prussia. His Prussian liaison was Major Tiedwiss, former Commandant of the Schernen and Aszecken camps. The king's reply and the treatment of the refugees needs to be placed in a larger context that includes the kings cabinet order of September 6, 1831; the complaints of the Polish émigré community in the west; public sympathy for the Polish cause in Prussia; and the imminent fall of Warsaw with an unexpected refugee problem on the Prussian Polish border. The king replied:

> To the Polish General Chłapowski's petition of the 25th of the previous month ... that my terms of February 11 of this year were only instructions for the commanders of our border stations.... I could not have foreseen the extensive number of troops seeking refuge in our territory that has occurred. With the defection of individuals or small detachments, as is assumed in my instructions, the commanders of the border stations have allowed them to return to their homeland. It was not intended for such a massive number of troops of many thousands of men. The measures for the distribution of officers and troops have already been made. The Imperial Russian side requested the extradition of Polish officers and privates ... there is not found to be a sufficient indication according to the existing treaties for this, and the return of the same during the remaining of the war, is quite inadmissible.
>
> Charlottenburg, 5 September 1831.
> (Signed) Frederick William.[100]

According to the king, his original order in February was only in reference to small detachments of men that could be easily cleared by local commanders at the various border stations. He indicated that he never foresaw thousands of Polish soldiers crossing the border. He did not address directly Chłapowski's complaint about Polish soldiers having to surrender their arms. However, from earlier agreements, which he referred to as "existing treaties," Prussia would honor those agreements. But he stipulated that Prussia had decided that nothing in the treaties forced Prussia to turn over the soldiers seeking refuge in Prussia and so they would not do so. By a prior agreement made on December 30, 1830, the Prussian government "ordered all Prussian authorities not to allow the passage of ammunition, to arrest those who set foot on their territory and allow no relationship between the Polish insurgents and their partisans outside the Polish territory." As far as Prussia was concerned, it was honoring its agreements, even in its refusal to turn over Polish insurgents to the Russian authorities. For example, General Chłapowski was specifically named as one of the chiefs of the insurrection in Poland. Baron Maltitz, the czar's ambassador in Berlin, requested he be extradited to Russia in a dispatch dated July 13, 1831.[101]

As for the refugees being held in a quarantine camp, it was a matter of public opinion that their health conditions be communicated to the public and this policy of quarantine was integral to the government's medical policy. It was no coincidence that Dr. Albers, who had been sent earlier to Russia as part of the Prussian Medical Commission, was appointed Camp Commandant and Quarantine Director of Packmohnen. It was his signature that appeared on the health certificates of the Schernen and Aszecken camps too. According to Dr. Lorinser, Dr. Albers was President Rust's "trusted servant" and was undoubtedly appointed to ensure that all sanitary regulations and policies were followed.[102]

Even the king up until September 6, 1831, had not wished to interfere in the actions of the Immediate Commission and (as we have seen this commission coordinated both civilian and military cholera regulations). As late as September 1, 1831, the king had informed Dr. Balz that he did not believe the cholera was infectious but that he had to "yield to the laws and the regulations given to the public." The king's hesitancy in modifying the regulations can partly be explained by the following three factors; Rust's obstinacy as head of the Medical Administration; the disease was perceived as a medical emergency combined with a medical community with limited experience with this new disease; and according to Dr. Lorinser, President Rust was a powerful adversary even for the king because it was known that "the sphere of influence under such a President … was not pleasant or desirable … [his] … intrigues inspired disgust and contempt."[103]

The king finally had enough and in his cabinet order of September 6, 1831, ordered the "Immediate Commission with further orders to publish immediately the subsequent alterations necessary to the decrees and directions already issued…." The new instructions included letting local police enforce cholera regulations, removing the interior military lines and shortening quarantine time.[104]

The king had also made arrangements as part of the refugee policy not to turn over Polish soldiers to the Russians but to maintain them until the war was concluded. The proposal to quarter the soldiers in the towns and cities of East Prussia did not contradict any earlier agreements. As the direction of the war changed and as the theater of war came closer to the border, the policy was designed to prevent "the opportunity for insurrection and insubordination" on the part of the Polish and Lithuanian soldiers in Prussia.[105] This decision was fraught with complications (especially after the fall of Warsaw and the acceptance of even more military refugees into Prussia). In some respects it earned Prussia the greater enmity of the Polish émigrés in the west than of those soldiers that had been held in the quarantine camps.[106]

Finally as for the treatment the soldiers received in the camps, according to a number of sources there was a general "sympathy and friendship" on the part of the junior Prussian officers. Gaszyński as well as others were critical of the upper ranks of the Prussian military. He wrote, Prussian officers below the rank of major showed the "refugees true sympathy and friendship but from the rank of major on up, they were all servants of Nicolas." Others noted the senior Prussian officers were distinguished by their "hostility toward the Polish cause."[107]

Others, especially during the second half of August, following the "health inspection" when the soldiers were able to establish contact with the local population, noted their "initial surprise and disbelief" that not only did Polish officers receive sympathy from the junior Prussian officers but the public referred to the "Polish people as warm and friendly.[108]

This relationship between the public and the wounded and sick soldiers in the camp was demonstrated by a thank you note from General Rohland while residing in the Packmohnen camp. It was published in a Königsberg newspaper. The note referred to a gift of linens and bandages from an "unknown lady in Konigsberg." Rohland wrote, he and his troops "had nothing to desire in respect to our sick and wounded since our arrival in the Prussia, thanks to the king. We have enjoyed all possible care, so it surprised us as a pleasant gift." But "we feel such gratitude for the sympathy that was given to us wretches here." He no doubt he chose the word "wretches" to convey the demoralized feelings of those men fit and able to fight but instead had to remain in the quarantine camps.[109]

Prussia Accepts More Refugees

With the storming of Warsaw on September 6–7, one of the major concerns of the Prussian military was to secure the borders and especially to "protect individual districts against cholera." The cholera still carried the weight of being an "eerie disease" that filled the world with "horror" and caused "whole garrisons to be gripped with panic and terror." The worst problem for the military when it broke out was resulting "disorder" which could lead to a catastrophe.[110]

Controlling the borders became very difficult for the Prussian government after the fall of Warsaw. Refugee flight became a significant problem. On September 8, 1831, the Polish army was pushed to the Prussian border and great "trains of Polish refugees, senators, and other dignitaries, all of which had been compromised in the insurrection sought safety in Prussia.[111] Prussian Major, von Brandt was sent to the border to deal with the refugee problem, including quarantining refugees before they mixed with the Prussian population. However, many of these refugees simply by passed quarantine.[112]

The local Prussian military were massed at what was expected to be a main refugee crossing point into Prussia, an area between Lautenburg and Krümmungen along the Vistula stretching about 75 to 80 miles. The army purchased food, established a magazine, a bivouac area and continued to insist on proper sanitary measures. It erected a lazaret and "took precautions against cholera, in a word nothing was omitted."[113]

However, the majority of refugees headed for the small and unprepared city of Strasburg (today the Polish city of Brodnica). General Brandt described the situation. Each day the city of Strasburg was filled with all manner of refugees, many hiding outside of the city. Those with money were able to stay in the city until they could continue their journey. By the middle of September conditions deteriorated further, supplies were expensive and merchants were exploiting the situation. The number of guards in the city increased. They began patrolling the streets. It was like "being in a war, but with no war." The frustration level was so high that, "there was no more talk of observing the quarantine measures, because the disease had broken out everywhere, Posen Danzig and Thorn. In addition, there was a lack of funds to maintain the regulations." Strasburg, you would have to "shoot the people to enforce the cholera measures." With the huge crowds even that "would change nothing." And, "it would have been a hundred times easier to be in actual war circumstances than between cholera and the inconvenience of trying to satisfy three governments ... [Poland, Russia and Prussia]" and a "crowd of people running wild on the rocks and sand without equipment or supplies."[114]

The Defection of the Polish Army

With the surrender of Warsaw and the fall of the Polish government the military had lost its leaders. There was conflict among the Polish generals. The Polish army under General Rybinski withdrew to the Prussian border. Naturally, the Prussians were concerned that the Polish army might cross the border into Poznan or in one of the other areas bordering Poland and continue the insurrection. However, without food, ammunition and other supplies the Polish military and parliament (that had withdrawn from Warsaw) asked to "retire to Prussia."[115]

On October 5, 1831, the Polish army under Rybinski crossed into Prussia. The army consisted of 20,891 men, with over 2,000 officers or those who held the rank of officer. The combined number of men in the Polish army that withdrew to Prussia including Gielgud's and Rybinski's troops totaled 27,639.[116] The Prussian king allowed this major influx of refugees to enter Prussia but his government naturally wished to exercise some control. This was necessary to secure the border areas to prevent insurrectionary activities not only from occurring on the border but also prevent the Polish cause from spreading into Prussia. General Brandt put it more bluntly: "it was the duty of the government to resort to these measures to maintain peace in East and West Prussia and protect inhabitants against the unrestrained insolence of free soldiers and to ensure against any unrest that that might result in neighboring countries."[117]

At the same time measures to ensure sanitary control were not neglected and continued to be important. Sanitary measures were clearly enumerated in two of the seven articles in the negotiated agreement to allow the military to cross into Prussia. The third article stated sanitary conditions required the officers and men be placed under "a strict five day quarantine ... and that the bivouac site be guarded by the military during the quarantine period."[118] The fifth article stated that "Polish soldiers had to follow the instructions of the Prussian sentries and patrols during the quarantine period or the full force of Prussian weapons would be used against them."[119]

In article six, like Gielgud's men who had been held earlier in quarantine and dispersed to other parts of Prussia, the Polish generals had to agree that after five days of quarantine they and their troops "on the subject of their future residence, will inevitably comply with and not leave this place without the command of His Majesty the King of Prussia."[120]

The resettlement of Rybinski's troops was "peaceful and orderly" and completed by the middle of November. The regular troops were quartered in the districts of Danzig, Marienburg, Stuhm and Elbing. Officers were quartered in Marienwerder, Rosenberg and Mohrungen.[121]

Although unrelated to cholera directly, a word should be said about the result of Prussia taking in so many military refugees and the consequences to Prussia's reputation. The peaceful settlement soon began to deteriorate. According to General Brandt, instead of being grateful to Prussia for its "hospitality and thoughtfulness," the Poles began to prove "most ungrateful" and "began to commit mischief and fell into conflict with the authorities.[122]

Brandt wrote, the trouble was "entirely in the hands of a few intriguers" seeking to prevent the soldiers from returning to Poland and working against the acceptance of a Russian amnesty.[123] According to the émigré publication *Polonia* many of the Polish soldiers chose to be exiles "rather than enjoy the benefits and amnesty held out by the czar." The question of trying to get the Poles to either return to Poland or to emigrate to France or other places continued to perplex the Prussian government.

Once amnesty from Russia had been proclaimed, on orders from Berlin, a Civilian and Military Commission was established to gauge the level of compromise of the various refugees. The commission even sought the views of Polish authorities to help establish the basis for these categories.[124] Accordingly, three meetings were held. The first meeting was held in Elbing on December 22, the second in Neutiech on December 29, and the third in Dirschau on January 3, 1832. They occurred "without bloodshed but not without the use of force."[125] However the culmination of an undercurrent of rebellion occurred in the city of Fischau on January 27, 1832. When the commission arrived, the situation was developing into an unpleasant one. The Prussian military was removed and only a few soldiers remained while the commission continued its work.[126] The Polish soldiers and local population had arrived early and had been drinking in the taverns all day. This led to fights and questions about the role of the committee. "What were they doing here" and "we are all compromised" were some of the more notable criticisms. Eventually fights broke out. Finally, the local Prussian commander gave the order to fire. Nine men fell dead and others were wounded.[127]

The fugitives attempted to escape but were rounded up by locals using "clubs, pitchforks and guns." The fugitives were handed over to the court in Marienburg. This event made a poor impression outside of Prussia. It was written up in the foreign press as another example of Prussian ruthlessness. In the émigré press, it was referred to as a "massacre," sarcastically described as Poles revolting "against Prussian authorities, armed only with sticks, conspiring against the safety of the state."[128]

As a result of the uprising, the classification system was abandoned at the beginning of February. The question of how to deal with the refugees continued to frustrate the Prussian government and led to a number of different decrees throughout the spring of 1832. In March, the king even offered a two month grant to soldiers and civilians who were seriously compromised to leave for France and England.[129]

Finally on May 25, 1832, the king decided to "end this drawn out relationship with Polish refugees" and those who refused to return to their homeland or to leave for abroad. They were to be "strictly supervised and ordered to work to receive food and other necessities." They were ordered to do excavation work in Prussian military fortresses. In order to avoid complaints of mistreatment they were expected to do the same work as civilian convicts located in these fortresses but were to be "kept apart in all other aspects."[130]

At the end of July the "refugee business" was ended. This was demonstrated by the following results; of the 3,972 refugees still in Prussia, 3,221 had returned to the Polish Kingdom or Imperial Russia; 592 refugees were relocated to the fortress at Danzig or Graudenz and 114 wealthy refugees were awaiting a decision from the czar.[131]

Unlike the cholera measures, which were enacted independent of any thought of the Polish insurrection and based on known medical procedures, the humanitarian gesture of accepting thousands of refugees in the middle of a cholera epidemic was not without considerable medical risk. In return, the Prussian government attempted to exercise control over the refugees during the entire course of the epidemic.

Ironically, both the attempt to prevent the cholera and to accept the Polish refugees led to later complaints against Prussian policy during and immediately following the insurrection from the Poles and sympathetic western governments. So much so, that early on it was reported with regard to the Polish refugee situation that the king wished for a "a true representation of this entire odious Polish story ... supported by documents" from the Foreign Office.[132]

Even the Russians expected more cooperation from Prussia than they received. Prussia's strict cholera quarantine measures during the war and the unexpectedly pro–Polish refugee policy were unacceptable to Nicolas. In September 1832, Nicolas found himself confounded by Prussia's attitude once again with regard to reimbursing Prussia for having taken in the Polish refugees. In the midst of the Belgian question, about measures to be taken against liberalism, as well as several other minor issues, there developed "a significant difference of opinion between the Russian government and the one in Berlin." In one notable aspect, given the background I have provided, it was probably not unexpected that Nicolas "lost his temper." This happened when the Prussian ministers replied they were "not satisfied with a sum of nearly 800,000 talers" to be paid to Prussia from the Russian treasury "for the Polish insurgents who had found a refuge in Prussia." The Emperor maintained this was "so contrary to all sense of justice, I would say even of delicacy" that he was reluctant to believe the answer had been approved by the Prussian government.[133]

12. Prussia, Cholera and the Polish Refugee Crisis

As we have seen, throughout the Russian-Polish war it appears the czar was sometimes as frustrated with Prussia's cholera policy as with the revolutionary government in Poland. As for the western powers, Prussia was continually criticized for its cholera policy during the Polish insurrection and criticism from everyone, for its handling of the Polish refugees during the revolt and after the fall of Warsaw.

Conclusion

On the eve of the cholera epidemic in Prussia, medical officials were actively trying to discover the nature of cholera and to decide whether or not it was contagious. They looked to the Russian experience for immediate guidance. A Doctor's Commission was dispatched to Russia to determine whether the cholera was contagious and how best to treat the new disease. If it was deemed contagious, they could look to their own past that included the Prussian Plague Regulations of 1709. For Dr. Rust, an Austrian by birth and the architect of Prussia's initial policy, he admitted the highly successful and more contemporary Austrian plague regulations and infrastructure along the Turkish border served as a successful model. This model worked for Austria and would most likely for Prussia too. However, Prussian officials proceeded with caution. They wanted assurance the disease was contagious before imposing a land and water quarantine. They were acutely aware of the financial burden that would be placed on their own government. Of the four doctors that traveled to Russia on the Doctor's Commission to observe cholera there, on their return three reported the cholera contagious. As a result, the Immediate Commission implemented a strict quarantine based sanitary policy.

Cholera entered Prussia by two routes. The first was in early May 1831, in the government district of Gumbinnen on the Prussian-Russian border. The second occurred at the end of May by way of the city of Danzig. Prior to the second incursion the Prussian government had already begun taking measures to prevent cholera from making any further inroads into Prussia. On May 5, the government called the first meeting of an Immediate Commission to investigate and prevent cholera. The Immediate Commission under the medical leadership of Doctor Rust and headed by General Thile ordered extraordinary and detailed prophylactic measures to prevent cholera from entering Prussia. These measures included a military cordon spanning the approximate 550 mile Prussian border with Russia and Poland. Inspection offices and quarantine facilities were ordered as well. Ships had to undergo quarantine at Prussian seaports and along Prussian rivers. Travelers were issued health passes by the authorities. Money, goods and people were inspected and disinfected in quarantine stations at towns and border crossings.

One major question raised by Ackerknecht and most recently by Baldwin, in the case of Prussia in 1831, was can one speak of a "prophylactic strategy" based on ideology?" The answer is that in Prussia there was no long term commitment to an ideological "prophylactic strategy." There was no "pertinent distinction ... between conservative interventionism and laissez-faire." Instead there was a more pragmatic approach in which the degree of intervention was modified in stages as Prussian officials gained more experience with the cholera. They noted the failure of the initial policy and experienced the unrest resulting from the strict measures first ordered by the Immediate Commission. Ironically, opposition to the initial reactionary interventionism was not championed by prominent state physicians but by non-medical local officials, independent physicians and state officials (including the king), who were faced with the economic and social consequences of what quickly came to be seen as an ineffective quarantine policy. The struggle was played out even in "despotic Prussia" not over many years but over the course of the first cholera epidemic. It became clear to the Central government that the strict interventionist sanitary policies promoted by the Immediate Commission were ineffective, costly and socially destabilizing.

Prior to the cholera epidemic, Prussia did not have a centralized "medical police" super structure. During the "reform era," the government decentralized the administration of the state and this included the medical administration. Stein's City Ordinance of November 1808 transferred public health matters from the state to city administrations. In 1815, new provincial medical boards and sanitary commissions were established, subordinate to the local governments but not answerable to a central medical authority. They now answered to the new office of the provincial president. In 1817, with the creation of the Ministry of Religion, Education and Medical Affairs, all medical matters were transferred to one ministry. Unfortunately this led to conflicts due overlapping areas of medical and public health authority between the new Ministry and the Ministry of the Interior. The inability to administratively resolve these issues by re-organization within one ministry placed the medical departments under the scrutiny of an Immediate Commission to reform the state budget with a mandate to cut costs.

Rather than emerging with a solution to the paralysis plaguing the Prussian medical administration the opposite occurred. The budget reform commission made its cost cutting recommendations in 1824. In 1825, the medical police and related public health responsibilities were transferred out of the Ministry of Religion, Education and Medical Affairs to the Ministry of the Interior. As a result, medical education and research were separated from the policing of public health and medicine. What this meant in 1831, on the eve of the first cholera epidemic in Prussia was that there was no unified medical administration within the government to oversee a response to the cholera. There were two departments within two ministries with overlapping areas of responsibility.

The problem was temporarily resolved with the first meeting of the Immediate Commission on May 5, 1831. The purpose of this commission was to centralize the administrative response and provide immediate communication among all critical Prussian ministries including the military. By including medical representatives from both Ministries it temporarily resolved the overt conflict over areas of responsibility the two departments had continued to wage before and after 1825. The open conflicts of overlapping areas of responsibility were temporarily resolved, but with the dissolution of the Immediate Commission in January 1832, conflict between the two ministries resumed. It was not to be resolved until the two departments were unified under the authority of the Ministry of Religion, Education and Medical Affairs in 1848.

Once cholera was considered contagious the response of the Prussian government and medical administration was to model the regulations on the Prussian Plague regulations of 1709. This included border security, health passes, house quarantines and so forth.[1] It was the local decentralized government organizations and medical organizations made up of private physicians from the reform era that later opposed these regulations issued by the central authorities in Berlin and helped overturn these strict interventionist measures.

Following the end of the cholera epidemic in January 1832, the Prussia government initiated a comprehensive policy to deal with cholera and other contagious diseases. The need for a policy was partly a result of the confusion and conflict created by the strict measures imposed in Prussia over the course of the epidemic in the prior year. In addition, Prussia had no previous contagious diseases laws except for the earlier plague legislation of 1709.[2] Any future policy would need to serve as the basis for legislation and for pragmatic medically based administrative measures concerning plague, cholera and other contagious diseases. Because of the experience gained from the partially discredited interventionist approach during the cholera epidemic in 1831, it quickly became obvious cholera did not seem as contagious nor did it to spread in the same way as plague. This approach was reflected in the Prussian Cholera Act of February 2, 1832, and the later Contagious Diseases Law of August 8, 1835. Ironically, the two most important infectious diseases laws in Germany followed in the wake of two national disasters. The 1835 law in Prussia followed the cholera epidemic of 1831. The *Reichsseuchengesetz* of June 30, 1900, in Germany followed the cholera epidemic in Hamburg 1892.[3]

Impact on the Social Question

It is important to be clear that this sanitary policy did not address the developing "social question" in Prussia and did not reflect any improvement for the health or welfare of the lower classes in Prussia. It addressed the congruent needs of government officials sympathetic to the economic interests of the middle class that they saw as critical to the future economic welfare of the state. For the Prussian bourgeoisie the highest priorities at the time were political and economic in nature. They demanded that elusive constitution that would give them political participation in the state. They supported a liberal ideology that promoted more personal and economic freedom. The middle class was not prepared to support an interventionist medically based social policy that they would have seen as leading to more State interference and required coercive enforcement.

As for the bureaucracy, some members were sympathetic to free trade but it had not evolved to face the "social question." Any chance of reforms being introduced at the bureaucratic level following the cholera epidemic were unlikely because the linkage between the educational and research divisions of the medical administration and the medical police departments in Prussia was not resolved until the two departments were unified in 1848. Secondly, the bureaucracy continued to operate with outmoded prescriptive "camaralist" sanitary policies based on "increasing the population" for the state rather than combining social reforms with political reforms. Doctor Rudolph Virchow summed up this approach of the state bureaucracy even in 1848 with reference to the victims of the typhus epidemic in Silesia. His sentiment would not have seemed foreign to members of the middle class in the 1830's, "civil servants had not been appointed to serve their [typhus victims] interests rather they were appointed by the police state to serve the interests of the state."[4] However, to be fair, even Virchow's ideas advocating higher wages, improved working conditions, better housing and sanitary policies for the population known as "social medicine" were not acceptable to the liberals let alone the bureaucrats in the late 1840's and it would not be until the 1860's that "social medicine" policies under a more conservative leadership in Prussia took hold.[5]

Unlike the more famous Silesian Weaver Revolt in 1844, the uprising in Königsberg in July 1831 did not set off a "major public discussion of the social question in Germany."[6] The question was virtually ignored following the urban cholera riot in Königsberg in 1831. Both events did involve hundreds of rioters. In the Weaver Revolt, there were 12 deaths reported and in the cholera uprising eight deaths were reported.

However, the context was quite different in 1831. The French July Revolution of 1830 struck fear into the conservatives in Europe. It was viewed as a destabilizing event. The fear inspired by cholera raging in Russia and Poland, and then the outbreak of cholera in Prussia became linked with the uprising in Poland. The Prussian government initially feared the 'tumult' in Königsberg as possibly a political conspiracy rather than a "worker's revolt" or a populace dissatisfied with their general conditions. This issue was investigated during the trials following the riot with particular attention being paid to whether it was a political conspiracy. It was not that Prussian officials feared a popular uprising as much as they feared that "revolutionaries might capitalize on the popular discontent to advance their conspiracies." A fear that had its origins in the year's following the Congress of Vienna.[7]

Initially, the *Prussian Gazette* reported the "tumult" as a "misunderstanding of the interpretation of the measures against the cholera" between the local authorities who ordered a modification of the strict regulations and the police who had not received the new orders and implemented the harsher measures. Additionally, the paper reported the public felt the "physicians instead of healing them were trying to poison them." The misunderstanding of the timing of the repeal of the strict cholera measures sparked the riot among journeyman artisans and quickly spread to the lower classes. The result was eight deaths, numerous injuries, imprisonments and the destruction of property throughout the city and suburbs. The accounts presented at the trial of the rioters showed evidence that most of culprits were basically confined to the poorest elements in the city. The other classes did not demonstrate sympathy toward the rioters. The mob attacked officials and physicians as well as local militia members who tried to quell the riot and protect property. The workers, artisans and upper classes supported the government soon after the riots began once they were notified that the strict quarantine regulations had been lifted. The new regulations were no longer a threat to the economy of the city or the individual livelihood of most of the working population of the city. In order to provide employment during this difficult time and to avoid the chance of more riots, the president of the province ordered public works projects in the city.

Although there were over 500 arrests resulting from the riot the number of individuals eventually tried and punished was much reduced. The conclusion was that there was no conspiracy and there were no "ringleaders" tied to any revolutionary movement. The riot was a confluence of the "mob." Some rioters were simply fearful of the economic impact of the strict cholera measures on their livelihood and attempted to destroy police records. Others attacked lazarets to free comrades and family members. In addition, doctors, medical personnel as well as pharmacies were threatened because the rioters saw them as part of an overall conspiracy to poison them. Others simply took advantage of the situation to riot, destroy property and commit theft.

Once the government communicated the new regulations to the public, trust in the government was restored. This gave people the confidence to lead a "normal life" in the midst of the epidemic. The riot in Königsberg was never perceived as related to the "social question" or injustices regarding the poor, but as a protest against the government's harsh cholera regulations.

The tumult's most significant role was that it marked the beginning of an official opposition movement to the harsh regulations ordered by the Central government. The opposition was led by the Chief President Schön of the Province of Prussia, who challenged the sanitary measures of the Immediate Commission. The tumult confirmed his belief that the Immediate Commission's measures were dangerous and economically ruinous. His example illustrating the end result of these policies was the on-going misery in Danzig, because the city was forced to slavishly follow the government's strict sanitary policy.

The change in Prussian cholera policy began in Königsberg as a consequence of Schön's opposition and the example of the riot in Königsberg. As the cholera inexorably moved toward Berlin, more doctors, government and city officials became familiar with the disease and began to complain of the enormous costs, coupled with the major failures of the centralized sanitary policy. They demanded that a more realistic and cost effective approach be implemented based on local initiative and control.

The pressures on the king and his advisors began to constitute a serious threat to peace and stability in the Kingdom. Normally the king's intervention in state matters was limited and policy matters were left to his civil servants. However, in this crisis the king took actions which would normally have been left to the bureaucratic apparatus of the state, in this case his medical experts. The king's councilors and city officials had been advising him against implementing the Immediate Commission's strict interventionist policy in Berlin. On September 6, 1831, he issued a cabinet order and subsequent royal proclamation independent of the Immediate Commission that moderated the strict cholera regulations ordered by the commission.

As a result of this crisis, the king took on the more traditional role of the one legitimate authority in the state by supporting "stability and order." He was the "protector of the land from foreign conquest or sickness and defending his people from destitution." The proclamation ordered by the king during this crisis caused him momentarily to be seen as the "sacred and omnipotent figure" of the past, rather than in his contemporary, weaker role as the first servant in a bureaucratic state. With this action the king restored a sense of order and stability to the country during this crisis. He was later criticized by his medical officials for overstepping his authority. On the other hand, by displaying his "legitimate authority" decisively during this crisis he undoubtedly "gained the support of an enormous sector of the masses."[8]

During the epidemic, the Prussian government relied on its medical authorities to plan a response to the cholera. The military lines on the borders and in the interior were part of the medical response. It was not until the cholera erupted in Berlin that the king and his councilors found it necessary to reverse the Immediate Commission's policy. This was not related to any change in the status of the Polish revolt but originated in the practical experience of officials in Berlin, who now recognized the impracticality and exorbitant costs of quarantine and military cordons and the impact on trade and commerce. It was also recognized that if the latter policies were imposed it would have placed Prussia in a weak military and economic position. After all there was the possibility of more popular unrest. It occurred in Königsberg and Memel in July and in Stettin on September 2, 1831. A riot in in Berlin as a result of the strict cholera policy was not out of the question. Prussian officials and military elites undoubtedly saw that Prussia would be weakened and if necessary, would not be able to repel a feared French invasion if tensions continued to escalate among the lower classes.

This fear was palpable when the cholera arrived in Berlin. The city administration and the Prussian government had learned a hard lesson from Königsberg of the potential for unrest from the on-going interventionist cholera policy. The king modified the Immediate Commission's strict regulations and advocated a series of positive measures that he wanted introduced. He further warned he would not tolerate those who acted against the interests of the state.

To prevent a Königsberg type of riot, the Central Government, the city government of Berlin and the middle classes of Berlin all participated in providing relief to the poor in Berlin during the epidemic. The king ordered public works construction to provide temporary work for the unemployed in Berlin. The city organized a Chief Sanitary Committee as well as 61 local protection commissions based on the "poor relief" districts in Berlin. They were ordered to support hospitals, provide medicine, transportation and supplies for the sick. Local rate payers were taxed to support them. Middle class charity organizations and other volunteers jumped into the breach on behalf of the victims by collecting clothing, opening soup kitchens and providing for the orphaned children of cholera victims.

There is no doubt that the official and charitable approach to dealing with the cholera in 1831 was entirely palliative and limited to the crisis. The medical view on both sides of the debate was that the cause of cholera was a combination of diet and morality. This view inhibited any attempt to address the contributing social issues of high unemployment, sanitation, overpopulation and poverty.

The modification of official government policy at the beginning of the cholera epidemic in Berlin was accomplished by the king without regard to a resolution of the medical debate between interventionists and the non-interventionists. It was based on the pragmatic understanding of the failure of the cholera quarantine, the on-going exorbitant financial cost to the state, the negative impact on trade and the potential for popular unrest and the impact on the power and stability of the Kingdom.

Prussian Cholera Policy's Effect on Russian and Polish War Efforts

While Prussia's sanitary policy was intended for the protection of its own people, it quickly came to have unintended consequences affecting Prussia's ability to assist the Russian war effort as well as Poland's war effort. Much of the anxiety among elites in Prussia was due to the foreign policy matters that the king, his officials and the military had to consider in the midst of the cholera epidemic in Prussia. They were concerned about the domestic impact of cholera and anxious about Prussia's ability to fight a war with France alone or fight a two front war with France and Poland. The fear of France resulted from the July days of 1830 and directly affected Prussia's reaction to events in 1831. The public's tension and distrust of the government, the outright approval of revolutionary ideas emanating from France and sympathy for the Polish insurrection were recognized at the highest levels by Prussian officials and motivated the government's actions.

While Prussia was in the midst of examining the nature of cholera and determining what policy it would implement, cholera broke out in Poland. The initial Polish response was to fall back on interventionist polices established in the past for plague and impose quarantine. The General Medical Council of the Polish kingdom supported an interventionist policy but it was soon overruled by the newly appointed Central Health Committee established by the Polish revolutionary government. The latter followed the non-contagion views of the Moscow doctors and suspended the original regulations. This decision served two purposes, first the Polish government realized that in the midst of war a non-interventionist policy was impossible and would only impede the war effort. Second, it could later use this policy to its advantage to level international criticism at Prussia. To the western powers, the Polish government, military and medical establishment appeared to be united in the view that cholera was not contagious. The Polish government was able to take advantage of this united front and vigorously complain that the Prussian *cordon sanitaire* on the Polish border was simply a ploy to prevent aid from France, England and the smaller German states from reaching Poland and thus undermine the Polish insurrection.

However, sanitary policy in Poland was actually more nuanced. The almost immediate decision to accept the idea that "the cholera was not contagious" based on the experience and the judgment of doctors in Moscow was made without investigating the disease further. It was opposed in some measure by two important military men, the Governor General of Warsaw and the Chief Medical officer of the Polish army as well as a number of foreign doctors who arrived in Poland to observe and assist Polish doctors in treating the disease and who advocated for contagion and quarantine.

The Polish Foreign Office's general complaints about Prussian policy with regard to Prussian support of the Russian war effort in Poland did not take into account Prussia's nuanced interpretation of international law and "legitimacy." That aside, the initial interventionist sanitary-medical policy introduced in Prussia was based on agreed upon medical practice among medical officials of the Prussian kingdom and not based on or used as a hostile act toward Poland during the insurrection. Nevertheless, the strict quarantine measures enacted by the Prussian government were seen at the time an excuse to close the Polish borders and stop Polish inhabitants and their goods from crossing the Prussian border. The belief the cordon against Poland was part of a political plot to offer support to Russia and hinder the Polish insurrection has continued to this day.

However, as the evidence shows, once cholera broke out in Prussia and the Immediate Commission took charge of the situation there was a serious effort to create policies, administer the Prussian borders and develop internal policies to prevent the spread of cholera in Prussia. Initially, the Prussian government under the leadership of the commission was almost excessive in its medical administrative measures. These measures included minute and detailed regulations concerning boundary cordons, quarantine establishments, the isolation of the sick, trade restrictions, travel restrictions, and the establishment of cholera hospitals. These regulations were consistent with an overwhelming amount of public documentation showing how seriously Prussian officials were in attempting to prevent the disease from entering and spreading in Prussia among its inhabitants.

The outbreak of the Polish rebellion in November 1830, and the Russian response in the spring of 1830, facilitated the spread of cholera into Poland. Prussia was prepared to aid the Russians by providing a port for foodstuffs for the Russian army. As late as May 13, 1831, Frederick William III had given orders to allow the Russian army to buy supplies in East and West Prussia. This cooperation quickly cooled off following the outbreak of cholera in Danzig at the end of May.

Had cholera not broken out in Poland, the free movement of goods and other supplies across the border to the Russian troops would not have been delayed to the extent that it affected the fighting effectiveness of the Russian army in Poland. Prussia would have been freer to support the Russians more effectively although public opinion in support of the Poles would still have had to be taken into consideration. The outbreak of cholera, with the strict domestic sanitary response and Prussian public sympathy for the Polish cause, were factors that combined to inhibit Prussia from providing the level of aid Russia expected. The czar and his ministers complained bitterly about the lack of assistance from Prussia throughout the campaign. Some historians have written that individual Prussian officials sympathetic to the Poles on the border made supplying the Russian army difficult by being overzealous in their support of the cholera measures. However, this was not necessarily the case, but was part of an on-going policy directed from the highest levels of the Prussian government.[9] As the cholera spread into Prussia, the government was forced to concern itself with not only protecting the public from the disease but preventing unrest in the country as well.

Cholera Policy, Quarantine Camps and Polish Refugee Asylum in Prussia

On July 13, 1831, General Gielgud's Polish army corps crossed into Prussia. After the fall of Warsaw on September 6, 1831, a mass exodus of Polish civilians and government officials also crossed into Prussia. The subsequent defection of the main Polish army under General Rybinski into Prussia on October 5, 1831, as refugees, was a continuing humanitarian gesture on the part of Prussia. In the middle of the cholera epidemic this humanitarian gesture of taking in all these Polish refugees was not without considerable medical risk to Prussia.

At first, the Prussian government made extraordinary efforts to prevent the spread of cholera in Prussia by initially settling Gielgud's soldiers in cholera quarantine camps. Later after they had undergone a suitable quarantine, the government publically announced they were free of cholera so that the soldiers could be temporarily settled in East Prussia without incident. As for the later refugees, Prussia implemented medical procedures and quarantine facilities along the border to process them, however, the wave of Polish refugees was simply too great to handle them successfully.

Nevertheless, it was the cholera regulations and the humanitarian gesture of accepting Polish refugees that placed Prussia in an awkward domestic and international position following the end of the epidemic. These policies also affected Prussia's standing with Russia during and after the insurrection and generated the heaviest criticism from France, England and the Polish emigré communities in the west. The criticism was so intense that the king later ordered a full inquiry by the Prussian Foreign Office.

The Prussian government's treatment of the Polish refugees was not without controversial aspects following the settlements in Prussia. In the cases where Polish soldiers committed thefts, did not remain in their assigned areas or were a threat to public safety the government dealt harshly with them. However, the majority of military refugees that came to Prussia in July and the second wave of civilian and military refugees that came in early October were given the possibility of settling in Prussian cities or traveling onward to other locations. Most importantly, the soldiers and Polish government officials as well as officials who made it to Prussia were not turned over to the Russians even after the Russians demanded them. In a secret agreement between Prussia and Russia in 1830, Nicolas had added a statement that Prussia would deliver any rebels to Russia. The Prussian government refused, saying "it was impossible for them to execute the latter requirement."[10] Prussia continued its historic policy of giving asylum to political refugees.[11] In addition, Prussia initially absorbed the Polish refugees with no guarantee that it would be reimbursed for its efforts.

There was little doubt that Poland was upper most as a matter of Prussian foreign policy and Russian success was a desirable objective on the part of Prussia. However, Prussian sanitary policy during the cholera epidemic should not be seen as an excuse by Prussia to limit Poland's options and extend aid to the Russian army during the Polish uprising.

The Russians initially were given to expect more cooperation from Prussia than they received and were surprised by Prussia's frustratingly strict cholera quarantine measures during the war and the unexpectedly pro–Polish refugee policy. As we have seen repeatedly during the Polish insurrection it seems the czar was just as stymied by Prussia's attitude and policy toward Russia as the revolutionary government in Poland felt about Prussia's attitude toward it.

Finally, the Prussian experience with cholera demonstrated the need for a comprehensive approach to contagious diseases in Prussia. What was required next was a medically based solution that would bridge this gulf and serve as a foundation for a future policy that would meet the needs of the Prussian medical community, while satisfying the economic needs of the Prussian government and the developing economic power of the middle class with its emphasis on laissez-faire. The king established a commission immediately following the cholera outbreak to write a law for contagious diseases. The commission recommended a separate study of plague and therefore plague was not included in what would become the Prussian Contagious Diseases Law of August 8, 1835. This law remained on the books as the only infectious diseases law in Prussia until it was superseded in Germany by the Contagious Diseases Law of 1905.

Epilogue

Cholera continued to be a deadly disease of the nineteenth century, striking Europe as a pandemic with deadly consequences three more times. In Germany, the Hamburg epidemic in 1892 was especially devastating, killing in excess of 8,000 people. Nevertheless, over the century the various governments of Europe began to respond to cholera epidemics, eventually giving rise to sanitary policies that would improve mortality rates and contribute to a longer life expectancy for their populations.

Ironically, it was in Germany that the argument over contagion versus anti-contagionism was finally settled. Robert Koch, a German doctor, identified the cholera bacillus in 1884. He proved that particular microorganisms reproduce in the body and cause specific diseases, including cholera. The German hygienist, Max Joseph Pettenkoffer, one of the more famous supporters of anti-contagionism at the end of the nineteenth century, was not convinced by Robert Koch's research and continued to adhere to the belief cholera was spread through the air. Nevertheless, supporters of anticontagionism began to lose credibility in the scientific community as the evidence in support of Koch's findings mounted. Within the scientific and medical community the theory of anti-contagion began a quick and precipitous decline.[12] It was replaced by the germ theory of disease. The latter theory came to dominate medical science and provides the basis for today's public health measures and on-going medical research into epidemic disease.

Although cholera is considered a classic disease of the nineteenth century even today it can strike with devastating consequences. When water and sanitation systems are compromised or lacking and the government does not adequately support a sanitary infrastructure, cholera can be introduced into the water supply. Food and water become contaminated. The method for treating cholera is well known and fairly simple. It includes administering fluids with small amounts of salts to replace lost fluids. Nevertheless, cholera is a dangerous disease especially when the water supply is contaminated. It can quickly overwhelm a local population as well as the medical authorities attempting to treat the victims. The most recent example of cholera's ability to spread rapidly through an unsuspecting population and overwhelm medical authorities occurred in Haiti in October 2010, following a devastating earthquake in January of that year. As of February 2014, the United Nations reported 698,893 cholera cases in Haiti, with 8,540 deaths.[13]

Chapter Notes

Introduction

1. William H. McNeil, *Plagues and People* (New York: Anchor Press, 1977) and Alfred W. Crosby, *The Columbian Exchange* (Westport, CT: Greenwood Press, 1972). Even intellectual history, which would appear to be far removed from the impact of epidemic disease, suffered a severe blow especially in Prussia with the untimely deaths of philosopher, Georg Wilhelm Friedrich Hegel, and military theorist Carl von Clausewitz, whose writings have directly influenced intellectuals from the nineteenth to the twenty first century. Both men were victims of the 1831 cholera epidemic in Prussia.

2. Good examples of the social impact of cholera can be found in the following works, Louis Chevalier, *Le Cholera: la première épidémie du XIX siècle* (La Roche-sur-Yon: Impr. Centrale de l'Ouest, 1958); Michael Durey, *The Return of the Plague: British Society and the Cholera* (Dublin: Gill and Macmillan, 1979); R.J. Morris, *Cholera 1832: The Social Response to the Epidemic* (New York: Holmes & Meier, 1976); and for the psychological impact see Charles E. Rosenberg, *The Cholera Years: The United States in 1832, 1849, and 1866* (Chicago: University of Chicago Press, 1962).

3. On the variety of responses see Richard J. Evans, "Epidemics and Revolutions: Cholera in Nineteenth Century Europe," *Past and Present*, no. 121 (1988), 127. An early attempt to link the cholera to the English Great Reform Bill of 1832 can be found in David Eversley, "Le Cholera en Angleterre," in Chevalier, *Le Cholera*, 157–188. For developments in public health and administrative history for England see C. Fraser Brockington, "The Cholera 1831," *Medical Officer* 96 (1956) and C. Fraser Brockington, "Public Health at the Privy Council 1831–34," *Journal of the History of Medicine* 16 (1961),161–185; Margaret Pelling, *Cholera, Fever and English Medicine 1825–1865* (New York: Oxford University Press, 1978); for Russia see Roderick McGrew, *Russia and the Cholera 1823–1831* (Madison, University of Wisconsin Press, 1965) and for France, Francois Delaporte, *Disease and Civilization: The Cholera in Paris, 1832* (Cambridge: MIT Press, 1986). For the most recent work on this topic see Peter Baldwin, *Contagion and the State in Europe, 1830–1930* (New York: Cambridge University Press, 1999).

4. See Chevalier, *Le Cholera*; Delaporte, *Disease and Civilization*; Durey, *The Return of the Plague*; Richard Evans, *Death in Hamburg: Society and Politics in the Cholera Years 1830–1910* (New York: Oxford University Press, 1987); McGrew, *Russia and the Cholera*; Morris, *Cholera 1832*; Rosenberg, *The Cholera Years*; and George D. Sussman, "From Yellow Fever to Cholera: A Study of French Government Policy, Medical Professionalism and Popular Movements in the Epidemic" (PhD. diss., Yale University, 1971).

5. Barbara Dettke, *Die Asiatische Hydra: Die Cholera von 1831/31 in Berlin und den preussischen Provinzen Posen, Preussen und Schlesien* (Berlin: De Gruyter, 1995), 11–13; Werner Conze "Sozialgeschichte 1800–1850," in Hermann Aubin und Wolfgang Zorn, Hg. *Handbuch Der Deutschen Wirtschafts und Sozialgeschichte* 2 (Stuttgart: Klett-Cotta, 1976), 454; Ute Frevert, *Krankheit als politisches Problem 1770–1880* (Göttingen: Vandenhoeck & Ruprecht, 1984), 369 and see footnote 6. Two earlier works of limited value are Dietrich Helm, *Die Cholera in Lübeck* (Neumunster: Wachholtz, 1979). The latter is a brief work that provides no information on Prussia. However, see Dr. Georg Fleischer, *Die Choleraepidemien in Düsseldorf* (Düsseldorf: Triltsch, 1977), which provides some limited information on cholera in Prussia.

6. Dettke, *Die Asiatische Hydra* and Olaf Briese, *Angst in den Zeiten der Cholera* I–IV (Berlin: Akademie Verlag, 2003).

7. Richard S. Ross, "The Prussian Administrative Response to the First Cholera Epidemic in Prussia in 1831" (PhD. diss. Boston College, 1991) and Baldwin, *Contagion and the State in Europe*.

8. Dettke, 10–12.

9. Evans, *Death in Hamburg*, VIII, 258–259; Dettke, 13.

10. Dr. Ernst Horn, "Die Contagiosität der Asiatischen Cholera; aus Gruenden der Wissenschaft und Erfahrung nachgewiesen," in *Cholera- Archiv mit Benutzung amtlicher Quellen*, J.C. Albers et al. ed., 2 (Berlin: Enslin, 1832), 18.

11. J. Westland, *Report of the district of Jessore: its antiquities, its history & its commerce* 2nd ed. (Calcutta: Bengal Secretariat Office, 1874), 140; Erwin H. Ackerknecht, *History and Geography of the Most Important Diseases* (New York: Hafner, 1972), in which he wrote "the 'cholera' described by Hippocrates, much like the '*cholera nostras*' or '*cholera infantum*' of early medical authors, has nothing to do with the disease we are discussing here, except for diarrhea, which all have in common," 23.

12. Horn, 18.

13. Dr. J. Rehmann, a Russian official who corresponded with the famous Prussian physician, Dr. Christoph Wilhelm Hufeland wrote that the cholera prevailed in the northern parts of Persia in the summer of 1822 and

even in Tauris near the Russian border. Through newspaper reports he learned that the "disease which had raged so terribly in India" also prevailed in some southern regions of Persia and Turkey and had spread from Baghdad to Aleppo. People laughed at those "who predicted that probably this new plague with crushing dysentery would likely come to our part of the world." Rehman wrote he believed the disease "to be contagious." That there was "no doubt that it came by boat to Astrakhan" and was "conveyed by men and their goods from one place to another." Interestingly, he noted that "even when it erupts, it is not as contagious as the plague. The latter would later be adopted by those who were against official Prussian interventionist policy. Dr. J. Rehmann, "Die Ankunfts der orientalischen Cholera am Mittelländischen und Kaspischen Meere: Ausbreitung der Cholera in den Russischen Provinzen am Kaspischen Meere bis nach Astrachan," *Hufelands Journal der Practischen Heilkunde* III Stück, September, 1824:, 4; Horn, 23.

14. Ibid., 21.

15. The history of cholera on a broad scale has been undertaken usually in conjunction with other diseases. There are a number of important general histories including Heinrich Haeser, *Lehrbuch der Geschichte der Medicin und der epidemischen Krankheiten* 3rd ed., 3 (Jena: Dufft, 1875–82); Dr. August Hirsch, *Handbook of Geographical and Historical Pathology; Acute Infective Diseases* 2 (London: New Sydenham Society, 1883); George Sticker, *Abhandlungen aus der Seuchengeschichte und Seuchenlehre: Die Cholera* 2 (Geissen: Töpelmann, 1912); and R. Pollitzer, *Cholera* (Geneva: World Health Organization, 1959). For the epidemic in Hamburg see Evans, *Death in Hamburg.*

16. McNeil, *Plagues and People*, in which he discussed the ecological relationship between man and the ecology of microbes; and Aiden Cockburn, *The Evolution and Eradication of Infectious Diseases* (Baltimore: Johns Hopkins Press, 1963), 175.

17. This did not mean the automatic acceptance of Robert Koch's germ theory of disease by the medical establishment. In Germany, the physician, Max von Pettenkopfer, continued to receive support for his anti-contagionist theories even after Robert Koch's published findings on cholera. See C.A. Winslow, *The Conquest of Epidemic Disease* (Princeton: Princeton University Press, 1943), 326–327; For example see Hirsch, *Handbook of Geographical*, vol. 1. He stressed that the causal agent for cholera was based on Dr. Max Pettenkopfer's theory on the characteristics of the soil, 451; and Charles Creighton, *A History of Epidemics in Great Britain* 2 vols. (Cambridge: Cambridge University Press, 1894; 2nd ed., 1965). Charles Creighton continued to be a notorious anti-contagionist until his death.

18. Delaporte, 14.

19. Winslow, 1.

20. E.R. Ackerknecht, "AntiContagionism between 1821 and 1867," *Bulletin of the History of Medicine* 22 (1948), 568.

21. Delaporte, 14.

22. Dr. F.W. Becker, *Letters of the Cholera in Prussia: Letter I to Dr. John Thomson* (London: J. Murray, 1832), 2.

23. Ibid.

24. Dr. Schlegel,"Darstellung der im Regierungs-Bezirk Leignitz vorgekommenen Faelle von asiatischer Cholera," in *Cholera-Archiv* 2, 392.

25. Ackerknecht, "Anticontagionism…," 567. For a contrary view of what may of caused the more reactionary governments of Europe like Austria, Prussia, and Russia to react immediately with quarantines while the more liberal governments like France and England approached the cholera more cautiously see *Baldwin,* Ch. 6. For the purposes of this discussion, see especially 529–530. Baldwin disagrees that there is a "correspondence between politics and prophylaxis" when it come to public health and ideology.

26. Ibid., 567.

27. Delaporte, 141.

28. Delaporte, 190.

29. Dettke, 8.

30. Mack Walker, *Germany and the Emigration, 1816–1885* (Cambridge: Harvard University Press, 1964); Wilhelm Abel, *Agricultural Fluctuations in Europe: From the Thirteenth to the Twelfth Century* (New York: Methuen, 1980); Wilhelm Abel, *Massenarmut und Hungerkrisen im Vorindustriellen Deutschland* (Hamburg: Parey, 1974); and Wilhelm Abel, *Der Pauperismus in Deutschland am Vorabend der Industriellen Revolution* (Dortmund: Gesellschaft für Westfälische Wirtschaftsgeschichte, 1966).

31. It has been noted by Dettke, 7–8, that the Silesian Weaver's Revolt in 1844 is generally seen as the "event of the *Vormärz*" that raised the middle classes from their *Biedermier* lethargy. However one anonymous author looking back on the cholera epidemic in Germany in 1831 wrote that the "fear" of the cholera was much greater and had a "greater" grip on the people in general than even the revolution of 1848 seventeen years later. However, it seems that in the 1848, with most epidemics, they were quickly forgotten and it quickly becomes a distant memory. Those left moved on with their lives. For cholera and related events in Königsberg in July 1831, see for example, Fritze Gause, *Die Geschichte der Stadt Königsberg in Preussen* 2 (Köln: Ostmitteleuropa in Vergangenheit und Gegenwart, 1968), 497.

32. Agatha Ramm, Germany 1789–1919 (Oxford, Oxford University Press, 1967), 167; and Werne Conze, *The Shaping of the German Nation: A Historical Analysis* (New York: George Prior Publishing, 1979), 33; and Lawrence J. Baack, *Christian Bernstorff and Prussia* (New Brunswick, NJ: Rutgers University Press, 1980), 165–204.

33. Chad to Palmerston, August 2, 1831, PRO FO 64/174, Ackerknecht, 63.

34. Becker, 43.

35. Dr. Fr. Klug,"Geschichtliche Zusammenstellung derjenigen wissenschaftlichen Erörterungen über die Cholera, welche den von der Verwaltungsbehörde getroffenen früheren Massregeln zum Grunde gelegt worden sind..," in *Cholera-Archiv*, 1, 18.

36. Becker, 43.

Chapter 1

1. Ethne Barnes, *Diseases and Human Evolution* (Albuquerque: University of New Mexico Press, 2005), 281. See Haeser, *Lehrbuch der Geschichte der Medicin*, 877–878; *Hufeland's Journal der praktischen Heilkunde* in 1822 ran a series of abstracts on English physicians and the cholera in India, especially focusing on James Jameson's, *Report on the Epidemic Cholera morbus, as it visited the Territories subject to the Presidency of Bengal in the years 1817–1819* (Calcutta: Printed at the Government Gazette Press, by A.G. Balfour, 1820) this would have been available to Prussian physicians; Dettke, 71.

Notes. Chapter 1

2. Rosenberg, *The Cholera Years the United States*, 2–3.
3. Barnes, 282–283; Ackerknecht, *History and Geography*, 23; A.W. Woodruff and S. Bell, *Synopsis of Infectious Tropical Diseases* (Baltimore, William and Wilkins, 1968), 103–104.
4. Dr. W. Eck, "Schilderung der hinsichtlich der Erscheinungen, Ursachen und Behandlung der asiatischen Cholera in Berlin gemachten Erfahrungen," in *Cholera-Archiv*, 3, 13.
5. Carl von Grolman, *Leben und Wirken des General der Infanterie und kommandirenden Generals des V. Armeekorps Carl von Grolman*, ed. C. von Conrady III (Berlin: Mittler, 1896), 110.
6. Adolph Streckfuss, *500 Jahre Berliner Geschichte Vom Fischerdorf zur Weltstadt* 2 (Berlin: Albert Goldschmidt, 1886), 782.
7. D.J. Lanska, "The Mad Cow Problem in the UK: Risk Perceptions, Risk Management, Health and Policy Development," *Journal of Public Health Policy* 19, no. 2 (1998), 164, 170.
8. Thomas Stamm-Kuhlmann "Die Cholera of 1831 Herausforderungen an Wissenschaft und Staatliche Verwaltung," *Sudoffs Acrhiv* 73 (1989), 179.
9. Gunther E. Rothenberg, "The *Austrian Sanitary Cordon and Control of the Bubonic Plague*," The Journal of the History of Medicine and Allied Health 26 (1973), 15–23.
10. Immediatebericht des Ministers der geistlichen, Unterrichts- und Medizalangelegenheiten Karl Sigmund Freiherr vom Stein zum Altenstein, Berlin, 4. December 1830. ZSTA Merseberg [GStA PK] Geheimes Zivilkabinett 2.2.1 Nr. 24496 f. 1–2 in *Stamm-Kuhlmann*, 180.
11. Ibid., 180.
12. M. Pistor, "Geschichte der Preussen Medizinalverwaltung Erster Teil: Die Medizinalverwaltung in Preussen von 1809 bis end 1907," in *Deutsche Vierteljahresschrift für öffentliche Gesundheits Pflege,* 40 (Berlin, 1907), 764–765.
13. Ibid.
14. Ackerknecht, "Anti-contagionism between 1821 and 1867."
15. Ibid., 567.
16. Ibid.
17. Hirsch, v. 1, 394–396; Sticker, II, 119.
18. Klug, *Cholera-Archiv*, 1, 2.
19. Ibid.
20. Ibid.
21. Dettke, 65.
22. GStA PK, Rep. 77, Tit 247, Nr.1 Bd.1 Bl.3. in Dettke, 66.
23. Klug, 4.
24. Dettke, 67; Brenn to Altenstein, November 9, 1830, ZSA Me, [GStA PK] Rep. 76 IXA, Nr. 3018. Bl. 36–37; Altenstein 3.10.1832 an Innenminister Gustav v. Brenn, in I. Ha, Rep. 77 Ti 182 Nr. 46 1, Bl. 208–213, *passim*, in Bärbel Holtz, *Das preußische Kultusministerium als Staatsbehörde und gesellschaftlicherAgentur (1817–1934)* Bd.1 (Berlin: Akademie Verlag 2009), 29.
25. Altenstein 3.10.1832 an Innenminister Gustav v. Brenn, in I. Ha, Rep. 77 Ti 182 Nr. 46 1, Bl. 208–213, die Zitate Bl. 209 in *Holtz*, 29.
26. Klug, 5–6.
27. Ibid., 3.
28. Brenn to Altenstein, November 15, 1830, GStA PK, Rep. 76 IXA, Nr. 3018 Bl. 36–37.
29. Dettke, 67.
30. Ibid.
31. Klug, 3.
32. Ibid., 4.
33. Protokol Königliche Wissenschaftliche Medizinal deputation, November 24, 1830, GTSA PK, Rep. IXA, Nr. 3018, Bl. 44; Rust to Brenn, November 24, 1830, GTSA PK, Rep. 76 IXA, Nr. 3018. Bl. 40–41; Klug, 4.
34. Klug, 5–6.
35. Idid., 6.
36. Idid., 8.
37. Ibid., 9–10.
38. Ibid., 11–12.
39. Dettke, 66.
40. Rothenberg, 17; see pages 16 and 23 regarding this controversy.
41. Ibid.,19.
42. Ibid., 18.
43. *Mémoires du Marechal Marmont, Duc de Raguse, de 1792 à 1841*, 3rd ed. 3 (Paris: Perrotin, 1857), 378–379.
and Drzavni Archiv, Zagreb, Gkdo. Zagreb F-30-31 in Rothenberg, 21.
44. Klug, 13.
45. J. N. Rust, "Sendschreiben des Praesidenten Dr. Rust an Se. Excellenz koenigl. preuss. Wirklichen Geheimen Rath und Kammerherrn Freyherrn Alexander v. Humboldt in Paris," *Cholera-Archiv*, 3, 66.
46. Klug, 15–16.
47. The reports by Steuart and Phillips were included in K. Searle ueber die Natur, die Ursachen und die Behandlung der Cholera (Berlin: Duncker & Humblot 1831) from an English edition with a forward by C.F. v. Graefe.
48. See Promemoria, o. D., o U, GStA, PK, 2.2.1 Nr. 24496 f.9, in *Stamm-Kuhlmann*, 180.
49. Klug, 4.
50. Immediatebericht des Ministers der geistlichen, Unterrichts- und Medizinalangelegenheiten Karl Sigmund vom Stein zum Altenstein. Berlin 4. Dezember 1830., Geheimes Zivilkabinett,GtSA PK, 2.2.1. Nr. F. 1–2 in *Stamm-Kuhlmann*, 180.
51. Konzept der Kabinettsorder, abgegangen den December 10, 1830, GtSA PK, 2.2.1, Nr. 24496 in *Stamm-Kuhlmann*, 180.
52. Klug, 17.
53. Dettke, 71.
54. Pistor, 765.
55. Dettke, 70–71.
56. Rust, 66.
57. *Allgemeine Deutsche Biographie* (Leipzig: Duncker & Humblot, 1890), 30, 26.
58. Schön to Altenstein and Innenminister von Brenn, Koenigsberg, December 3, 1830 (Abschrift) GtSA PK, 2.2.1, Nr. 24496 f. 5–6 in *Stamm-Kuhlmann*, 180.
59. Erna Lesky, "*Die Oesterreicheische Pestfront an der KK Militaergrenze*," v.8, *Saeculum* (1957), 86.
60. Klug, 15.
61. Ibid.
62. Ibid.
63. See August Geradin et Paul Gaimard *Du Choléra-Morbus en Russie en Prusse et en Autriche pendant les années 1831 et 1832* 3rd. ed. (Paris: F. G. Levrault,1833); Morris, *Cholera 1832*, 23–25; *Ackerknecht,* "Anti-contagionism between 1821 and 1867," 567. Although Prussia sent one of the first commissions, Ackerknecht ignores this in his seminal article. He probably did this for two reasons: he had a low opinion of German medicine and he was making the

point that other European commissions returned home recommending that quarantine was useless. The majority of doctors on the Prussian commission recommended that cholera was contagious. Ackerknecht, 576.

64. Dettke, 69.
65. The three diseases were considered contagious but for each there was a different degree of contagiousness. However, in the case of typhus the doctors of that time were actually discussing both typhus (human louse borne and this was not identified until 1909, the causative agent not until 1916) and typhoid fever (transmitted through oral-fecal matter from human to human) as the two were not sufficiently distinguished until much later. Ackerknecht, "Anti-contagionism...," 586 and *Barnes*, 260 and 289.
66. GtSA Pk, Rep. IXA, Nr. 3018, Bl. 118–119.
67. GtSA PK, Rep. IXA, Nr. 3018, Bl. 118–122.
68. Ibid.
69. Dr. Edmund Dann, "Bericht über die im Auftrage Eines Hohen Königl. Preuss. Ministerii Behufs der Untersuchung der Cholera nach Russland unternomme Reise," *Archiv für medizinische Erfahrung* (January–February, 1832), 119.
70. GtSA PK, Rep. IXA, Nr.3021. Bl. 98–99; Dann, 120.
71. Dann, 128.
72. Ibid., 127.
73. Ibid., 141.
74. Ibid., 123, 128.
75. Ibid., 152–153; for a discussion of Mudroff's views on cholera see McGrew, 137.
76. GtSA PK, Rep. IXA, Nr. 3021, Bl. 133–135.
77. Dann, 140.
78. McGrew, 137.
79. Bisset Hawkins, *History of the Epidemic Spasmodic Cholera...Official and Other Documents* (London: J. Murray, 1831), 291; "Report of Dr. Albers, A Prussian Physician at the head of a Commission sent by the Prussian Government to Moscow, to ascertain the nature of the Cholera under date March 9–21, 1831," in *Hawkins*, 287–291.
80. Carl Ignatius Lorinser, *Eine Selbstbiographie Vollendet und herausgegeben von seinem Sohne Franz Lorinser* (Regensburg, Manz, 1864), ii, 13.
81. D. Carl Venturini, *Chronik des neunzehnten Jahrhunderts. Das Jahr 1831* (Leipzig, 1833), 164.
82. Rust, "Sendschreiben," 60.
83. Dann, 183–184; McGrew, 100–105; Klug, 18.
84. Klug, 18.
85. Dann, 184.
86. Ibid., 185.
87. Ibid.
88. Ibid., 186.
89. Ibid., 188–208.
90. Curiously, Michael Drury in his book *The Return of the Plague*, 11, cites an instance where Dr. Walker noted that Dr. Albers' had made non-contagionist remarks. This would have been most unlikely and is further evidence of the confusion that Dr. Walker appears to have sown back in England. Dr. Albers maintained in his report of March 9–21, 1831 that cholera was spread person to person but could describe "no instance which could render it at all possible that the Cholera is disseminated by inanimate objects." Hawkins, 291. His support of "person to person" infection was enough for Rust to order quarantine and cordons.

91. Lorinser, ii, 25 and 28.
92. Horn, "Die Contagiostät der Asiatischen," *Cholera Archiv*, 2, 2; Klug, 19–26.
93. Ewald, "Aus den Erlebnissen der Preussen i. J. 1831 beim ersten Auftreten der Cholera," *Altpreussische Monatschrift* 21 (1884), 9; Dr. Ernst Barchewitz, *Über die Cholera. Nach eigener Beobachtung in Russland und Preussen* (Danzig: F.S. Gerhard, 1832), 61.
94. Rust, "Sendschreiben" 61. This was a strong defense of the contagionist position taken by the government under Rust's leadership during the cholera epidemic. It also reveals the depth of the animosity which Rust felt toward the anticontagionists. As late as 1833, one chronicler of the times, still gave the official government position that there were four doctors sent to Russia and they reported back to the Prussian government that the "sickness belonged to the kind which was infectious (contagious) and can only be prevented through mass regulations." Venturini, 164. This was not accurate, because Barchewitz's opinion was well known and in his own published account he claimed he had early on become an anticontagionist.
95. Theodor von Schön, *Weitere Beträge und Nachträge zu den Papieren des Ministers und Burgrafen von Marienburg Theodor von Schön* (Berlin: Leonhard Simeon, 1881), vii; Ewald, 9; Zbigniew Olkowski, "Epidemia Cholery Azjatyckiej W. Prusach Wschodnich W. Latacj 1831–1832," *Komunikaty Mazursko-Warmińskie* 102 (1968), 548.
96. Schön, 264.
97. Schön, 264–265; *Ewald*, 11.
98. Olkowski, 548 and *Amtsblatts der Königl. Preuß. Regierung zu Königsberg*, VIII, 1831, 99–101.
99. Schön, 270–271.
100. Barchewitz, x. See for example *Beilage zur Allgemeine Zeitung München*, August 2, 1831, 1138. On the international level Barchewitz found his views vigorously attacked by Dr. Becker, a contagionist physician in Berlin who advised the English ambassador to Prussia, George Edward Chad, on matters relating to the cholera in Berlin. Chad to Palmerston, October 18, 1831, PRO FO 64/174, 233; "Memorandum der Central-Gesundheits-Behörde in London die Quarantainen gegen die Cholera betreffend," *Cholera-Archiv*, 1, 122; Becker, 19.

Chapter 2

1. Dr. Formey, a member of the Ober-Collegium Medicum et Sanitatis (Chief Medical and Sanitary Board) corresponded with Intendat Bignon during the Napoleonic occupation of Berlin to secure the salaries of the members of the Board "in these difficult times." Ragnild Münch, *Gesundheitswesen im 18. und 19. Jahrhundert: Das Berliner Beispiel* (Berlin: Akademie-Verlag, 1995), 47.
2. Münch, 66
3. Oberpräsident (1808), Wissenschaftliche Deputation für Medizinalwesen (1808), MedizinalKollegium (1815), Sanitätskommission (1815) and Kultusministerium (1817).
4. George Rosen, "Cameralism and the Concept of Medical Police," *Bulletin of the History of Medicine* 27 (1953), 21–42; George Rosen, "The Fate of the Concept of Medical Police, 1780–1890," *Centaurus* 5 (1957), 97–113; Ute Frevert, *Krankheit als politisches Problem 1770–1880* (Göttingen: Vandenhoeck & Ruprecht, 1984).
5. Werner Conze, "Das Spannungsfeld von Staat und

Gesellschaft im Vormärz," in *Staat und Gesellschaft im Deutschen Vormärz*, Werner Conze ed. (Stuttgart: E. Klett, 1962), 246–261; Reinhart Koselleck, *Preussen zwischen Reform und Revolution: Allgemeines Landrecht, Verwaltung und soziale Bewegung von 1791 bis 1848* (Stuttgart: Ernst Klett, 1981), 331.

6. Münch, with regard to the dissolution of the Chief Medical and Sanitary Board, 47; *Lancet* (1844), 579–580.

7. Baldwin, 30.

8. Baldwin, 30; Dettke; Ross; Olaf Briese, *Angst in den Zeiten der Cholera* 1 (Berlin:Akademie Verlag, 2003), 255–257. Briese sees the primary support for quarantine and cordons coming from the Crown, the nobility and the military with some support among those who saw this as "bulwark against an Asiatic invasion."

9. Watts, Sheldon, *Epidemics and History: Disease, Power and Imperialism* (New Haven, CT: Yale University Press, 1997), 16.

10. Reinhold Dorwart, *The Prussian Welfare State before 1740* (Cambridge, Mass.: Harvard University Press, 1971), 3–5, 12–22; Marc Raeff, *The Well Ordered Police State; Social and Institutional Change through Law in the Germanies and Russia 1600–1800* (New Haven: Yale University Press, 1983), 5; Münch, 9–12.

11. Rosen, "Cameralism," 21–24.

12. Ibid., 23.

13. Rosen, "The Fate of the Concept," 98.

14. Münch,, 10.

15. Ibid., 21.

16. Rosen, "The Fate of the Concept," 98

17. Ibid., 111; Otto Hintze, *Acta Borussica: Die Behördenorganization*, VI, in Dorwart, 17; Münch, 19.

18. Rosen, "The Fate of the Concept," 110.

19. Ibid., 111.

20. Münch, 26.

21. Thomas Nipperdey, *Germany from Napoleon to Bismarck, 1800–1866* (Princeton, NJ: Princeton University Press, 1996), 21.

22. Münch, 50–53.

23. Ibid., 53.

24. Rosen, "The Fate of the Concept," 98.

25. Ross, Chp. 2: 4; Münch, 57.

26. Frevert, 40–44; "Claudia Huerkamp, "Ärzte und Professionalisierung in Deutschland: Überlegungen zum Wandel des Arztberufs im 19. Jahrhundert, "*Geschichte und Gesellschaft* (1982), 350–351.

27. Ludwig von Rönne and Heinrich Simon, *Das Medicinal-wesen Preussischen Staates*. 1 (Breslau: Aderholz, 1844), 13 and Dorwart, 240.

28. Rönne, 14–15.

29. *Medicinal Edict vom 1725*, in Rönne, 15–20; J. N. Rust, *Die Medizinal-Verfassung Preussens, wie sie war und wie sie ist* (Berlin:Enslin, 1838), 42–43.

30. Rönne, 16–17.

31. Dorwart, 252.

32. Frevert, 43

33. Ibid.

34. Plague had devastated East Prussia in 1709–1710. This combined with famine led to the deaths of approximately 250,000 people or "more than a third of the East Prussian population." Christopher M. Clark, *Iron Kingdom: The Rise and Downfall of Prussia, 1600–1947* (Cambridge, MA.: Belknap Press of Harvard University Press, 2006), 86.

35. Rönne, 50.

36. Ibid., 50–51.

37. The General Directory was the chief governing body in Prussia. It was founded in 1722 and lasted until 1806. Initially it was made up of four provincial departments, each with a director. In 1786 Frederick the Great added five more departments. Departments represented in the General Directory had access to the King. W.H. Bruford, *Germany in the Eighteenth Century: The Social Background of the Literary Revival* (Cambridge: Cambridge University Press, 1965), 24–29.

38. Rönne, 56.

39. Münch, 133.

40. Rönne, 51.

41. Rust, 66.

42. Nipperdey, 22–23.

43. Koselleck, 331.

44. Nipperdey, 25–26.

45. Ibid., 44–45.

46. Münch, 50.

47. Nipperdey, 24.

48. Alfons Fischer, *Geschichte des Deutschen Gesundheitswesens*, 2 (Berlin: F. A. Herbig, 1932), 287.

49. Münch, 48.

50. Ibid.

51. In the *Riga Memorandum* Altenstein had envisioned an independent medical officialdom united with the police (for public health purposes) and recommended the transformation of the Chief Medical and Sanitary Board into a research organization rather than have it continue in a purely administrative capacity.

52. Münch, 50.

53. Nipperdey, 23; Willard R. Fann, "The Consolidation of Bureaucratic Absolutism in Prussia, 1815–1827," (PhD diss. University of California, 1965), 11–24.

54. Münch, 58–59.

55. Ibid., 52.

56. Ernst Müsebeck, *Das Preussische Kultusministerium vor hundert Jahren* (Stuttgart u.a.: Cotta, 1918), 75–76.

57. Rönne, 66 and Rust, 73.

58. Bruno Gebhart, *Wilhelm von Humboldt als Staatsman*, Bd. 1 (Stuttgart: Verlag Aalen, 1965), 338; Rust, 67.

59. Münch, 133–134.

60. "Memorandum September 11, 1807," in Georg Winter, ed., *Die Reorganisation des preussischen Staats unter Stein und Hardenberg. Erster Teil: Allgemeine Verwaltungs- und Behördenreform* (Leipzig: S. Hirzel, 1931), 533.

61. Münch, p. 58-59

62. Ibid., 59

63. Ibid.

64. Ibid.

65. Münch, 60; Müsebeck, 45.

66. Münch, 60.

67. Ibid.

68. Gebhart, 339; Rust, 67; Rönne, 57.

69. Münch, 69.

70. Müsebeck, 115–116.

71. The office actually fell into disuse after 1810 but was later revived by the order of April 30, 1815 and the later regulations of 1817 and 1825. See Fann, 220.

72. The office of the Oberpräsident was a controversial one within the bureaucratic organization of the governmen Its creation had brought to the forefront opposition between "bureaucrats and regionalists," "hierarchs and collegialists,"and "liberals and reactionaries." The Oberpräsi-

dent was a compromise between those with "Statist demands" and those with "regional desires." Koselleck, 221.

73. Rönne, 79.
74. Münch, 48–49.
75. Ibid., 57.
76. The provinces include Prussia, Brandenburg, Silesia, Pomerania, Posen, Saxony, Westphalia and the Rhine province.
77. Rönne, 83.
78. Ibid.
79. SanitätsKommission were established at Gumbinnen, Marienwerder, Koslin, Reichenbach, Leignitz, Oppeln, Bromberg, Merseberg, Erfurt, Minden, Hamm, Kleve, Koblenz and Trier. Rönne, 83.
80. The Kreis physician and Kreis surgeon prior to the nineteenth century had been local offices. They were appointed and paid by the local commune. In 1812 the Kreis physician became a paid state office. Rust saw this as another step in the progress of the medical estate in Prussia. Rus 56; The Kreis surgeon position was similarly established in 1816. Rönne, 117.
81. Rönne, 112.
82. Münch, 52–53.
83. "Schuckmann an Altenstein vom Dezember 21, 1817," GstA PK, Rep. 76 VIII A, Nr. 5, Bl. 8–10, in Münch, 56.
84. Ibid., 63.
85. Ibid.
86. Ibid., 64.
87. Rust, 73, 75–76.
88. Freiherr von Altenstein, "*Denkschrift Über den Zusammenung des Kultusministeriums mit der Staatverwaltung s.d. Ende April bis Anfang Mai 1819,*" in Müsebeck, 279–292.
89. Ibid., 289.
90. The school of surgery was later scrapped. Ibid., 290.
91. Ibid.
92. Ibid.
93. Ibid., 292.
94. Ibid.
95. Ibid.; Fischer wrote that as a result of Stein's "City Ordinance of 1808" public health was made a local concern, and that much would be done in the next sixty years of investing in sewer systems and the laying of water pipes. This would benefit the entire population. The same sense of civic sacrifice was missing when it concerned the needs of the poor alone. This was Altenstein's complaint in 1819. Fischer, 287.
96. Münch, 64–65.
97. Ibid., 66.
98. Ibid.
99. Ibid., 69.
100. Koselleck, 231–233.
101. Münch, 66.
102. Rust, 78–79 and Rönne, 59–61.
103. "Rücksichtlich der dem Min. der G.,U. u. Med. Ang. Verbleibenden Angelegenheiten concurrirt das Min. Innern," March 25, 1825, in Rönne, 63.
104. Koselleck, 232.
105. Rust, 81–82
106. Müsebeck,. 69.
107. Münch, 66.
108. Ibid., 69
109. Rust, 81–82.

Chapter 3

1. Theodor Schiemann, "Die Sendung des Feldmarschalls Diebitsch nach Berlin September-November 1830," *Zeitschrift fuer osteuropaeische Geschichte* Bd.1, 2. (1910/11), 2–22.
2. Baack, 168–169.
3. Baack, 173.
4. Schiemann, 13.
5. Ibid.,7.
6. Ibid., 9.
7. Ibid., 13–14; Baack, 169.
8. Ibid., 14.
9. Baack, 176.
10. Major von Felgermann, *General W.J. von Krauseneck* (Berlin: Reimer, 1851), 159.
11. Schiemann, 18.
12. Ibid.
13. Ibid.
14. Baack, 186.
15. Ibid., 187.
16. Schiemann, 18.
17. Baack, 187.
18. Ibid., 177.
19. Schiemann, 20–21.
20. Ibid., 21.
21. Schiemann, 21; Heinrich Treitschke, *Treitschke's History of Germany in the Nineteenth Century*, vol. 5 (New York: McBride, Nast & Co. 1919), 66–67.
22. Victor Adolf Riecke, *Mittheilungen über die morgenländische Brechruhr* 3 (Stuttgart: Hoffmann, 1832), 44, 117, 119–120.
23. Baack, 195.
24. Ibid., 197.
25. Ibid., 198.
26. McGrew, 101–102.
27. Anneliese Gerecke, *Das Deutsche Echo Auf Die Polnische Erhebung Von 1830* (Wiesbaden: Harrassowitz, 1964), 10.
28. Ibid.
29. Theodor Schiemann, *Geschichte Russlands unter Kaiser Nikolaus I*, 3 (Berlin: G. Reimer, 1913), 41–42.
30. Treitschke, 71.
31. Gerecke, 12.
32. "Notes des Berliner Gesandten Grafen Alopeus vol. 19 Dez. 1830 an den Minister des Auswärtigen, Grafen Bernstorff," in Manfred Laubert,"Beiträge zu Preussens Stellung gegenüber dem Warschauer Novemberaufstand V.J. 1830," *Jahrbucher fuer Kulture und Geschichte* (1929), 381.
33. Ibid., 381.
34. Ibid., 382.
35. Ibid.
36. Schiemann, *Geschichte Russlands*, 3, 43, 45.
37. Friedrich von Raumer, "Preussens Verhältnisse zu Polen in den Jahren 1831 bis 1832, aus amtlichen Quellen dargestellt," *Vermischte Schriften* 2 (Leipzig, Brockhaus, 1853), 505.
38. Baack, 197.
39. Treitschke, 73.
40. Ibid., 73.
41. Ibid., 103.
42. Frederyk Wilhelm III cara Mikolaja I kwiecien 1831, GStK, PK, AA I Rep I, 2333, in Henryk Kocój, "Wladze pruski oraz opinia publiczna Prus I Niemiec wobec pow-

stania listopadowego," *Roczniki Histororyczne* 30 (1964), 95.
43. Kocój, passim.
44. Kocój, 106.
45. Schiemann, *Geschichte Russlands,* 3, 120–121.
46. Ibid., 121–122; *McGrew,* 105; R. F. Leslie, *Polish Politics and the Revolution of November 1830* (London: Athlone Press, 1956), 213.
47. Schiemann, *Geschichte Russlands,* 3, 122–123.
48. Riecke, 117–118.
49. Zbigniew Olkowski,"Epidemia Cholery Azjatyckiej w Prusach Wschodnich w Latacj 1831–1832," *Komunikaty Mazursko-Warminskie,* 102 (1968), 531.
50. "Note Officielle ... de Pologne au Cabinet de Berlin," in, *La Pologne et La Prusse en 1831* (Paris, 1832), 15–16.
51. Piotr Władysław Goździk, *Cholera W Królestwie Polskim w 1831 Roku* (Warszawa: Lekarz Wojskowy, 1938), 33.
52. Goździk, 38; Riecke,127.
53. Laubert, 386–387.
54. Goździk, 36.
55. Riecke, 127.
56. Carl Julius Remer, *Beobachtungen über die epidemische Cholera gesammelt in Folge einer in amtlichem Auftrage gemachten Reise nach Warschau* (Breslau: Max, 1831), 44–45, 57.
57. Dr. Leopold Leo was born in Königsberg and moved to Warsaw in 1825. He developed one of the most famous cholera cures during this first epidemic in Europe, the "bismuth treatment." McGrew, 140–141.
58. Olkowski, 531; Goździk, 8.
59. Riecke, 127.
60. Riecke, 127–128; Goździk, 10–11.
61. Goździk, 7; Remer, 122; F. E. Fodere, *Recherches Historiques et Critiques sur la Nature, Les Causes et Traitment du Choléra-morbus de L'inde, de Russie, de Pologne, at autres contrées* (Paris: Levrault, 1831), 317–319.
62. Goździk, 7.
63. Ibid., 8.
64. Ibid.
65. Polish doctors did not base their knowledge of the cholera on personal observation but on the written reports of Dr. Andrzej Wysokinski. Dr. Wysokinski observed an earlier cholera outbreak on the Persian frontier. He returned to Vilna and published his book entitled the *Dissertatio inauguralis medico-practica de cholera epidemica Indorum* (1828). Goździk, 37.
66. A. Brierre de Boismont, *Relation Historique et Médicale du Cholera Morbus de Pologne* (Paris: Germer-Baillière, 1832), 244.
67. Olkowski, 532.
68. Goździk, 8.
69. Ibid.
70. Boismont, 244.
71. Goździk, 8.
72. Boismont, 244; Goździk, 9.
73. Goździk, 8.
74. Goździk, 9; Riecke, 135.
75. Riecke, 135; Remer, 49.
76. Franciszek Giedroyć, *Rada Lekarska Księstwa Warszawskiego i Królestwa Polskiego 1809–1867* (Warszawa: E. Wende, 1913), in *Olkowski,* 532; Dr. K. Chr. Hille, *Beobachtungen über die asiatische Cholera, gesammelt auf einer nach Warschau im Auftrage der K. Sach* (Leipzig: Barth, 1831), 8.

77. Remer, 122.
78. Riecke, 136.
79. Ibid.
80. Fodere, 317.
81. Goździk, 22–27.
82. "Acts Du Comite Central," in Boisemont, 245–252.
83. Riecke, 137.
84. Remer, 48; Riecke, 131.
85. Goździk, 9; Remer, 44.
86. Goździk, 10.
87. Riecke, 131
88. Goździk, 10.
89. Boisemont, 245.
90. Goździk, 14.
91. Ibid.
92. Karol Kaczkowski, *Wspomnienia z papierów pozostałych po ś.p. Karolu Kaczkowskim, General Sztab-Lekarzu wojsk Poliskich,* ułożył, Tadeusz Oksza Orzechowski, I (Lwów: Gubrynowicza i Schmidta, 1876), 246; Goździk, 62.
93. Goździk, 23–24
94. Ibid., 24–25.
95. Goździk, 25.
96. Ibid.
97. "Akta Komisji Rzadowej Wewntęrznych i Policji tyzące się cholera morbus i innych chorób epidemicznych," nr. vol. 5207 a-e, raport Kaczkowskiego z dnia 28 czerwca, in Goździk, 25.
98. Goździk, 38; Kaczkowski, 246.
99. Goździk, 27.
100. Kaczkowski, 246.
101. Goździk, 39.
102. Dr. Remer reported at the time that he did not believe the death reports to be accurate "due to a great reluctance on the part of the government." Remer, 9.
103. The term miasma as it was understood at the time referred to a given area, its temperature, soil conditions, humidity and topography, which combined to create effluvia conducive to the disease. Adherents of the miasmic theory did not look for a single causative agent.
104. "La Comité Central de Sante la Commission de l'Interior et de la Police," April 29, 1831, GStA PK, Rep. 76 VIII C, Nr. 25. Bl. 10. See the statistics reported by Kaczkowski from the hospital at Mienia for April 13–27, 1831. Of the 886 military patients admitted to the hospital, 218 died. Up to that date, he reported 336 patients were discharged or recovering in Minsk. On May 11/12, he reported the hospital had received 1,506 patients, 399 died and 720 had been discharged. The rest remained in the hospital under observation.The recovery rate was fairly high and can most likely be attributed to Kaczkowski's more traditional hygienic procedures. "Akta Komisji Rządowej...," in Goździk, 26.
105. Remer, 49.
106. Remer, 57; 117.
107. Olkowski, 532.
108. B. Sawicki, "Luźna notatka z dawnych naszych stosunków lekarskich," *Gazeta Lekarska* (1912), nr. 27, in Goździk, 34.
109. B. Pawlowski, *Źródła do dziejów wojny polskorosyjskiej 1830–1831* (Warszawa: Wojskowe Biuro Historyczne, 1931), i,198; Goździk, 34.
110. Fr. Giedroyc, "Lekarze cudzoziemcy w Polsce w roku 1831," *Archiwum Historji I Filozofji Medycyny* 2 (1925),

4–5; S. Kunowski, "Deutsche Aerzte im Polenaufstand 1831," *Die Medizinische Welt* (Dezember, 1931), 1805; Goździk, 34–36.

111. Reports of this evidently supported the Prussian claim by Flottwell that "Under the alleged study of cholera, French doctors found themselves traveling to Warsaw. They were evidently French officers, who were there to take part in the uprising. An examination of their personnel effects was wholly correct." See Laubert, 388.

112. Kunowski, 1805.

113. Louis Blanc, *The History of Ten Years 1830–1840; or France Under Louis Philippe*, Translated by Walter Kelley, I (Philadelphia: Lea and Blanchard, 1848), 437; "Circular of the Polish Government respecting the Cholera Morbus," in Hawkins, 273.

114. "Note Officielle ... de Pologne au Cabinet de Berlin," in *La Pologne*..., 14

115. "Circular of the Polish," in Hawkins, 274.

116. Ibid.

117. Ibid.

118. Note Officielle ... de Pologne au Cabinet de Berlin," in *La Pologne*, 15.

119. Baack, 194–198; see "Skrzynecki to Friedrich Wilhelm III, June 19, 1831," in Leonard Chodzko, ed., *Recueil des Traités, Conventions et Actes Diplomatiques concernant La Pologne 1762–1862* (Paris: Amyot, 1862), 825–826. There were many complaints about Prussians assisting the Russians and even fighting on their side. These were later refuted. See Raumer, 509

120. "Note Officielle ... de Pologne au Cabinet de Berlin," in *La Pologne*..., 15–16.

121. Laubert, 387. The quote is from a response that Privy Councilor Eichhorn in the Prussian Foreign Office requested from Provincial President Flottwell to refute the Polish Minister of Foreign Affairs complaints against the Prussian Government on July 18, 1831. Flottwell's handwritten response was delivered on October 3, 1831. It was meant to be used diplomatically to counter the Polish Government's complaints and appears not to have been published. Laubert, 385; Raumer, 504–505.

122. Klug,18.

123. Olkowski, 534.

124. Gneisenau to Roder, April 27, 1831, Zeither, and Kraft, GStA PK, Rep. 76 VIII C, Nr. 23, Bl. 5.

125. Gneisenau to Kraft, May 3, 1831, GStA PK., Rep. 76 VIII C, Nr. 23, Bl. 5.

126. "Skizze zür Organisation einer Grenz Cordons im Grossherzogtum Posen," Gneisenau to Witzleben, April 29, 1831, GStA PK, Rep. 76 VIII C, Nr. 23, Bl. 5.

127. Gneisenau to Kraft, May 3, 1831, GStA PK, Rep. 76 VIII C, Nr. 23, Bl. 5.

128. "Skizze zür Organisation einer Grenz ..." Gneisenau to General von Witzleben, April 29, 1831, GStA PK, Rep. VIII C, Nr. 23. Bl. 5.

129. Gneisenau to General Witzleben, May 3,1831, GStA PK, Rep. 76 VIII C, Nr.23, Bl. 5.

130. Hille, 122.

131. Gneisenau to General von Witzleben, May 3, 1831, GStA PK, Rep. 76 VIII C, Nr.23, Bl. 5.

132. Laubert, 384.

133. Ibid., 382, 384.

134. Ibid., 385.

135. Ibid.

136. Franciszek z Blociszewa Gajewski, *Pamietniki*, II, 136, cited in Wieslaw Stembrowicz, "Pruski Kordon Sanitarny W Okresie Wojny Polsko-Rosyjskiej (1830–1831)," *Archiwum Historii Medycyny* 45 (1982), 43; Kocój, *Wladze Pruski Oraz Opinia*..., where he wrote the "vigorous closure of the East Prussian border was political in nature" and was one of a number of measures that contributed to the "smothering of the November insurrection," 127–128; Stembrowicz, 43; McGrew, 104.

Chapter 4

1. Baack, 98.
2. Fedor I. Smitt, *Geschichte des polnischen Aufstandes, in den Jahren 1830 und 1831 und Kriegs* (Berlin: Duncker und Humblot, 1848), iii, 171.
3. Pistor, 766.
4. Dettke, 74–75.
5. *Allgemeine Deutsche Biographie*, 38. (Leipzig: Duncker & Humblot, 1890), 38–42; and *ADB*, 30, 25–29.
6. Wissman to Stägemann, 13 June 1831, in F.A. von Stägemann, *Briefe und Aktenstucke zur Geschichte Preussens unter Friedrich Wilhelm III*, ed. Franz Rühl, 3 (Leipzig: Duncker u. Humblot, 1902), 486.
7. Schön, 287.
8. *Allgemeine Zeitung*, May 25, 1831, 581.
9. Klug, 17.
10. Immediat Commission zur Abwehrungen der Cholera Acta betreffn Conferenz Protokol, May 5, 1831, GStA PK, Rep. 76 VIII C, Nr.2, Bl. 2–3.
11. F. de Martens, *Recueil des traités et conventions, conclus par la Russie avec les puissances étrangères:Traités Avec L'Allemagne, 1825–1888*, VIII (SPetersbourg: Impr. du Ministère des voies de communication, 1888), 317; Baack, 196.
12. May 5, 1831, GStA PK, Rep. 76 VIII C, Nr. 2, Bl. 2.
13. Preuth to Bernstorff, May 10, 1831; and Count Malachowski of Poland to the Prussian Minister of Foreign Affairs, May 9, 1831, GStA PK, Rep. 76 VIII C, Nr. 43, Bl. 90.
14. Conferenz Protokol, May 27, 1831, GStA PK, Rep. 76 VIII C, Nr. 2, Bl. 6–7.
15. Conferenz Protokol, May 16, 1831, GStA PK, Rep. 76 VIII C, Nr. 2. Bl. 5.
16. Thile to Flottwell, Schön and Merkel, May 8, 1831, GStA PK, Rep. 76 VIII C, Nr. 43, Bl. 53–54.
17. Dr. Wagner, "Die Verbreitung der Cholera in Preussischen Staate: ein Beweis ihrer Contagiosität," *Cholera-Archiv*, 2, 200–202
18. John Hamett, M.D., "Extracts From Medical Reports, Founded On Actual Observation, And Communicated To The Government, On The Cholera Morbus which Prevailed at Danzig Between the End of May and the First Part of September 1931," *The Medico-Chirurgical Review and Journal of Practical Medicin*, New Series, vol. 16 (London, 1832), 306–308; and Wagner, 131.
19. Ewald, 15.
20. "Amtliche Bericht über die Wirkung der Sperr-Massregeln gegen die Cholera enthaltend," in *Verhandlungen der Physikalischen-Medicinische Gesellschaft zu Königsberg über Die Cholera*,"(Königsberg, 1831), 441.
21. Hamett, 305.
22. "Amtliche Bericht," 425–426.
23. "Epidemic Cholera," *American Journal of the Medical Sciences*, vol. 9 (1831), 465.

Notes. Chapter 4

24. "Amtliche Bericht," 426–427.
25. Conferenz Protokol, June 1, 1831, GStA PK Rep. 76 VIII C, Nr. 2. Bl. 8–9; *Allgemeine medizinische Zeitung mit Berücksichtigung des Neuesten und...,"* (Altenberg, 1831) 928; and Wagner, 136.
26. Conferenz Protokol, June 1, 1831, GStA PK, Rep. 76 VIII C, Nr. 2. Bl. 8–9; and Ewald, 56. Ships and people had to pass through the quaratine station at Dirschau where a military blockade was established. See "Verordnungen der Königl. Regierung, Den Verkehr mit Danzig und der Umgegend betreffend, June 17, 1831" *Amtsblatt der Konigl. Preuss. Regierung zu Marienwerde,* June 23, 1831, 245. See Thile to Schön, June 25, 1831, GStA PK., Rep. 76 VIII C, Nr. 24. Bl. 33–34, where Thile informs Schön that ships along the Vistula will have to subscibe to a 20 day quarantine in Dirschau; that a Contumaz was established there for all vessels; and the responsibility for internal shipping will fall under the military control (General Lieutenant Krafft), Bl. 32 & 34. Dirschau was part of the "great waterway of the Vistula" that included "the cities of Stargard, Caldone Dirschau, Elbing and Danzig." *Sachs Repertorisches Jahrbuch für die neuesten und vorzüglichsten Leistungen der...,* ed. Dr. L. Posner, XVII (Berlin: 1850), 206.
27. "Bericht aus dem Regierungsbezirke Marienwerder für den Monat August 1831," *Preussische Provinzial-Blätter,* 5 (Königsberg, 1831), 476.
28. "Amtliche Bericht," 451.
29. *Allgemeine Handlungs-Zeitung Nuernberg,* July 29, 1831, 388.
30. Dr. Louis Stromeyer, *Skizzen und Bemerkungen von einer Reise nach Danzig und dessen Umgegend* (Hanover: Hahn, 1832), 5.
31. Ewald, 18.
32. Stromeyer, 5.
33. Wagner, 134.
34. Ibid., 133–135.
35. "Amtliche Bericht," 426.
36. He noted the frequency that the Polish Jews crossed the border without control. This information was sent to Ewald on June 3, 1831. Ewald was ordered to pay strict attention to travelers and to make sure they had health certificates. Olkowski, 544.
37. Wagner, 135.
38. Stromeyer, 5.
39. Ibid., 6.
40. Ibid., 5; "Amtliche Bericht," 429.
41. Ibid., 6.
42. Ibid.; "Amtliche Bericht," 436.
43. Ibid., 7.
44. Ibid.
45. "Instruction für den Dienst in den Cholera-Lazarethen," *Acta betreffend den Ausbruch und den Fortgang der Cholera in den Stadt Posen und die Correspondence mit der dortigen Regierungen,* GStA PK., Rep. 76 VIII C., Nr. 83, Bl. 17.
46. *"Allgemeine medizinische Zeitung"* 928.
47. Stromeyer, 7.
48. "Amtliche Bericht," 429–30.
49. Ibid., 436. This could also have been attributed to the fact that those with severe cases died before they reached the lazarets.
50. Ewald, 19.
51. Ibid.
52. "Amtlicher Bericht " 435.
53. Ewald, 19.
54. Ibid.
55. Ibid.
56. "Amtliche Bericht," 427.
57. "Amtliche Bericht," 440.
58. Ewald, 22.
59. "Amtliche Bericht," 432.
60. Ibid., 444.
61. Ibid., 443
62. Conferenz Protokol, June 21, 1831, GStA PK., Rep. 76 VIII C, Nr.2. Bl. 20.
63. Schön, 268.
64. Conferenz Protokol, June 21, 1831, GStA PK., Rep. 76 VIII C, Nr. 2. Bl. 21.
65. Ibid.
66. Schön, 269–270.
67. Ibid., 270–271.
68. Schön, 279
69. Schön, 265–266.
70. Ibid., 280.
71. Ibid.
72. Schön, 281.
73. Ibid., 281–283.
74. Ibid., 283.
75. Conferenz Protokol, July 4, 1831, GStA PK., Rep. VIII C, Nr. 2. Bl. 33.
76. Conferenz Protokol, July 8, 1831, GStA PK., Rep. VIII C, Nr. 2. Bl. 36.
77. Ibid.; and Conferenz Protokol, July 15, 1831, GStA PK., Rep. VIII C, Nr. 2 Bl. 43.
78. Schön, 283.
79. In fact these measures had caused an uprising in St. Petersburg. A June 30, 1831, letter in the Prussian archives from there refers to the uneasiness of the lower classes there as a result of strict regulations regarding quarantine. It reported "one hospital has been devastated. The doctors were attacked ... victims of the fury of assailants." The writer wrote that troops were called in and the Czar helped restore order by his presence. Schön, as well as other members of the government had to be concerned. See *Circulaire, St. Petersbourg,* June 30, 1831, GStA PK., Rep. 76 VIII C, Acta generalia, Nr.1. Bl. 193–195.
80. Schön, 284.
81. Ibid.
82. "Amtliche Bericht," 444.
83. Conferenz Protokol, July 17, 1831, GStA PK., Rep. VIII C, Nr. 2 Bl. 44.
84. Ibid.
85. Ewald, 29; and R. Eylert, ed. *Charakter-Zuege Friedrich Willhelm III,* 2 (Madgeburg: Heinrichshofen, 1847), 339.
86. Stromeyer, 8.
87. Ibid.
88. Ibid., 9.
89. Ibid.
90. "Amtliche Bericht," 443–444.
91. Stromeyer, 10.
92. Ibid.
93. "Amtliche Bericht," 439.
94. "Amtliche Bericht," 438.
95. Ibid,. 440.
96. Ibid.
97. Conferenz Protokol, July 18, 1831, GStA PK, Rep. VIII C, Nr. 2 Bl. 47.
98. Olkowski, 561–562.

99. "Amtliche Bericht," 440.
100. Schön, 319–320; and see Amtliche Bericht," 424, where the authors indicate that they have "duly executed" the central government's instructions and this Sanitary Commission would "report on the blunders they believed had been committed" as a result.

Chapter 5

1. Joseph Hordynski, *History of the Late Polish Revolution and the Events of the Campaign,* 4th ed. (Boston: Printed for subscribers, 1833), 318.
2. Smitt, *Geschichte des...Aufstandes,* 3, 40.
3. Smitt, *Geschichte des...Aufstandes,* 2, 3, 40, 347; Kocój, 117.
4. For General Graf Toll, see "Feldmarschall Diebitsch.Vertrauliche Berichte über seinen Feldzug in Polen 1831," in F. Smitt, ed., *Feldherrn-Stimmen aus und über den Polnischen Krieg vom Jahr 1831* (Leipzig: Winter, 1858), 206 and *Le Messager Polonais,* June 27, 1831, 130.
5. L. Tegoborick, to Consular General Russie, Danzig, May 17, 1831, GStA PK, Rep. 76, VIII C, Nr. 1. Bl. 46–47.
6. Ibid.
7. Ibid.
8. Chad to Palmerston, July 5, 1831, PRO FO 64/173, 47.
9. Ibid., 47–48.
10. *Allgemeine Preussische Staats-Zeitung,* June 27, 1831, 1103.
11. Smitt, *Feldherrn-Stimmen aus ... vom Jahr 1831,* 206.
12. Adalbert Cohnfeld, *Ausführliche Lebens- und Regierungs-Geschichte Friedrich Wilhelms III: Königs von Preussen* 3 (Berlin: Lewen, 1842), 624.
13. *Preussische Staats-Zeitung,* June 21 1831, 1084.
14. *Amtsblatt Königlich Preussen Regierung zu Marienwerder,* July 1, 1831, 266.
15. Schön, 267.
16. Ignacy Prądzyński, *Pamiętniki generała Prądzyńskiego,* III (Krakowie: Spólka wydawn, 1909), 29; and *Le Messager Polonais,* June 27, 1831, 130.
17. Karol Forster, *Powstanie Narodu Polskiego, wr. 1830–31* (Berlin: Wydawnictwo polskie, 1873), 57. Forster does not document this. I could find no evidence for this in the minutes of the Immediate Commission.
18. Ewald, 12.
19. Schön, 274.
20. Ewald, 13; *The Journal de SPetersbourg,* June 20/July 2, 183, in McGrew, 108; and Schön, 270–271.
21. Ewald, 13. For a description of quarantine of Danzig and environs see, *Amtsblatt... zu Marienwerder* June, 24, 1831, 244–245.
22. Conferenz Protokol, June 21, 1831, GStA PK, Rep. 76, VIII C., Nr. 2. Bl. 19–20.
23. F. Smitt, *Geschichte... Aufstandes,* 3, 171.
24. "General Intendant Pogodin, über die Verpflegung des Russiche Armee unter dem Grafen Paskewitz" in F. Smitt (ed.), *Feldherrn-Stimmen aus ...vom Jahr 1831,* 249; "Feldmarschall Paskewitz, Umrisse das Feldzugs in Polen," in *Feldherrn-Stimmen ... Jahr 1831,* 365; and Général Prince Shcherbatov, *Le Feld-Marechal Prince Paskévitsch sa Vie eMilitaire d'a près des Documents,* 3 (SPétersbourg: Trenke et Fusnot, 1893), 33.

25. Aleksandr Shcherbatov, *Kampania polska księcia Paskiewicza w 1831 r.* (Warszawa: skł. gł. w księgarni Jana Fiszera, 1899), 53; and Kocój, 118.
26. Shcherbatov, *Le Feld-Marechal,* 33.
27. "Bekanntmachung," July, 6, 1831, *Amtsblatt ... zu Marienwerder,* July 15, 1831, 286.
28. Shcherbatov, *Le Feld-Marechal,* 54.
29. Shcherbatov, 55–56.
30. Smitt, *Feldherrn-Stimmen,* 216.
31. Ewald, 13.
32. Ibid.
33. "Bekanntmachung des König. Ober Prasidium," June 18, 1831, in *Amtsblatt ... zu Königsberg,* no. 26, June 29, 1831, 200.
34. Ewald, 17
35. Dr. Mährlan, *Polens Kampfe um Seine Wiedergeburim Jahre 1831,* 2 (Stuttgart: Schweizerbart's Verlagshandlung, 1832), 22–23.
36. Ewald, 13–14
37. Schön, 267
38. Ibid.
39. Ewald, 13.
40. Ibid., 14.
41. Ibid.; Schön, 268
42. Schön, 269–270.
43. Ibid.., 269.
44. Ibid., 264–265.
45. Karl Faber, *Die Haupt- und Residenz-StadKönigsberg in Preussen* (Königsberg: Gräfe und Unzer, 1840), 269; and "Address des magistrats de la Ville de Königsberg au roi de Prusse Frederic-Guilliame III en se plaignant," in Chodzko, 833–834.
46. Dr. v. Baer, "Geschichte der Cholera Epidemie zu Königsberg im J. 1831," *Verhandlungen der physikalischmedicinischen Gesellschafzu Königsberg, über Die Cholera* (Königsberg: Bornträger, 1832), 335.
47. Chad to Palmerston, July 5, 1831, PRO FO 64/173, 47–48.
48. Conferenz Protokol, June 21, 1831, GStA PK, Rep. 76, VIII C., Nr. 2. Bl. 20.
49. Ibid.
50. Ibid. June 24, 1831, Bl. 23–24.
51. Cohnfeld, 624.
52. Chad to Palmerston, July 13, 1831, PRO FO 64/173, 87–88.
53. Ibid.
54. Richard Otto Spazier, *Historja Powstania Narodu Polskiego w Roku 1830–1831,* 3 (Paryzu, 1855), 190.
55. "Address des magistrats...," in Chodzko, 833–834.
56. Ibid. and *La Pologne eLa Prusse en 1831* (Paris: Pinard, 1831), 33–34.
57. Chad to Palmerston, July 13, 1831, PRO FO 64/173, 87.
58. Conferenz Protokol, July 8, 1831, GStA PK, Rep. 76, VIII C., Nr. 2. Bl. 35; and Conferenz Protokol, July 11, 1831, GStA PK, Rep. 76, VIII C, Nr.2. Bl. 38
59. Schön, 270.
60. Thile to Schön, June 25, 1831, GStA PK, Rep. 76, VIII C., Nr. 24. Bl. 33–34.
61. Conferenz Protokol, July 8, 1831, GStA PK, Rep. 76, VIII C., Bl. 35.
62. Treitschke, vol. 5, 254.
63. Spazier, *Historja Powstania,* 3, 180.
64. Chad to Palmerston, July 13, 1831, PRO FO 64/173, 87–88.

65. "The Polish-Russian border from Thorn to Nimmersatt was closed. Quarantine was established in eighlocalities." These areas were all near Königsberg. *Faber*, 269
66. Chad to Palmerston, July 25, 1831, PRO FO 64/173, 143-44.
67. Raumer, 506 and 508.
68. "Manifeste du gouvernement" in Chodzko, *Recueil*, 837-839; and Raumer, 507-508.
69. Hamett, 306.
70. Carl von Clausewitz to Marie von Clausewitz, July 26, 1831 in Karl Schwartz, *Leben des Generals Carl von Clausewitz und der Frau Marie von Clausewitz*, 2 (Berlin: Ferd. Dümmlers, 1878), 372
71. *Raumer*, 508-509.
72. The quarantine policy was an attemp to thwart the Polish rebellion. See *McGrew*, 104.
73. Shcherbatov, 33.
74. See Smitt, *Geschichte...Aufstandes*, 3, 171, for an early corrective that Prussia had completely supported the Russians on the border to the exclusion of the insurgents during the cholera epidemic. Smitt also wrote that Lithuanian insurgents received their supply of "powder and shot" during this time from inside Prussia.

Chapter 6

1. *Note Officielle du Ministère des Affaires Etrangerès*, in *Nouvelles de Pologne* (Paris: Pinard, 1831), 16; Chodzko, 838.
2. *Hordynski*, 318.
3. *Prądzyński*, 3, 29. The Polish General wrote in his diary, "Huge stocks of ammunition and food were brought to Danzig, which were then transported further to the Russian army." See also General Graf Toll (interim Commander of the Russian army). He wrote that supplies arrived from Danzig until the quarantine. By June 18, 1831, there was "no less than a six week delay of provisions" due to quarantine restrictions. Smitt, *Feldherrn-Stimmen*, 206.
4. Smitt, *Geschichte...Aufstandes*, 3, 40.
5. John Shelton Curtiss, *The Russian Army Under Czar Nicholas I, 1825-1855* (Durham, NC: Duke University Press, 1965), 80-81.
6. Schiemann, *Geschichte Russland,* 3, 107; *Curtiss*, 82
7. Aleksandr K. Puzyrevskii, *Wojna Polska-Ruska 1831* (Warszawa: nakł. Maurycego Orgelbranda, 1899), 231-234.
8. Schiemann, 3, 110.
9. Ibid.; and Puzyrevskii, 214.
10. Schiemann, 3, 110.
11. Jozef Frejlich, "Operacje rosyjskie między Narwią a Dolną Wisłą w lipcu 1831 roku," *Kwartalnik Historyczny*, 43 (1929), 189.
12. Schiemann, 3, 110; "Dépêche du comte Alopéus du 16 mai 1831," in Martens, *Recueil des traités*, 173.
13. Martens, *Recueil des traités*, 174, 183.
14. Schiemann, 3, 109.
15. Shcherbatov, *Le Feld-Maréchal*, 4, 16.
16. Ibid., 19.
17. Frejlich, 190; and for a general description of the Russian army supply problems see Puzyrevskii, 370-374.
18. Smitt, ii, iii, 40, 347. During the month of May the *Preussische Provinzial-Blätter 1831*, reported from the Government District of Gumbinnen: "This past month there have been major purchases and transports especially of flour, rye and oats to provision the Czar's troops," in Kocój, 117.
19. Smitt, *Feldherrn*, 189.
20. Ibid., 193-194.
21. Ibid., 205, 210.
22. *Dziennik Powszechny Krajowy,* 10 V 1831, and 26 VI 1831 in Wiesław Stembrowicz, "Pruski Kordon Sanitarny W Okresie Wojny Polsko-Rosyjskiej (1830-1831)," *Archiwum Historii Medycyny*, 45 (1982), 41.
23. Puzyrevskii, 297.
24. Richard Otto Spazier, *Ein Geschichte des Aufstandes des Polnischen Volkes in den Jahren 1830 und 1831* (Stuttgart: Fr. Brodhagsche, 1832), 91; Schiemann, 3, 123.
25. Hans Delbrück und G.H. Pertz, *Das Leben des Feldmarschalls Grafen Neidhardt von Gneisenau* (Berlin: Hermann Walther, 1895), 678; Theodor Stürmer, *Der Tod des Russisch Kaiserlichen General-Feldmarschalls Grafen Diebitsch Sabalkansky* (Posen: Bromberg Mittler, 1832); *passim* and Brandt, 122-123.
26. He argued that even though his doctors diagnosed him with the cholera, the doctors under Russian authority could not "provide irrefutable evidence" and a pharmacist had been arrested. Spazier, *Ein Geschichte*, 297; Smitt, ii, 350, for a defense of the Emperor in this event see Puzyrevski, 297; and for Orloff's other purported poisonings, Brandt, 122-123.
27. Schiemann, 3, 124; Frejlich, 192.
28. Le Vte. De Beaumont-Vassy, *Histoire de mon temps: premier serie: Regne De Louis Philipe-Seconde Republic 1830-1834* (Paris: Perrotin, 1855), 360; and see also Forster, *Powastanie*, 57. It is unlikely that this and a number of other points he cited were agreed to at the time as the following will show. Also, neither Beaumont-Vassey nor Forster document this. I could find no evidence for this in the minutes of the Immediate Commission.
29. Schiemann, 3, 123.
30. Ibid.; Frejlich, 200.
31. Schwartz, *Leben*, 2, 360.
32. Schiemann, 3, 123; Schwartz, *Leben*, 2, 360. At the end of April 1831, Palmerston informed Prussia that if it invaded Poland and France attacked the Rhine Province, "it would be impossible for England to help Prussia." Müller, 78.
33. Chodzko, 826.
34. *Staats und Gelehrte Zeitung des Hamburgischen unpartheiishen Correspondenten*, No. 174, Juli, 26, 1831, 3; and Peter Paret, *Clausewitz and the State* (New York: Oxford University Press, 1976), 418-419.
35. Prądzyński, iii, 29.
36. Shcherbatov, *Le feld-maréchal*, 4, 13.
37. Paret, 411.
38. "Bekanntmachung des König. Ober Prasidium," June 18, 1831, in *Amtsblatt ... zu Königsberg*, no. 26, June 29, 1831, 200.
39. Ewald, 12.
40. Raumer, *Vermischte Schriften*, 2, 501-509; Laubert, "Beiträge zu Preussen," 386-388.
41. Ewald, 13; McGrew, 108; Schön, 270-271.
42. Schön, 274.
43. Shcherbatov, *Le feld-maréchal*, 4, 43; Smitt, *Feldherrn-Stimmen* 249, 365.
44. Shcherbatov, *Kampania* 53.
45. Ibid., 55-56
46. Smitt, *Feldherrn-Stimmen*, 216.
47. Puzyrevskii, 108.

48. "Manifeste du gouvernement," Chodzko, 837–839.
49. Lettre en date de Tsarskoé-Selo 15 (27) juillet 1831. 20 pièces de siège (dont 12 mortiers) furent ainsi expédiées au moyen de chevaux loués à cet effet. In Shcherbatov, *Le feld-maréchal*, 4, 51–52.
50. General von Auer to General Lieutenant von Krauseneck, June, 22, 1831, in Fejlich, 193–194. The anti-contagionist doctor, Barchewitz was one of the doctors on board the steamship *Isara*.
51. Shcherbatov, *Le Feld-Maréchal*, 4, 26; Frejlich, 194.
52. Frejlich, 200.
53. Shcherbatov, *Kampania*, 53.
54. Shcherbatov, *Le Feld-Maréchal*, 4, 43.
55. Ibid., 34–35.
56. Frejlich, 214.
57. Heinrich D. Brandt, *Aus Dem Leben des Generals der Infanterie Dr. Heinrich von Brandt* (Berlin: Ernst Siegfried Mittler und Sohn, 1869), ii, 134.
58. Frejlich, 214.
59. Ibid., 210, 215.
60. Kojóc, 122.
61. Conferenz Protokol, July 17, 1831, GStA PK, Rep. VIII C., Nr. 2. Bl. 1–2.
62. Brandt, 135 and Paret, 413.
63. Schwartz, *Leben*, 2, 372.
64. Delbrück, 679.
65. Schwartz, *Leben*, 2, 357, 378; and Paret, 422.
66. Conferenz Protokol, July 17, 1831, GStA PK., Rep. VIII C., Nr. 2, Bl. 1–2. See footnote 104, the mission also entailed smoothing out relations between the civilian and military authorities at Thorn.
67. Brandt, 112–116; and Sixième circulaire... par l'empereur Nicolas I," du médecin russe à Varsovie, et aux motifs qui ont obligé le gouvernement polonais de ne pas le recevoir, Varsovie, le juin 16, 1831, in Chodzko, 824–825.
68. Brandt, 130.
69. Frejlich, 200.
70. Brandt, 116.
71. *Instruktion für den Major v. Brandt vom Generalstabe, Posen, den 17. July 1831*, in Brandt, 117–118. However, according to a communication to the Immediate Commission [Brandt] it was understood that in Bromberg and Thorn the existing regulations were being adhered to. In Thorn, he was to ensure that the proper procedures for quarantine were adopted and to order the Commandant "to make measures for maintaining the strict regulations compulsory." See Conferenz Protokol, July 17. 1831, GStA PK, Rep. VIII C., Nr. 2. Bl. 1–2.
72. Brandt, 119.
73. Shcherbatov, *Le Feld-Maréchal Prince*, 4, 58–59.
74. Brandt, 119.
75. H. V. Hansen, *Zwei Kriegsjahre Erinnerungen eines alten Soldaten an den Feldzug der Russen gegen die Türken 1828 und den polnischen Aufstand 1831* (Berlin: Ernst Miller und Sohn, 1881), 272.
76. Frejlich, 210–212.
77. Chad to Palmerston, July 25, 1831, PRO FO 64/173, 114–115.
78. Dettke, 141–142.; Schwartz, *Leben*, 2, 370.
79. Brandt, 120.
80. *Cholera Archiv*, 2, 218–219.
81. "Immediate Zeitung Berichte der Königliche Regierung zu Marienwerder von Juli, 1831," in *Cholera Archiv*, 2, 164.
82. Brandt, 127.
83. Ibid., 135–136
84. Shcherbatov, *Kompania*, 54.
85. Shcherbatov, *Le Feld-Maréchal*, iv, 52–53.
86. Ibid., 53–54.
87. *Cholera-Archiv*, 2, 166.
88. Ibid., 162.
89. Dr. Weese "Über Entstehung, Erkennung, Schutz- und Heilmittel der cholera. Sendschreibung. Des Herren Kreisphysikus Dr. Weese zu Thorn vom October 17, 1831 an Hrn. Prof. Cerutti zu Leipzig," *Allgemeine Cholera-Zeitung: Mittheilungen des Neuesten und... von Justus Radius* 1, no. 21 (November 9, 1831), 161–164 and No. 22 (November 12, 1831), 169–172.
90. *Cholera-Archiv*, 2, 164–166, 218; and *Weese*, 161
91. Ibid.
92. Ibid., 164.
93. Ibid., 161.
94. *Cholera-Archiv*, 2, 167.
95. Ibid.
96. General von Thile to Frederick William, October 18, 1831, GStA PK, Rep. 76, VIII C., Nr. 20.
97. Walter Krehnke *Der Gang der Cholera in Deutschland seit ihrem ersten Auftreten bis heute* (Berlin: Schoetz, 1937), 6–18, *passim*.
98. *Cholera Archiv*, 1, 264.
99. On the role of the military in many of these districts see [Johann Gottfried] Hoffman,"Die Wirkungen der asiatischen Cholera im preussischen Staate wärend des Jahres 1831. Nach den bei dem statistischen Bureau eingegangenen Nachrichten," *Historisch-Philologische Abhandlungen der Koniglichen Akademie der Wissenschaften zur Berlin Aus dem Jahr 1832* (Berlin, 1834), 77; *Cholera Archiv*, 1, 217–218.
100. *Cholera Archiv*, 1, 217–218.
101. Ibid., ii, 171–172
102. Paret, 411.
103. Dettke, 156.
104. Conferenz Protokol, July 17, 1831, GStA PK, Rep. 76, VIII C., Nr. 2 Bl. 1–2.
105. Chad to Palmerston, PRO FO 64/173, 114–115.
106. Dettke, 141.
107. Brandt, 126
108. *Cholera Archiv*, 2, 161–162.
109. Schwartz, *Leben*, 2, 370.
110. Ibid.; Joseph Samter, "Zur Geschichte der Cholera-Epidemien in der Stadt Posen (1831–1873)," *Zeitschrift der Historischen Gesellschaft für die Provinz Posen*, 2 (1886), 285.
111. Conferenz Protokol, July 17, 1831, GStA PK, Rep. 76, VIII C., Nr. 2, Bl. 1.
112. "Instruktion für die Herren Aertzte der Stadt Posen" July 17 1831, in Immediat Commission Acta Betreffend Ausbruch und den Fortgang der Cholera in der Stadt Posen und die Correspondence mit der dortigen Regierung vom July 11 bis November 12, 1831, in GStA PK, Rep. 76, VIII C., Nr. 83, Bl. 12. The quick organization of the medical community in Posen was important. Samter wrote that "the epidemic reached such a level in Bromberg that in spite of the sparse number of doctors in Posen, the Oberpräsident made arrangements to remain there." Samter, 288.
113. "Instruktion für die Herren Bezirks-Versteher" July 17, 1831, in Immediat Commission Acta Betreffend Ausbruch und den Fortgang der Cholera in der Stadt Posen ..." GStA PK, Rep. 76, VIII C, Nr. 83, Bl. 13–14.
114. "Bekanntmachung über die Instruktion der Stadt

Posen durch die Asiatische Cholera und die Cirnirung derselben mit ihrer Umgegend im Umkreise von drei meilen," July 18, 1831, in Immediat Commission Acta Betreffend Ausbruch und den Fortgang der Cholera in der Stadt Posen...," GStA PK, Rep. 76, VIII C, Nr. 83, Bl. 15–16.
115. *Cholera Zeitung*, Königsberg, 1832, 97–98.
116. Dettke, 157.
117. *Cholera-Archiv*, 2, 162.
118. *Cholera Zeitung*, Königsberg, 1832, 69–70.
119. Dettke, 142.
120. Brandt, 151–152.
121. See Samter, 285 on Tatzler; Brandt, 138–140, gives an eyewitness account; Pertz, 687–689, describes his last few hours; Schwartz, 386–389, for Clausewitz's eyewitness account of his death and his complaint that for such a great man the king had only issued two cursory reports; and Paret, 425–426.
122. Schwartz, *Leben*, 2, 580 and 581; Brandt, 512, "the reports from Warsaw were sparse."
123. *Cholera Archiv*, 2, 162–163.
124. *Archiv für medizinische Erfahrung im Gebiete der praktischen Medizin, Chirugie, Geburtshülfe und Staatsarzneikunde*, Juli, August (Berlin, 1832), 726.
125. Krehnke, 14–15
126. *Cholera Archiv*, 1, 220–221; for the death rate per thousand, see Krehnke, 15.
127. Ibid., 222.
128. Brandt, George "Die Epidemien in der Provinz Posen in der ersten Hälfte des Jahrhunderts," *Zeitschrift Historische Gesellschaft für Posen*, 16. (1901), 117.
129. General Skrzynecki, "Letter Du Généralissime Polonais au Roi De Prusse, Juin 19, 1831," *La Pologne et la Prusse*, 29.
130. "Interview with Mr. Ancillon," Chad to Palmerston, July 31, 1831, PRO FO 64/173, 187–188.
131. "Manifest de Gouvernement Polonais," and "Note Officielle," in *La Pologne und Prusse*, 3–27, 53–56.
132. *Staats und Gelehrten...Correspondenten*, No. 174, July 26, 1831, 3; Paret, 418–419.
133. Schwartz, 376.
134. Ibid., 375–376; Schwartz, 384.
135. Paret, 419. Cholera broke out in Breslau on September 20, 1831 and lasted until December 28, 1831. The first case occurred in the All Saints Hospital in Breslau. A beggar woman, Joahnne Karlsdorf died. Others who had slept in the same room with her also became sick. A laundress who had "accidentally washed Karlsdorf's clothing" became ill as well. This started the epidemic in the city. It lasted for 3 months. 1,347 people became sick and 795 died out of a population of 90,000. See R. Kayser, *Zur Geschichte der Cholera, special der Choleraepidemien in Breslau* (Breslau: Preuss u. Jünger, 1884), 8.
136. Chad to Palmerston, July 31, 1831, PRO FO 64/173, 185; and "Article de la Gazette D'Etat de Prusse Relatif a la letter du Generalissime Polonais," in *La Pologne und Prusse*, 30–32.
137. Laubert, 384–385
138. Chad to Palmerston, July 31, 1831, PRO FO 64/173, 188–189.
139. Chad to Palmerston, August 11, 1831, PRO FO 64/173, 241.
140. Ibid., 242.
141. Paret, 418.
142. Chad to Palmerston, July 20, 1831, PRO FO 64/173, 120.

143. "Manifest de Gouvernment Polonais," in *La Pologne und Prusse*, 55.
144. "Note Officielle," in *La Pologne und Prusse*, 15, 16. See pages 16–22, devoted to complaints concerning the cordon sanitaire on the Prussian-Polish border. They comprise nearly 30 percent of this document.
145. McGrew, 104.
146. Later one medical official wrote in reference to the strict quarantine that as long as the "disease spared in Europe all expected the immediately threatened Prussia to take this measure of protection." Moreover, "Prussia saw it as a sacred duty even if the consequences were questionable Horn, "Die Contagiosität der Asiatischen Cholera," in *Cholera- Archiv*, 2, 84; *Morgenblatt für gebildete Stände*, 25 (July 1831), 900; Dettke, 65.
147. Chad to Palmerston, July 20, 1831, PRO FO 64/173, 121.
148. Shcherbatov, *Kompania*, 55.
149. Ibid., 55–56.

Chapter 7

1. *Zamknięcie granicy ku Polsce i Litwie Rossyiskiey z powodu Cholery*, facsimile notice in Olkowski, 534–35.
2. Ibid.
3. Stembrowicz, 42.
4. Olkowski, 536.
5. H. Bonk, *Geschichte der Stadt Allenstein* (Allenstein: Danehl, 1914), 4, 223; Olkowski, 536.
6. "Zur Ausführung der Instruktion über das bei dem Ausbruch der Cholera zu beobachtende Verfahren vom 5. April (June 1) 1831, Für die Provinzen Preußen, Posen und den auf rechten Oder-Ufer gelegenen Theil von Schlesien."*Amtsblatts der Königl. Preuss. Regierung Frankfurth a. d. Oder*, nr. 34, August 24, 1831, in *Amtsblatts ... zu Frankfurth a. d. Oder (Trowitzsch und Sohn, Frankfurth an der Oder)*, 286.
7. Stembrowicz, 42.
8. "Note Officielle," in *La Pologne*, 18–22.
9. "Instruktion für die Königlichen Kontumaz-Beamten," in *Amtsblatts... zu Frankfurth a. d. Oder*, 156.
10. *Amtsblatt ... zu Marienwerder*, Nr. 26, July 1, 1831, 256.
11. Stembrowicz, 41.
12. Stembrowicz, 41–42. For these regulations see "Anweisung über das Desinfections-Verfahren bei den aus Gegenden, wo die Cholera herrscht, kommenden Reisenden, Waaren und Thieren," in *Amtsblatts... zu Frankfurth a. d. Oder*, 156.
13. Ibid.
14. J. U. Niemcewicz, *Pamietniki z 1830–1831* (Krakow, 1909), 155; Stembrowicz, 42.
15. Boismont, 167–169.
16. Stembrowicz, 42–43.
17. Stembrowicz, 41.
18. Johannes Sembritzki, *Memel im Neunzehnten Jahrhundert: Geschichte der Königlich Preussischen, See— und Handelsstadt* 2 (Memel: F.W. Siebert, 1900), 122.
19. Stromeyer, 2.
20. Olkowski, 545.
21. Boismont, 164–165.
22. Ibid., 165.
23. Ibid.

24. *Amtsblatt ... zu Königsberg,* 29 VI n. 26, 1831, 195–198.
25. Polish Jews were seen as a particular problem on the Polish-Prussian border. See "Instruktion für die Königlichen Kontumaz-Beamten," in *Amtsblatt ... zu Frankfurth a. d. Oder,* 156; also see June 3, 1831, order by Regierung President Meding of Königsberg, issued on the recommendation of Provincial President Schön, forbidding Jews from Poland to enter East Prussia without a certificate of health. It directed that those Jews who were already in the country without proper certificates were to be arrested and deported, Olkowski, 545; and finally even the French physician Brierre De Boismont recommended that the heads of the quarantine stations especially supervise "Jewish peddlers and their bundles," Boismont, 168.
26. Olkowski, 544.
27. Ibid.
28. Stromeyer, 2, 16–17.
29. Laubert, 387–388.
30. Wagner, 137.
31. Olkowski, 545.
32. Wagner, 138.
33. Ibid.
34. Ibid., 139.
35. Ibid.
36. For more information on the cholera epidemic in Elbing see R. Burdach, "Über den Ursprung der Cholera-Epidemie in Elbing," *Cholera-Zeitung* (Königsberg), 45–46; the latter was published in Königsberg August 6–October 1, 1831, and was known for its anti-contagion opinions.
37. Wagner, 144.
38. R. Burdach, "Verbreitung und Tödlichkeit der Cholera in Königsberg im Jahr 1831," *Cholera-Zeitung* (Königsberg), 142–143.
39. A.B. Granville, *Travels to S Petersburg: A Journey To and From That Capital; Through Flanders, the Rhenish Provinces, Prussia, Poland, Silesia, and Saxony, The Federated States of Germany and France,* vol. 1 (London: Longman, 1828), 347.
40. D. Brewster, *The Edinburgh Encyclopedia,* vol. 12 (Edinburgh: William Blackwood, 1830), 481.
41. Karl Friedrich Burdach, *Rückblick auf mein Leben. Selbstbiographie* 3 (Leipzig: Voss, 1844), 396.
42. Burdach, *Rückblick auf mein Leben,* 387.
43. Marion Gray, "Prussia in Transition: Society and Politics under the Stein Reform Ministry," *Transactions of the American Philosophical Society* vol. 76, Part I (1986), 108.
44. Gray, 108–109.
45. Wagner, 208.
46. Burdach, "Über die Verbreitung," 114–116.
47. Ibid., 115.
48. Ewald, 33.
49. For Memel and Stettin see Evans, 244; Sembritzki,122; and for Memel and for Stettin see also the report in the *Staats und Gelehrte...Correspondenten,* September, 9, 1831, 1.
50. Karl Faber, *Die Haupt-und Residenz-Stadt Königsberg in Preussen* (Königsberg: Grafe und Unzer, 1840), 269.
51. Faber, 269–270.
52. "Bekanntmachung," Königliche Preussische Regierung, Abteilung des Innern, GstA PK, Rep. 76, VIII C, Nr. 42. Bl. 109.
53. *Cholera Zeitung* (Königsberg), 92.
54. Stromeyer also noted a general non-belief in contagion among the common people. Stromeyer, 8.
55. *Cholera Zeitung* (Königsberg), 92.
56. Ibid., 93.
57. Schön, 272–273. See also Frevert, 125–128 on the attitude of the middle class towards the relationship between the poor and sickness. Poverty was regarded as a two-fold danger from both the social and sanitary aspects.
58. Fear of the government and doctors as agents of the government, as well as the fear of the upper classes by the lower classes is not only anchored in economic terms but can also be seen in fears against middle class acceptance of Malthusian ideas. Malthus was translated into German as early as 1807, however, there was no actual debate in Germany until a decade later. Frevert, 118–119. The best example of the influence of Malthusian ideas in Germany is found in Prussian Medical Councilor, C.A. Weinhold's book, *Von den Überbevölkerungen in Mittel Europa und deren Folgen auf die Staaten und ihr Civilization* published in 1827. He wrote, "war, plague, hunger and emigration were not enough to decrease overpopulation. The poorer classes had to be prevented from begetting children, *Weinhold,* 41. However, not everyone supported his ideas on sterilization, because he also advocated harsh measures like castration and infanticide. *Fischer,* 460–461; One can easily imagine that by 1831 these Malthusian ideas (or at least Malthusian inspired) had been altered to feed the fears of the poor about the higher classes wanting to be rid of them; Werner Conze wrote that the governments of Germany passed legislation forbidding "male servants, journeymen and apprentices in the cities and in the country to marry...," unless they could support a wife and children. This legislation to limit the increase of the socially undesirable was common in the Germanies in the thirties. See Werner Conze, "Vom Pöbel zum Proletaria Sozialgeschichtliche Voraussetzungen für den Sozialismus in Deutschland," *VSWG,* vol. 41 (1954), 339.
59. Schön did not agree with the central government's methods because they were essentially plague prevention measures. He complained that the April 5 and June 1 regulations were simply "modified Russian plague instructions." Olkowski, 549.
60. Ewald, 29–30.
61. Ewald, 30; "Amtliche Bericht," 440.
62. Karl Friederich Burdach (1776–1847) was a physiologist, physician and professor at the University of Königsberg. Burdach supported the Polish revolution in 1830 and made a short trip back to Poland "his homeland" dreaming of its liberation. His sympathy toward the Polish uprising colored his attitude toward the Prussian Government's response to cholera. This included his harsh criticism of Schön in his autobiography. See Fritze Gause, *Die Geschichte der Stadt Königsberg in Preussen,* 2 (Köln: Ostmitteleuropa in Vergangenheit und Gegenwart, 1968), 494; and Burdach, *Rückblick auf mein Leben,* 390.
63. Burdach, *Rückblick auf mein Leben,* 385
64. Faber, 269.
65. Ewald, 31; "Amtliche Bericht," i–v.
66. Burdach, *Rückblick auf mein Leben,* 386–387.
67. Ibid., 390.
68. Ibid.
69. Burdach, *Rückblick auf mein Leben,* 388–390; for the Prussian Court and the Immediate Commission see the previous chapter; Schön expressed his concern regarding the accusations of compliance on his part in support

of the Russian army to Thile. He wrote, this was "entirely repugnant to him. "Should this land be harmed as a result of the measures...[that he has taken]... he would let the entire Russian army go to the ground." Schön, 269–270.

70. Burdach, *Rückblick auf mein Leben*, 390; "Amtliche Bericht," i–v; Ewald, 31; and Schön where he noted that Burdach simply wanted "to lead the cause." Initially Schön had to support the Berlin measures. After the decision of the Conference held in Königsberg on July 26, 1831, he was convinced to suspend them. In addition and contrary to Burdach's contention that only the physicians from the local medical society were advising him, Schön stated he was being advised by three physicians who were his technical advisors, Dr. Karl Ernst von Baer, Regierungsmedizinrath Dr. Kessel and Dr. Christoph Elsner who all happened to agree with Burdach. However, Burdach was not part of this team and continued to accuse Schön, of "official rigidness" and of opposing physicians like himself. Schön, 326.

71. The latter in direct response to misinformation published in an unnamed *Königsberg* newspaper quoting Schön. The doctors believed this misinformation contributed to mob violence against the doctors. Burdach, *Rückblick auf mein Leben*, 393–394.

72. Ewald, 31.
73. Ibid. 31.
74. Dettke, 125; Wagner, 143.
75. Prof. V. Baer, "Bericht über die Veranlassung zum Ausbruch der Cholera in Königsberg," *Cholera Zeitung* (Königsberg, 1832), 36.
76. *Wagner*, 144.
77. Emil Schnippel "Leichenwasser und Geisterglaube in Ostpreussen," *Zeitschrift der Verein für Volkskunde*, vol. 20 (Berlin, 1910): 394–398. Schnippel focuses on East Prussian beliefs concerning "corpse-water" (i.e. water in which the corpse was washed), which was scattered or poured upon people as a good omen. The water was kept in a bowl in the death chamber to be later broken on the wheel of the wagon or hearse scattering the water. Otherwise the "dead will find no rest." There is the distinct possibility that some contaminated water might have been in the contaminated bedclothes, and water might have gotten on the women from their customary washing of the dead. The water sprinkled on the bier could have helped spread cholera.

78. Dettke, 125.
79. Wagner, 145; Dettke, 126.
80. Ewald, 32; Dettke, 126.
81. Burdach, *Rückblick auf mein Leben*, 391.
82. R. Baehrel, "La Haine de Classe en Temps D'Épidémie," *Annales* 7 (1952), 358–360. He references poisoning accusations against doctors and pharmacists throughout Europe during the cholera epidemic of 1831–1832.
83. Baer, 28.
84. Ibid., 28–29.
85. Ewald, 32.
86. Baer, 29–31.
87. Ibid., 26.
88. Ibid., 32–34; Wagner, 159.
89. Baer, 31.
90. Ibid., 31–32.
91. Ibid., 33.
92. Ibid., 34.
93. Ibid., 35–36.
94. Ibid., 36.
95. Ibid., 36–37.
96. Ibid., 37–38.
97. Ibid., 26–39.
98. Wagner, 146–152.
99. This can be explained away by inexperience in diagnosing cholera, or that the physician did not initially want to panic the population. *Cholera Zeitung* (Königsberg), 36.
100. Officials provided the Meinert and the Brosche families with new beds. They chose to keep the old beds and considered the new beds a "luxury" and sold them. Ibid., 37.
101. Baehrel, 351–360; Chevalier, *passim*, including the widespread conviction that the "rich were assassinating the poor, even while they pretended to be helping." Sussman, 309.
102. Dirk Blasius, "Sozialprotest und Sozialkriminalität in Deutschland. Eine Problemstudie zum Vormärz Sozialprotest," in Heinrich Volkmann und Júrgen Bergmann (Hrsg.), *Sozialer Protest: Studien zu traditioneller Resistenz und kollektiver Gewalt in Deutschland vom Vormärz bis zur Reichsgründung* (Opladen Westdeutscher Verlag, 1984), 224; Sembritzki; 122–123; R.J. Evans, "Epidemics and Revolution in Nineteenth Century Europe," *Past and Present* CXX (1988), 138; and *Staats und Gelehrte...Correspondenten*, September 9, 1831, 1.
103. Baehrel, 359–360. Where Baehrel notes the poor in France blamed the doctors and pharmacists as instruments of the government in the service of the rich poisoning the poor. The Königsberg rioters do not incorporate hostility toward the rich as much as the government in Berlin as the cause of their misery. *Cholera Archiv*, 3 (1833), 245–246.
104. Schön, 289.
105. Schön, 326; Ewald, 32.
106. Schön, 289.
107. Ibid.
108. Ibid.
109. Ibid., 290.
110. Ewald, 33; Olkowski, 557.
111. Ewald, 33.
112. Schön, 320.
113. Olkowski, 547.
114. Schön, 312.
115. Ibid.
116. Schön, 296.
117. Ibid., 297
118. Schön, 306.
119. Conferenz Protokol, July 22, 1831, GStA PK, Rep. 76, VIII C, Nr.2, Bl. 48. (e.g. in Danzig).
120. *Verhandlungen der ... zu Königsberg*, v; Dettke, 132.
121. GStA PK, Rep. 76 VIII C, Nr. 115, Bl. 49 R. Bericht vom 27.7.1831. cited in Dettke, 132.
122. Burdach, *Rückblick auf mein Leben*, 391.
123. In some respects it is understandable that an immediate meeting was necessary as Hagen reported that both the Government and the Police had ordered newer and stricter quarantine measures for cholera infected dwellings on July 24, 1831. Schön, 305.
124. "Abschrift," July 25, 1831, *Ausserordentliche Beilage, Nr. 16. zu Nr. 31 des Amtsblatte der Königl. Ostpreuss Regierung*, 1831, 101–103 (supplement to the *Amtsblatts ... zu Königsberg*, 1831) for the results of the meeting and the signers of the proclamation, *Cholera Zeitung* (Königsberg), 92.

125. GStA PK, Rep. 76, VIII C, Nr. 96, Bl. 129, in Dettke, 132; Ewald clears up some confusion concerning what he calls the assembly of notables, Schön, 297.
126. *Ausserordentliche Beilage*, 91–106; Schön, 297, 306.
127. Schön, 318–319.
128. Ibid., 319–320.
129. Ibid., 320.
130. Ibid., 320.
131. "Verordnungen und Bekanntmachung der Königl Regierung," Abteilung des Innern, July 26, 1831 in *Ausserordentliche Beilage...*, 99–10: and Olkowski, 548–549.
132. Schön, 305–306.
133. Burdach, *Rückblick auf mein Leben*, 392.
134. Schön, 287, 289, and 290.
135. Burdach, *Rückblick auf mein Leben*, 392.
136. Schön, 325.
137. Burdach, *Rückblick auf mein Leben*, 392.
138. Ewald, 34.

Chapter 8

1. *Preussische Staats-Zeitung*, August 2, 1831, 1254.
2. "Der Volks-Auflauf in Königsberg am 28 Juli 1831," Mitgetheilt vom Kriminalrichter Richter, *Preussischer Provinzial Blätter* 7 (Königsberg, 1832), 160.
3. Richter wrote he did receive information that cow dung, and a type of fungus that grows on trees pulverized and mixed with chamomile tea was used as a household remedy for cholera. *Cholera Zeitung* (Königsberg), 16, comments on household remedies against cholera cautioning that "cow dung" was not an effective remedy against the cholera.
4. Richter, 161.
5. Ibid., 161–162.
6. Ibid., 163.
7. Ibid.
8. Ibid.
9. Faber, 272.
10. Ibid., 164–165.
11. Schmidt to Brenn, July 29, 1831, Ministerium des Innern Acta GStA PK, Vol. I. R77, Nr. 6, Vol. 1. Sec: Volksaufs und Tum. Provol. Preussen nr. 6. Bl. 24.
12. Schön, 321.
13. Schön, 298
14. Schön, 321.
15. Schmidt to Brenn, Juli 29, 1831, Bl. 22. However, this may have been a self-serving remark for Brenn's benefit because according to Ewald, Schmidt's daughter, a most "respectable woman ... had to be rescued by courageous men from the roof and thus protected from abuse." Ewald, 38.
16. Ibid.
17. Ibid.
18. Richter, 165.
19. Richter, 165; Schmidt to Brenn, July 29, 1831, Bl. 26; Faber, 273–274.
20. Schmidt to Brenn, Juli 29, 1831, Bl. 26; Olkowski, 558.
21. "Uebersicht von dem Dienstleben des am. Novol. 18, 1835 verstorbenen Herrn Polizeipräsident Schmidt" in *Vaterlandische Archiv für Wissenschaft, Kunst, Industrie und Agrikultur*, 15 (Konigsberg, 1836), 564; Ewald, 38.
22. Schmidt to Brenn, July 29, 1831, Bl. 26.
23. *Allgemeine Zeitung*, August 7, 1831, 1177; Ewald, 38.
24. Richter, 165.
25. Police President Schmidt, "Votum," August 15, 1831, GStA PK, Rep. 76, VIII C, Nr. 115, Bl. 69.
26. Ewald, 39–40.
27. Ibid., 40.
28. Schön, 299–300.
29. Faber, 274.
30. Ewald, 40–41.
31. Schön, 307; Faber, 274.
32. Schmidt to Brenn, JulY 29, 1831, Bl. 26.
33. Faber, 272–275.
34. Ewald, 41.
35. Faber, 272–275.
36. Richter, 166.
37. Schmidt to Brenn, July 29, 1831, Bl. 27; Olkowski, 558.
38. Ibid.
39. Faber, 276–277.
40. Olkowski, 558; *Allgemeine Zeitung*, August 7, 1831, 1177; *Preussische Staats-Zeitung*, August 2, 1831, 1254. *Allgemeine Zeitung*, August 14, 1831, 902; and Chad to Palmerston, August 2, 1831, PRO FO 64/173, 195.
41. Faber, 276–277.
42. Richter, 167.
43. Ibid., 167–170.
44. Ibid., 263–271.
45. Ibid., 272–278.
46. The liberation struggle in Poland was infamously compared to a disease. In an August 1, 1831, letter to the crown prince, Friedrich William III wrote these "revolutionary ideas were like a political plague from the west." In Thomas Stamm-Kuhlmann, *König in Preussens grosser Zeit Friedrich William III. Der Melancholiker auf dem Thron* (Berlin: Siedler,1992), 533.
47. J. Müller, *Die Polen in der Öffentlicher Meinung Deutschlands 1830–1832* (Marburg: L.G. Elwert, 1923), 64–65.
48. Gauss, 494.
49. Geheimes Staatsarchiv, Rep. 84a Nr. 4178, 4180, cited in *Blasius*, 224; for a facsimile of the circular see Dettke, 138.
50. Blasius, 224. "There was no political motivation hidden leadership or prior agreement that caused this turmoil." Faber, 277.
51. Richter, 158–159. This is the most complete published account on the uprising. For historical references with a variety of interpretations see Faber; and *Gauss* who mentions the riot in Königsberg but state it was quickly forgotten by the citizens. When the cholera receded the riot appeared "as an inexplicable dark, deep, evil dream, from an emotional underclass," Gauss, 497; Ewald; Wilhelm Martull "Anfange der Arbeiterbewegung in Ostpreussen," *Jahrbuch der Albertus-Universitaet zu Königsberg*, 14 (1964), 221–222, in Richard W. Reichard, *Crippled from Birth German Social Democracy 1844–1870* (Iowa State University Press, 1969); Alf Ludtke, "The Role of State Violence in the Period of Transition to Industrial Capitalism the example of Prussia from 1815–1848," *Social History*, 4 (May, 1979): 207; and *Blasius*, 212–227; Ross, The Prussian Administrative...," Chp. 5; Dettke, 134–140; and Wildrotter, *Das Grosse Sterben Seuchen*, 204–218.
52. Richter, 279.
53. Blasius, 224
54. Strangely enough "physical attacks and insults" against the authorities in pre–March Prussia were not uncommon. According to one historian, "insubordinate of-

fenses were directed against all levels of the Prussian administrative hierarchy" including all officials in contact with the public, "police, customs, tax, court officials and the higher civil servants." The "turmoil and disturbances were crimes no one was afraid of because large sections of the population during this period had lost faith in the "legitimacy of the legal norms" that had previously been respected. Blasius, 219.

55. See especially Police President Schmidt, *Votum*, August 15, 1831, GStA PK, Rep. 76, VIII C, Nr. 115, Bl. 69–71; and Faber, 271.

56. Schmidt, *Votum*, Bl. 69; and Ewald, 37 and 39. Ewald noted that at moments like this the "wildest tales easily entrance the deluded ignorant crowd." Other rumors were circulated including that it was the Jews poisoning the wells or the rich had bribed the doctors to "cure" the poor to death. Some Jews as well as doctors were roughed up during the riot.

57. Schmidt, *Votum*, Bl. 69; Wildrotter, 213.
58. Ewald, 37.
59. Sperber, 768–769.
60. Chevalier, *Le Cholera* (see introduction)
61. Weinhold, 41.
62. Schmidt to Brenn, July 29, 1831, Bl. 24.
63. Ibid.
64. Schön, 320.
65. Burdach, 393.
66. Chad to Palmerston, September 11, 1831, PRO FO 64/174, 63–64.
67. Chad to Palmerston, August 2, 1831, PRO FO 64/173, 195.
68. *Allgemeine Zeitung*, August 7, 1831, 1177.
69. Chad to Palmerston, August 2, 1831, PRO FO 64/173, 195.
70. See Weinhold above for Malthusian ideas in Prussia; John Aberth, *Plagues in World History* (New York: Rowman & Littlefield, 2011), 103.
71. Chad to Palmerston, September 11, 1831, PRO FO 64/174, 63–64.
72. Sembritzki, 122–123; and R. J. Evans, "Epidemics and Revolution in Nineteenth Century Europe," *Past and Present* CXX (1988): 138. Chad received a report that a revolt had broken out in Memel and it had "also been suppressed." Chad to Palmerston, August 2, 1831, PRO FO 64/173, 196.
73. *Staats und Gelehrte... Correspondenten*, September 9, 1831, 1.
74. *Cholera Archiv*, 3, 245–246.
75. Chad to Palmerston, September 11, 1831, PRO FO 64/174, 63–64; Charles C.F. Greville, *The Greville Memoirs*, vol. 2 (London: Longmans, Green and Co., 1874), 193. It is obvious that conspiracy theories were not unique to Prussia. Russia and France suffered from these conspiracy theories. For conspiracy theories in France and Europe see Baehrel, passim; Chevalier and Sussman for France and for Russia, McGrew.
76. Chad to Palmerston, September 11, 1831, PRO FO 64/174, 63–64.
77. Schmidt to Brenn, Juli 29, 1831, Bl. 26.
78. Chad to Palmerston, August 2, 1831, PRO., F.O. 64/173, 195.
79. Baer, 370.
80. Faber, 268–269.
81. Baer, 370; Gauss, 497.
82. George Rudé, *The Crowd in History A Study of Popular Disturbances in France and England 1730–1848* (New York, 1964), 254–255. The rioting in Königsberg followed the pattern of a common pre-industrial riot" in which there was a particular objective which the crowd wanted to achieve. As Rudé noted the destruction of lives by the crowd was not an objective of the crowd. Undoubtedly Police Chief, Schmidt, was never in danger of his life. Although the "tumult" may have gotten out of hand as even the trial document showed. The crowd attacked an apothecary shop along with assorted merchants. This was not a case of random violence but one directed toward those who had some aspect of medical authority over the people. See Geheimes Staatsarchive, Rep. 84a, Nr. 4180 in Blasius, 225; and Richter, 166.

83. *Allgemeine Zeitung*, August 7, 1831, 1177.
84. Schmidt, *Votum*, Bl. 70.
85. Schmidt to Brenn, July 29, 1831, Bl. 28
86. *Cholera Zeitung* (Königsberg), 32.
87. Baer, 370.
88. Traditionally Prussia was an unpoliced area. For example, in 1814 in Berlin, with a population of 150,000 there were only 127 police. In Gumbinnen in 1836 there were only 57 police for 300 square miles. The ratio for other areas of Prussia was not much better. During the pre–March period Prussia depended on "communal representatives" such as the Landrat, rather than state officials. Koselleck, 461–463.
89. Ibid., 463.
90. Schön, 284.
91. Schön, 320–321.
92. Ibid. 321.
93. Ibid.
94. Olkowski, 558.
95. Schmidt to Brenn, July 29, 1831, Bl 28.
96. Hans-Jürgen Belke *Die Preussische Regierung zu Königsberg 1818–1850* (Berlin: Grote, 1976), 49.
97. Belke, 49.
98. Olkowski, 558.
99. Schön, 292–293; Ewald, 46.
100. It would seem peculiar that a Prussian Oberpräsident would support these sentiments. However, Schön was one of the members of the reform party in 1807–1808 (which included General Boyen, General Gneisenau, and General von Clausewitz). Men like Schön supported more liberal views and had seen the army utilized as simply a tool of the government and were appalled by the "brutality with which the troops conducted themselves on occasion when they were, in fact, called out to preserve order ... as in the case of disturbances among the journeymen tailors in Berlin in 1830..." Gordon A. Craig, *The Politics of the Prussian Army 1640–1945* (New York: Clarendon Press, 1955), 81; Treitschke, vol. 4, 216, for a description of the "tailors revolt." For the military view see General von Rochow, "Aus den Briefen eines preussischen Militärs zur Zeit Juli Revolution," in *Historisch-Politische Blätter für das Catholische Deutschland*, redigirt Edmund Jörs und Franz Binder, 69 (München, 1872): 22–25. It is clear why Schön and the government of Königsberg harbored antipathy toward the army. It was not the people's army as the reformists had earlier wanted. By this time it was clear any reconciliation which had been done earlier during the reform era between the "military establishment with civilian society had been destroyed...." See Craig, 81.
101. Ewald, 45–46; Schön, 319.
102. Baer, 370.
103. *Cholera Zeitung* (Königsberg), 92.

Chapter 9

1. "Abändernde Bestimmungen zur Ausführung der Instruktion über das bei dem Ausbruche der Cholera zu beobachtende Verfahren vom 5. April (1. Juni)," Immediat Commission zur Abwehrung der Cholera, Berlin August 5, 1831; "Ausserordentliche...., 1-8, beobachtende Verfahren vom 5. April (1. Juni)," Immediat Commission zur Abwehrung der Cholera, Berlin, 5 August 1831, in *Ausserordentliche Beilage zum Amtsblatt No. 33 der Königliche Regierung*, 1-8, in *Amtsblatt für ... Marienwerder*, Bd. 21, August 19, 1831 [supplement follows page 174].
2. Ibid.; Olkowski, 550.
3. Olkowski, 550.
4. On September 5, 1831 the correspondent for a Hamburg Newspaper reported the king had informed his people that things could be done to alleviate any distress the cholera measures might entail and relieve the "distress among the working class so as not to induce a similar performance as occurred in Königsberg and Stettin." *Staats und Gelehrte ... Correspondenten*, September 9, 1831.
5. "Abändernde Bestimmungen..., August 5, 1831, *Ausserordentliche...*, 1-8. See also Olkowski, 550.
6. Schön, 317; and Ewald, 46.
7. Schön, 307 and Ewald, 46.
8. Ewald, 46; Schmidt, *Votum*, August 15, 1831.
9. Schön, 300-301; Ewald, 47.
10. Ewald, 47; Schmidt wrote that it was unlikely that even with these regulations that the dissatisfaction would rise to the same level of disobedience as on July 28. Even the citizens and craftsmen were not happy with regulations concerning travelers, trade with the provinces and internal trade within the city. However, interference with trade was a factor in agitating the "mob" and the working class," Schmidt, *Votum*.
11. Ewald, 47.
12. Ibid., 47-48.
13. Ibid., 49.
14. Becker, 48-49.
15. Schön, 314-315; Ewald, 51.
16. Conferenz Protokol, August 11, 1831, GStA PK Rep. 76, VIII C, Nr. 2. 61-2.
17. Schön, 312.
18. Ewald, 57.
19. Ibid.; And see Jacob von Gerlach ed. *Leopold von Gerlach, Aufzeichnungen aus seinem Leben und Wirken 1795-1877* Bd. 1 (Schwerin: Fr. Bahn, 1903), 198 and Nicolai I. Pirogow, *Lebensfragen Tagebuch eines Alten Arztes* (Stuttgart: Cotta, 1894), 397-398.
20. Paul Clausewitz, *Die Städteordnung von 1808 und die Stadt Berlin* (Berlin: Springer 1908), 183-184.
21. "Allerhöchstverordnetes Gesundheits-Comité für Berlin," *Berliner Cholera Zeitung*, October 18, 1831, 91.
22. Ibid., 91.
23. Ibid.
24. Ibid.
25. H. Scoutetten, *Relation historique et médicale de l'épidémie de choléra qui a Régné à Berlin en 1831*, 2nd ed. (Paris: Metz, 1832), 3-4.
26. Some of these recent events were known to the citizens of Berlin through the *Preussische Staatszeitung*. See Scoutetten, 9.
27. Chad to Palmerston, September 15, 1831, PRO FO 64/174, 88.
28. Conferenz Protokol, August 11, 1831, GStA PK, Rep. 76, VIII C, Nr. 2. 61.
29. Ibid.
30. Ibid., 61-62, 70-72; and *Berliner Cholera...*, October 18, 1831, 92.
31. Ibid., 61.
32. Chad wrote that the news regarding unrest in Memel was "suppressed." Chad to Palmerston, August 2, 1831, PRO FO 64/173, 197.
33. In a meeting on August 15th more troops were stationed on the Oder. Chad to Palmerston, August 17, 1831, PRO FO 64/174, 267; and Conferenz Protokol, August 11, 1831, GStA PK, Rep. 76, VIII C, Nr. 2. 61.
34. Conferenz Protokol, August 11, 1831, GStA PK, Rep. 76 VIII C, Nr. 2. 61; and Becker, 52.
35. Ibid.
36. Ibid.; and *Berliner Cholera*, October 22, 1831, 111.
37. *Allgemeine Preussische Staats-Zeitung*, August 30, 1831, 1369.
38. Conferenz Protokol, August 11, 1831 GStA PK, Rep. 76, VIII C, Nr. 2, 67-68.
39. Ibid.
40. Schön, 312.
41. Conferenz Protokol, August 11, 1831, GStA PK, Rep. 76, VIII C, Nr. 2. 69-70.
42. Ibid.
43. Ibid.
44. Acta der Königliche Civil Kabinett: Massregeln zur Abwehrung zur Cholera in der Haupt- und Residenz Stadt Berlin, August 13, 1831, GStA PK, Rep. 2.2.1, Nr. 24511. These were the questions the city deputies had raised through the Sanitary Committee of Berlin (especially Deputy Vetter) with regard to easing the regulations of August 5th concerning house quarantines and lazarets, noting that these would be especially costly and impractical in a city the size of Berlin. See Conferenz Protokol, August 11, 1831, GStA PK, Rep. 76, VIII C, Nr. 2. 67-70.
45. Ibid.
46. Ibid.
47. Ibid.
48. *Berliner Cholera*, 91.
49. Ibid., 91-92.
50. Ibid., 92 and Scoutetten, 9.
51. Scoutetten, 9.
52. *Berliner Cholera*, 92; and "Bestallung für die Communal Mitglieder der Schutz Commissionen," August, 1831; "Ober Bürgermeister, Bürgermeister, und Rath hiesiger Königlichen Residenzien, II. Bestallung für die Schutz Commissionsärzte," August 1831; and "Königlichen Verwaltungsbehörde des Gesundheits Comités für Berlin. III. Bestätigung der Schutz Commissionsvorsteher, August 1831," *Berliner Cholera*, October 22, 1831, 110-111.
53. *Preussischen Staats-Zeitung*, August, 30, 1831, 1370.
54. Becker, 10.
55. Conferenz Protokol, August 11, 1831; August 19, 1831, GStA PK, Rep. 76 VIII C, Nr. 2. 67-70,76; and Clausewitz, 183.
56. Dettke, 188-189.
57. Conferenz Protokol, August 11, 1831, GStA PK, Rep. 76 VIII C, Nr. 2. 61-2; and Dettke, 188.
58. Dettke,189.
59. John Snow, *On the mode of Communication of Cholera* 2nd ed. (London: J. Churchill, 1855); Berliner

Wasserwerke, *Die Wasserversorgung Berlins und die neuen Wasserwerke in ihrer Bedeutung für die Häuserlichkeit und das Familienwohl* (Berlin: Deckerschen,1857); and the British government blue book, John Simon, *Report on the Last Two Cholera Epidemics and their Spreading through the Consumption of Impure Water* (1856), 26.

60. *Die Wasserversorgung Berlins...,* 10 and 19.

61. Herman Werle, "Between Public Well-Being and Profit Interests: Experiences of the partial privatization of water supply in Berlin," *Brot fuer die Welt*, (2004): 4. (www.wasser-inbuergerhand.de/untersuchungen/berlin_water_privatisation.pdf).

62. *Die Wasserversorgung Berlins...,* 12–14.

63. Streckfuss, Bd. 2, 817; and Brian Ladd, *Urban Planning and Civic Order in Germany, 1860–1914* (Cambridge: Harvard University Press, 1990), 58.

64. Becker, 61.

65. Streckfuss, 777.

66. Scoutetten, 5.

67. Ibid., 6.

68. Becker, 62.

69. Stägemann, 487.

70. Dr. Albert Sachs ed., *Tagebuch über das Verhalten der bösartigen Cholera in Berlins* (Berlin: Fiackschen Buchhandlung, 1831), 131.

71. *Berliner Cholera,* September 24, 1831, 2.

72. Chad to Palmerston, August 29, 1831, PRO FO 64/173, 341; *Berliner Cholera,* 2; and *Scoutetten,* 20–21.

73. Chad to Palmerston, August 29, 1831, PRO FO 64/173, 346.

74. Ibid., 361.

75. *Preussische Staats-Zeitung,* August 30, 1831, 1370.

76. Chad to Palmerston, August 31, 1831, PRO FO 64/173, 361.

77. *Preussische Staats-Zeitung* , August 30, 1831, 1370.

78. *Staats und Gelehrte ... Correspondenten,* September 3, 1831.

79. *Berliner Cholera,* 2–3.

80. *Staats und Gelehrte ... Correspondenten,* September 3, 1831.

81. Ibid; Scoutetten, 23.

82. Ibid.

83. *Berliner Cholera,* 3.

84. *Berliner Cholera,* 3; Scoutetten, 25–26.

85. Ibid.

86. Theodor Friedrich Baltz, *Über diesjährige Brechruhr Cholera Epidemie in Berlin* (Berlin: Wohlgemuth's Buchhandlung, 1853), 13.

87. Scoutetten, 25–26.

88. "Protokol der Klausurtagung der Magistrates" am September 2, 1831, in Dettke, 189–190.

89. Von Arnim was used to taking command. When the butchers in Berlin raised prices on their meat and used the excuse of the cholera cordon, he went to the butchers. He told them that they had better lower their prices or by his authority under the "Freedom of Trade Act" he would establish a slaughter house and sell meat at a cheaper price. Consequently, they sold their meat at the usual price. In another case, a Berlin suburb did not want to be bothered with a cordon. The inhabitants signed a petition and presented it to Von Arnim. He replied that he was only a man and he could die tomorrow. If the petition was found it could cause much "inconvenience" for the undersigned. As a favor he said he would "destroy it before their eyes" to avoid any further trouble.

They were "happy" that he ripped it up in their presence. See Carl André Christian, ed. *Hesperus: Encyclopädische Zeitschrift für gebildete Leser* (Stuttgart,: Cotta,1832), 504.

90. Von Arnim addressed Rust directly on the matter of the blockade of Berlin and asked him if he would take responsibility for what might occur. Rust answered with a non-committal expression, and said, "I'd be very careful." Baltz. 12–13.

91. *Preussische Staats-Zeitung,* August 30, 1831, 1370.

92. Conferenz Protokol, August 19, 1831, GStA PK., Rep. 76 VIII C, Nr. 2. 76.

93. Conferenz Protokol, August 22, 1831; and September 2,1831, GStA PK., Rep. 76 VIII C, Nr. 2. 78 and 84.

94. *Augsburger Allgemeine Zeitung*, September 10, 1831, 1011. On censorship in see Prussia see Theodor Clemens Perthes, *Friedrich Perthes' Leben nach dessen schriftlichen und mündlichen Metteilungen aufgezeichnet* 6th ed. (Gotha: Perthes, 1872), Bd. 3, 348. On complaints concerning censorship on cholera matters see *Zeitung Für die Elegant Welt,* August 9, 1831, 1231; for the censorship of an article in Sach's *Tagebuch...,* by the battalion doctor Koch see Dettke, 198–200; and see Dr. Albert Sachs, *Tagebuch...,* 29 September 1831, 49 and October 4, 1831 65–66 for the publication of the censored article. Friederich Raumer in reference to the writing of the battalion Dr. Koch wrote, "The number of bans on books and magazines is growing...," And pointedly noted, "here a scientifically educated man is treated like an inexperienced child...," Friedrich von Raumer, *Lebenserinnerungen und Briefwechsel* t. 1 (Leipzig: Brockhaus, 1861), 397.

95. Baltz, 12 and Becker, 57.

96. Eylert, Bd. 2, 340.

97. "Lettre de Berlin," September 5, 1831 in *Staats und Gelehrte ... Correspondenten,* September 9, 1831, 6–7. According to Chad the king would came to Berlin everyday "but will receive no one." Chad to Palmerston, September 5, 1831, PRO FO 64/174, 43.

98. "Lettre de Berlin," September, 5, 1831.

99. Eylert, Bd. II, 340.

100. Becker, 22.

101. Conferenz Protokol, September 2, 1831, GStA PK., Rep. 76 VIII C, Nr. 2. 85–86.

102. Ibid., 84–85

103. *Cholera Archiv,* Bd. 2, 245.

104. *Nueste Conversations Lexicon oder Allgemeine deutsche Real Encyclopedie für gebildet Stande* Bd. 12, (Wien: Franz Ludwig, 1831), 339 and K.F.W. Dieterici, *Statistische Uebersicht der wichtigsten Gegenstände des Verkehrs und Verbrauchs in der Preussischen Staat* (Berlin: E.S. Mittler, 1842), 322.

105. *Zeitung Fuer die Elegant Welt*, Juli 26, 1831, 1151.

106. *Staats und gelehrte ... Correspondenten,* August 31, 1831 and September, 9, 1831; and *Preussische Staats-Zeitung,* September, 13, 1831, 1424.

107. Eylert, Bd. 2, 340; *Zeitung Fuer die Elegant Welt*, July 26, 1831, 1151; and Chad to Palmerston, September 17, 1831, PRO FO 64/174, 101.

108. K.A. von Kamptz, "Kabinetts Ordre Massregeln gegen die Verbreitung der Cholera 6 September 1831," *Annalen Preussischen Inner Staats-Verwaltung* Bd. 15 (Berlin, 1831), 609–612; the subsequent proclamation based on the Cabinet Order dated September 6, 1831 was

published on September 13, 1831 in the *Preussische Staats-Zeitung*. This appears to be the only Cabinet Order exclusively signed by the king that year with no reference to any other Ministry or Department. See Kamptz, Bd. 15, passim.

109. Conferenz Protokol, September 12, 1831, GStA PK., Rep. 76 VIII C, Nr. 2. 89 and the *Preussische Staats-Zeitung*, September, 13, 1831, 1424.

110. *Preussische Staats-Zeitung*, September, 13, 1831, 1424.

111. Rust, "Sendschreiben...," *Cholera-Archiv*, Bd. 3, 60.

112. Ibid., 58 and 60; and Becker, 52.

113. *Staats und Gelehrte ... Correspondenten*, September 12, 1831.

114. *Augsburger Allgemeine Zeitung*, 1059 and *Berliner Cholera*, 141.

115. Royal Proclamation of September 6, 1831, Chad to Palmerston, September 15, 1831, FO 64/174, 90; and the *Preussische Staats-Zeitung* September 13, 1831, 1424.

116. Chad to Palmerston, September 15, 1831, PRO FO 64/174, 88.

117. Schön, 312.

118. Becker, 44–45 and Wagner, 248.

119. Chad to Palmerston, September 15, 1831, PRO FO 64/174, 90.

120. Ibid., 90

121. Dr. Becker noted "it will give you pleasure to peruse the proclamation which the King of Prussia issued under these circumstances." Becker, 45.

122. Chad to Palmerston, September 15, 1831, PRO FO 64/174, 88.

123. Ibid., 91.

124. Ibid., 94–97; *Preussische Staats-Zeitung* September 13, 1831, 1424; Geradin, 257.

125. Becker, 48.

126. Ibid.

127. Although the government offered the cities of Prussia a revised City Ordinance in 1831, which ostensibly gave the cities more local control it did not come without certain administrative strings attached. The government could not force the cities to accept this new Ordinance. The "pressure of the July Revolution" forced the king to allow the "insecure cities of his free monarchy to opt for the old or new Ordinance." Most of the cities refused to accept it. They continued with the Stein Municipal Ordinance. Koselleck, 576–577.

128. Wagner, 268.

129. Ibid., 202, 208, 224.

130. Geradin, 83–84.

131. Ibid., 83–86.

132. Chad to Palmerston, September 15, 1831, PRO FO 64/174, 91.

133. *Berliner Cholera*, October 18, 1831, 92.

134. Becker, 50.

135. Ibid., 131.

136. Ibid., 50.

137. *Berliner Cholera*, 102.

138. Ibid., 131.

139. Chad to Palmerston, September, 15, 1831, PRO FO 64/174, 92.

140. Ibid., 101.

141. Ibid., 101–102.

142. Ibid., 102.

143. *Preussische Staats-Zeitung*, September, 13, 1831; and Chad to Palmerston, September 17, 1831, PRO FO 64/174, 101–102.

144. Chad to Palmerston, September 17, PRO FO 64/1741831, 101.

145. Briese, 166; and Chad to Palmerston, September 17, 1831, PRO FO 64/174, 101.

146. Chad to Palmerston, September 17, 1831, PRO FO 64/174, 101.

147. Ibid.

148. Chad to Palmerston, September 15, 1831, PRO FO 64/174, 93.

149. *Augsburger Allgemeine Zeitung*, September 10, 1831, 1011.

150. Dr. Haufsbrand, "Über die Cholera in Braunsberg," *Cholera-Archiv*, Bd. 3, 225–226.

151. Ibid.

152. Ibid.

153. Ibid.

154. Carl I. Lorinser, *Eine Selbstbiographie*, Franz Lorinser, ed. (Regensburg: Manz, 1864), Bd. 2, 16–17

155. Ibid., 17.

156. By removing quarantines the king gained the support of the middle classes of Prussia as well as the respect of the merchants and industrialists of the other German states. The idea of pacifying the middle classes through the support of a liberal economic program both within and outside Prussia was a central idea in Prussian Foreign Minister Bernstorff's *Denkschrift of January 29, 1831*. See Dr. C. Spielmann, "Regierungspraesident Karl von Ibell über die preussische Politik in den Jahren 1830 und 1831," *Annalen Des Vereins für Naussische Altertumskunde und Geschichtsforschung*, 37 (1896): 61–95; and "mentioned by the ministry in routine correspondence." Baack, 260–261.

157. Briese, 166–167. For a brief discussion on "conservative social protest" during the cholera years and later; the lack of political protest; and the rarity of actions against traditional scapegoats like Jews and foreigners in Prussia and the other German states during the cholera epidemic in 1831 see Briese,166–169.

158. Theodor Rochow, *Preussen und Frankreich zur Zeit der Julirevolution, Vertraute Briefe des preussischen General von Rochow an den preussischen Generalpostmeister von Nagler* (Leipzig: Brockhaus, 1871), 30.

159. Theodor Gottlieb von Hippel, *Beiträge zur Charakteristik Friedrich Wilhelms III* (Bromberg: Louis Levit, 1841), 185; and Koselleck, 420.

160. Koselleck, 420.

161. Hippel, 185.

Chapter 10

1. *Berliner Cholera*, September, 24, 1831, 9–11.
2. Becker, 8–9.
3. Ibid., 8.
4. Ibid., 8; *Berliner Cholera*, September, 24, 1831, 9.
5. Ibid., 9.
6. Ibid., 10.
7. Breise, 165.
8. Rudolph Skoda, *Die Rosenthaler Vorstadt. Wohnverhältnisse der Stadtarmut 1750-1850* (Berlin, 1985), 64 in Briese, 165; Becker, 10.
9. Dettke, 180–181.
10. Dettke, 182.

11. According to Bettine von Arnim there were "usually no factory workers, only day laborers and small businessmen" living in "Family houses," Briese, 166.

12. "Heinrich Ferdinand Wiesecke an das Polizeipräsidium, Berlin 27. Juli 1831," in Johann Friedrich Geist und Klaus Kurvers, *Das Berliner Miethaus 1740–1862* (München, 1980), 154 in Briese, 166.

13. *Berliner Cholera*, October 29, 1831, 135.

14. Sachs, 228; Dettke, 184.

15. *Berliner Cholera*, December 24, 1831, 288–289.

16. Sachs, 321.

17. Dettke, 182.

18. Becker, 10.

19. Dettke, 184–185.

20. Becker, 10–11.

21. *Berliner Cholera*, 300.

22. Becker, 21.

23. Ibid., 51.

24. Scoutetten, 9. For a detailed breakdown of duties and responsibilities see "Die Verwaltungs Behörde der Allerhöchstverordneten Gesundheits Comité für Berlin," V. Arnim. "Bekanntmachung," *Beilage Preussische Staats Zeitung*, no. 247, September, 4, 1831, 1–4 (this supplement also included a second notice with a breakdown of the sixty-one Berlin protection commission districts by number and street name).

25. Scoutetten, 11–12.

26. "Die Verwaltungs Behörde," *Beilage Preussischen Staats-Zeitung*, 1–3.

27. Becker, 37, 61.

28. *Berliner Cholera*, 131.

29. Die Verwaltungs Behörde der Allerhöchsteverordneten Gesundheits Comité für Berlin. V. Arnim. "Bekanntmachung: Einige Klassen...," Berlin, den 11 September 1831, *Preussische Staats-Zeitung*, September 12, 1831, 1421.

30. Ibid.; *Berliner Cholera*, 131–132.

31. *Berliner Cholera*, 132.

32. Ibid.

33. Ibid., 142.

34. Ibid.

35. Becker, 38–39.

36. Hospital I was headed by Dr. Romberg, hospital II was opened on September 9, headed by Dr. Behr, hospital III on September 30 under Dr. Bahn and later in October, hospital IV and V were opened headed by Dr. Casper and Dr. Thummel respectively.

37. Ibid., 102–106.

38. Scoutetten, 9; *Berliner Cholera*, 142.

39. *Berliner Cholera*, 142.

40. Eck, 100; Franz X Gietl, *Die Ergebnisse meiner Beobachtungen über die Cholera vom Jahre 1831–1874* (München: C. Kaiser, 1874), 1.

41. Becker, 15–16.

42. Eck, 102. A death rate of 60 percent appears to us to be excessive. However, one modern authority has stated that "As many as 50 percent to 75 percent of dehydrated cholera patients who are not appropriately treated die either from shock within the first day of the illness or from secondary effects after a week or so." Perhaps in individual instances some doctors did treat their patients and inadvertently hastened their deaths. However, on the average it would seem that the Prussian doctors in cholera hospitals probably could not have done anything for their patients nor did they do them much harm. See Abram. S. Benenson, "Cholera," in Franklin H. Top and Paul F Wehrle eds. *Communicable and Infectious Diseases* 8th ed. (Saint Louis: C.V. Mosby Co., 1981), 113; Drury, 128.

43. Eck,. 102

44. Becker, 54–55.

45. Ibid., 50–55.

46. *Berliner Cholera*, 142–143.

47. Eck, "Schilderung der hinsichtlich der Erscheinungen, Ursachen und Behandlung der asiatischen Cholera in Berlin...Heilanstalten No. I–V," *Cholera-Archiv*, Bd. 3, see especially 69–79. (Examples included various emetics, experimental steam baths with altered apparatuses, and irritating chemicals rubbed on the patient's skin.)

48. As far as experimental therapies during this period, some historians have attempted to look for and concern themselves with early attempts at experimental saline therapy for cholera. The closest experiments of this nature in Prussia were probably the experimental blood injections undertaken in cholera hospitals. However, as Drury noted, any type of injection into the body of a patient would not have been acceptable at this time because of poor equipment and aseptic techniques which could lead to the possibility of death by an "air embolism or septicemia." At this time, all therapeutic inquiries along this line would have undoubtedly led to failure. Drury, 129.

49. Eck, 33.

50. Ibid.

51. Rather, 185.

52. Ibid.

53. Dr. P. Phoebus," Cholera-Leichen-Öffnungen... Bericht über 69 Cholera-Sectionen," *Cholera-Archiv*, Bd.1, 405.

54. Rather, 192.

55. *Berliner Cholera*, September 24, 1831, 1.

56. Ibid.

57. *Berliner Cholera*, October 11, 1831, 68.

58. *Preussische Staats-Zeitung*, September 13, 1831, 1424; Becker, 52.

59. Sachs, 49, 159–160.

60. Ibid., 160–161.

61. Ibid., 163–165.

62. Becker, 52.

63. Ibid., 52–53.

64. Ibid., 53.

Chapter 11

1. Cholera appeared in Prussia in the summer and fall of 1832. In the government district of Merseberg there were 1,794 cases with 912 deaths. Cholera spread sporadically into neighboring districts including southeast Prussia and eventually died ou It did not spread throughout Prussia nor did it have the same impact as the first encounter in 1831. See Krehnke, 20–21.

2. By the end of the eighteenth century Berlin supported the greatest number of physicians approximately "40 to 50 doctors per 130,000 people." On the eve of the cholera epidemic there were 4,350 physicians in Prussia, Berlin had the greatest ratio of doctors to inhabitants 1:794 while the Department of Gumbinnen had an extremely low ratio of 1:10,734. Rönne and Simon, Bd. 2, 111.

3. Pistor, 515; Chad to Lord Palmerston, September 28, 1831, PRO FO 64/174, 163.

4. Ian Inkster discusses the role of local physicians who strived for individual status, and were members in a profession "yet in the making," see Ian Inkster, "Marginal Men: Aspects of the Social Role of the Medical Community in Sheffield, 1790–1850," ed. John Woodward and David Richards, *Health Care and Popular Medicine in the Nineteenth Century England* (New York: Holmes & Meier Publishers, 1977), 128. Michael Drury takes this concept and applies it directly to the doctors in England who were confronted "with this new and dangerous disease" This offered them the opportunity to gain prestige both for themselves and their profession." See Drury, 103. The same could be applied to Prussian doctors. See for example Dr. Lorinser's complaints regarding his lack of recognition by the government for his service during the cholera epidemic. Lorinser, Bd. II, 11.

5. "younger doctors who supported anti-contagion had never experienced the typhus and smallpox contagion of previous years, their closest experience to cholera was the intermittent fever in Germany in 1809, 1810 and 1811." Horn, "Die Contagiosität der Asiatischen Cholera...," *Cholera Archiv*, Bd. 2, 80, 84.

6. Becker, 13.
7. Sachs, 38.
8. Dettke, 301.
9. *Cholera Zeitung* (Königsberg), 56 and Sachs, 6.
10. "Extract of a Letter from Berlin," September 8, 1831, in Great Britain. Privy Council, *Papers relative to the disease called cholera spasmodica in India, Now Prevailing in the North of Europe (London, 1831)*, 59.
11. Rust, 56–57.
12. Dr. Hufeland, "Ein Wort an meine lieben Mitbürger über die Ansteckung der Cholera und die beste Verhütung derselben," *Preussen Staats-Zeitung*, September 11, 1831, 1419; See Heikki Lempa, *Beyond the Gymnasium: Educating the Middle-class Bodies in Classical Germany* (Lanham, Maryland: Lexington Books, 2007), 206. For a discussion on the role of diet and moral responsibility advocated by miasmists see Lempa, 206–209.
13. The reputation of Dr. Hufeland had declined because of his support of ideas verging on mysticism and mesmerism. See Lleland J. Rather ed., *Disease, Life and Man: Selected Essays by Rudolph Virchow* (Stanford, California: Stanford U.P. 1958), 180–181.
14. Dr.Hufeland, "Verwandtschaft der Cholera mit dem Wechselfieber,"*Journal der Practischen Heilkunden* Bd.73 (August, 1831): 126–127. See also Hufeland on the contagiousness of the common cold in Sachs, 82–83. Hufeland also references an earlier article written by him in which he distinguished between various degrees of contagion. Hufeland, "Atmosphärische Krankheiten und atmosphärische Ansteckung: Unterschied von Epidemie, Contagion und Infection; ein Beitrag zu den Untersuchungen über die Contagiosität des gelben Fiebers" *Hufeland's Journal*, Bd. 57 (July, 1823): 52–54 for a summary of his article.
15. *Cholera Zeitung* (Königsberg), 77–78.
16. For German dependence on rye as a staple of existence see Siegfried von Ciriacy-Wantrup, *Agrarkrisen und Stockungsspannen zur Frage der langen "Welle" in der Wirtschaftlichen Entwicklung* (Berlin: Parey,1936), 107. For rye prices prior to and during the cholera outbreak see *Amtsblatt der Regierung zu Potsdam und der Stadt Berlin*, for July see August 26, 1831, 179; for August see September 16, 1831, 231; for September see October 14, 1831, 283; for October see November 18, 1831, 329 and for November see December 16, 1831, 365.

17. See for example "Das Gesetz wegen Bestrafung derjenigen Vergehungen, welche die Übertretung der zur Abwendung der Cholera erlassenen Verordnungen betreffen. Von 15. June 1831," in *Amtsblatt der Königlichen Regierung zu Potsdam...*, June 24, 1831, 113–117.
18. Lorinser, Bd. II, 18.
19. Ibid., 18 and 20. Dr. Hufeland was an editor for the *Jahrbücher für wissenschaftliche Kritik* and was probably given Lorinser's article for review as a medical expert Lorinser in a number of places in his article made arguments similar to Hufeland's. In Lorinser, he probably found a likeminded young colleague.
20. Ibid.; see also George Gregory, M.D., "Lectures On The Eruptive Fevers, Delivered At S Thomas's Hospital In Jan. 1843" *The Medico-Chirurgical Review and Journal of Practical Medicine*, vol. 74 (January, 1844): 66.
21. Lorinser, Bd. II, 17–18.
22. *Preussische Staats-Zeitung*, October 4, 1831, 1515–1516; October 5, 1831, 1519–1520; October 6, 1831, 1523–1524; Lorinser Bd. II, 19.
23. Lorinser, 19; Chad provides a summary translation of the Royal Order to which Lorinser is referring. Chad to Palmerston, October 9 1831, PRO FO 64/174, 233.
24. Lorinser reviewed the following books; *Über die Ostindische Cholera, nach vielen eignen Beobachtungen und Leichen=Oeffnungen* by James Annesley; after a translation from the 2nd edition (1829) by Dr. Gustav Himln, Hannover 1831; *Über die Cholera=Krankhei Ein Sendschreiben*, J. Ch. Von Loder's (Königsberg 1831); *Beobachtungen über die epidemische Cholera* by, Dr. R. J. W. Remer. (Breslau, 1831), in the *Preussische Staats-Zeitung*, 1515.
25. Ibid., 1516.
26. Ibid., 1519.
27. Ibid., 1519–20.
28. Hufeland, "Verwandtschaft...", 126–127.
29. *Preussische Staats-Zeitung*, 1519–20
30. *Preussische Staats-Zeitung*, 1523–24.
31. Ibid., 1524.
32. It is taken from the play "Demetrius" by Schiller, and includes the line that "when the majority wins, ignorance decides." Lorinser expected his readers in the *Jahrbücher für wissenschaftliche Kritik* where his review was to be published to understand this reference. When his work was published without his knowledge in the *Preussische Staatszeitung* the individual (s) responsible for this clearly understood this criticism and recognized that it went to the heart of the debate as it was raging in Berlin. See Schillers *Sämmliche Schriften Historisch=Kritische Ausgabe Fünfzehten Theil. Zweiter Band. Nachlass. Demetrius.* Herausgeben Karl Goedeke (Stuttgart: Cotta, 1876), 457.
33. *Preussische Staats-Zeitung*, 1524.
34. Lorinser, Bd. II, 13; *Preussische Staats-Zeitung*, 1524.
35. *Preussische Staats-Zeitung*, 1524.
36. Lorinser, 19.
37. Ibid., 20.
38. Ibid.; Baack, 299–302; On Simrock, according to the Austrian ambassador, Werner, "Sogleich erliesen S. M. motu proprio eine Kabinettsorder," [His Majesty immediately issued a Cabinet Order on his own]. Werner an Metternich, Berlin, September 27, 1830. HHSta Staatskanzlei Preussen Karton, 135 Konv. 2 122. in *Stamm*, 719 and 53, 1–32.
39. Lorinser, 20–21.

Notes. Chapter 11

40. Rust, "Ein Wort zur Würdigung der Schutz Maßregeln gegen die Cholera," *Preussische Staats-Zeitung*, October 12, 1831, 1548.
41. Rust,"Sendschreiben des Präsidenten Dr. Rust...," 56 and 66.
42. Rust, 60.
43. Ibid., 59; Nipperdey, 282–283; on the Prussian bureaucrat's understanding of his role in the State system, see Fann, 301–303.
44. Rust, 58.
45. GStA PK, 2.2.1 Geh. Zivilkab., Nr. 15196, 2 und R. in Dettke, 303. Concerning unsuccessful attempts to censor writings contrary to the contagionist view during the epidemic see *Sachs, Tagebuch...*, September 27, 1831, 44 and October 4, 1831, 49.
46. Horn, 54–55; Lorinser, 21.
47. Horn, 54–55.
48. Lorinser, 12–13.
49. Horn, 57.
50. Ibid. 57.
51. Ibid., 58.
52. Ibid., 81.
53. Ibid., 83.
54. Ibid.
55. Lorinser, 21.
56. Ibid., 22.
57. Ibid., 23.
58. Ibid., 23.
59. Lorinser, 23; George Siegerist, "Zur Geschichte Medizin" *Archiv Brandenburgia Gesellschaft für Heimatkunde der provinz Brandenburg, Berlin* Bd. 7 (Berlin, 1901):33–34.
60. Lorinser, 24.
61. Dettke, 205.
62. *Amtsblatt der Regierung zu Potsdam und der Stadt Berlin*, October 21, 1831, 285.
63. Chad to Palmerston, September 28, 1831, PRO FO 164/74, 163. These reports were prepared and given to Chad by the ultra-conservative Prince Wilhelm Wittgenstein-Sayn. Dettke, 205; for morbidity and mortality statistics in October see the *Berlinische Cholera...*, 123.
64. Thile to King Frederick William, October 25, 1831, in Acta der Königliche Civil Kabinett: Massregln zur Abwehrung zur Cholera in der Haupt-und Residenz Stadt Berlin, GStA PK, Re 2.2.1, Nr. 24511, 143–146.
65. Ibid., 143–144.
66. Conferenz Protokol, October 17, 1831, GStA PK, Re 76 VIII C, Nr. 2, 96–98 for the discussion.
67. Thile to King Frederick William, October 25, 1831, in Acta der Königliche Civil Kabinet: Massregln..., GStA PK, Re 2.2.1, Nr. 24511, 144. See also September 12, 1831, *Preussische Staats-Zeitung*, 1421.
68. Ibid.
69. Ibid., 143–146.
70. "Bekanntmachung," October 25, 1831, in *Amtsblatt der Regierung zu Potsdam...*, November, 4 1831, 300–303.
71. "Dem Handel triebenden Publiko der Inn und Ausland...diesjahrige Martini Messe zu Frankfurt a/O.," Abteilung. Innern, 15 October, 1831, in *Amtsblatt...zu Marienwerder*, No. 43, October 28 1831, 532–33.
72. See "Das Gesetz wegen Bestrafung derjenigen Vergehungen, welche die Übertretung der zur Abwendung der Cholera erlassenen Verordnungen betreffen. Von 15. June 1831," in *Amtsblatt der Königlichen Regierung zu Potsdam...*, No. 24 June 24, 1831, 113–117; *Gesetzsammlung für die Königlichen Preussischen Staaten, 1831*, 61.
73. "Des Begnadigung derjenigen, welche die zur Abwehrung der Cholera erlassen Verordnungen übertreten haben," *Amtsblatt... zu Königsberg*, No. 51, December 21, 1831, 567; Olkowski, 551.
74. Hufeland, "Opinion of Hufeland on the Origin and Propagation of Cholera" *The London Medical Gazette*, Vol. IX (March 3, 1832), 860.
75. Chad to Palmerston, October 9 1831, PRO FO 64/174, 233.
76. Conferenz Protokol, December 20, 1831, DZA, Me., Re VIII C, Nr. 2, 100.
77. J. Rust, *Die Medicinal-Verfassung Preussens, wie sie war und wie sie ist* (Berlin, Enslin, 1838), 9
78. Conferenz Protokol, December 22, 1831, GStA PK, Re VIII C, Nr. 2, 101.
79. Ibid.
80. Ibid.
81. Dettke, 205.
82. *Gesetzsammlung...Staaten* (1831), 61.
83. Rust, 56–57; *Cholera Archiv*, Bd. 1- 3, passim.
84. Dr. Friedrich Bock, und Dr. Ludwig K. Hasenknopf, "Johann Nepomuk Rust" *Veröffentlichungen aus dem Gebiete des Militär-Sanitätswesens. Herausgegeben von der Medizinal—Abtheilung des Königlich Preussischen Kriegsministeriums; Kriegschirurgen und Feldärzte der ersten Hälfte des 19. Jahrhunderts (1795–1848), Heft 18, Bd. 2* (Berlin 1901). After all Rust's complaints he became personal physician to the Crown Prince in 1834 and later to King Frederick William IV. Two years later while taking a cure at Teplitz because of his arthritis he was invited by Prince Metternich to come to Vienna and become the successor of the late Imperial Physician there. Rust refused on the "grounds that he had strong ties to the King and to the city of Berlin." Bock, 306. Contrast Rust's treatment with that of Dr. Lorinser who wrote, "If ever anyone deserved public acknowledgement for the sacrifice he had recently made for the State" he did. The whole world was convinced that he could not miss receiving some recognition. Yet, all he received were travel expenses and not even a response to the "reports he had submitted." He felt the highest authorities were not satisfied with "his performance." He blamed a supervisor who was sick all the time for this "iniquity" and lack of recognition. He wrote, "now I could not read without bitter irony, the list of those promoted and decorated of which so many owe their elevation to chance." Lorinser, 11.
85. Ibid., 306.
86. *Gesetzsammlung...Staaten* (1832), 41.
87. Ibid., 43.
88. Ibid., 48.
89. Ibid.
90. Ibid., 53 and 55.
91. Ibid., 44.
92. Rönne, Bd. 2, 238; Pistor, 513.
93. Count Friedrich von Schuckman was the Minister of the Interior from 1819–1834. The Interior Ministry was a dual Ministry and the duties within the Ministry were divided. During these exchanges Brenn was serving as Interior Minister of Police, a section of the Interior Ministry. This explains his keen interest in retaining authority for his departmen In 1834, he was appointed Minister of the Interior, replacing Count Schuckman and served in that capacity until 1838.

94. Pistor., 515.
95. Pistor, 513.
96. Ibid., 514.
97. Ibid.
98. Ibid., 513; see Altenstein 3.10.1832 an Innenminister Gustav v. Brenn, in I. Ha, Re 77 Ti 182 Nr. 46 Bd. 1, 208–213, die Zitate 209v. passim, in Holtz, 29.
99. Pistor, 514; Holtz, 29.
100. Pistor, 513.
101. Holtz, 306.
102. Auszug auf Thile to King Frederick William III, June 17, 1835, in *Preussischen Gesetzsammlung 1835*, 240; Pistor, 750–51.
103. Ibid.
104. Ibid.
105. There are no detailed procedures for dealing with plague in the Prussian Infectious Disease Law of 1835. See Friedrich L. Augustin, *Die königlich Preussische Medicinalverfassung...Gesetze, Verordnungen und Einrichtungen* Bd. 6 (Potsdam, Horvath, 1838), 27–60. Later regulations for plague and yellow fever focused on Prussian harbors and maritime shipping. Dr. Wilhelm Horn, *Das Preussische Medicinalwesen: Aus amtlichen Quellen dargestellt* (Berlin: Hirschwald, 1857), 209–212.
106. Ibid.
107. Ibid.
108. Yellow fever and plague were treated separately. Yellow fever was not seen as a problem in Prussia for a variety of reasons and unlike cholera it had never really penetrated into Prussia. See Rönne, Bd. 2, 146 and 250; for plague, Rönne, 146.
109. Ibid., 238–239 and 251.
110. Ibid., 240.
111. Grafin Elise von Bernstorff, *Ein Bild aus der Zeit von 1789 bis 1835, Aus ihren Aufzeichnungen*, zweite auflage, Bd. 2 (Berlin: Mittler, 1896), 220. Although as Altenstein noted some of this could be attributed to outright criticism by private citizens, he was especially upset government censors were too lax and the editors of the newspapers were too "brash." He singled out a brochure by Dr. Albert Sachs "mocking" the decree of January 31, 1832. According to Altenstein, "In my view, in every case, it is dangerous to permit private opinion to influence the arrangements made by the State." Dettke, 303.
112. Charles Carrière, Marcel Courdurié, Ferréol Rebuffat, *Marseille Ville Morte: La Peste de 1720* (Marseille: Autres Temps Editions, 2008), passim.
113. Aside from an April 2, 1803, patent that applied to an infectious sickness of animals the only other legislation prior to 1835 for contagious diseases was for plague and the immediate past measures for cholera in 1831 and 1832. Rönne, Bd. 2, 253; Pistor, 767; Martin Kirchner, "Die Seuchenbekämpfung unter Berücksichtigung der einschlägigen deutschen und preussischen Gesetzgebung," in Dr.von Rapmund, ed. *Das Preussische Medizinal- und Gesundheitswesen in den Jahren 1883–1908* (Berlin: Fischer, 1908), 199. The *Reichsseuchengesetz* of June 30, 1900, was replaced in 1905 by the second Prussian law concerning the control of communicable diseases, on August 28, 1905. See A. Schmedding, *Die Gesetze betreffend Bekämpfung ansteckender Krankheiten: und zwar 1. Reichsgesetz betreffend die Bekämpfung gemeingefährlicher Krankheiten vom 30. Juni 1900, 2. Preussisches Gesetz betreffend die Bekämpfung übertragbarer Krankheiten vom 28. August 1905* (Münster: Aschendorf, 1905), 20.

114. Fleischer, 8–9; Ross, 207–211; Baldwin, 130; for an alternative view see Dettke, 304; on plague see above footnote 105 Augustin, *Die königlich Preussische...*, 27–60; Horn, *Das Preussische...*, 209–212.
115. See for example the contagionist *Cholera Archiv* Bd. 1–3 (1832–33), edited by Dr. Rust and his colleagues that continued to promote contagion.
116. Baldwin, p 124–125; Dettke, 309–311.
117. Ross, 207–211; Baldwin, 130.
118. Schmedding, 20.

Chapter 12

1. *Cholera Archiv*, Bd. 3, 248–249.
2. W. von Dankbahr, *Der Uebertritt der polnischen Corps von Gielgud, Chłapowski und Rybinski auf das Königlich Preussische Gebiet, ihr Aufenthalt daselbst und die angeordnete Entfernung derselben.Unter Benutzung amtlicher Quelle* (Königsberg: Bornträger, 1832), 13. The author specifically mentions the "strict cholera regulations" in force during the Gielgud Corps internment. Where cholera is mentioned but plays a minor role as the excuse for the internment see Kocój, 135–136; see Norbert Kasparek, Powstańczy *epilog: żołnierze listopadowi w dniach klęski i internowania 1831–1831* (Olsztyn: Uniwersytetu Warmińsko-Mazurskiego, 2001), 72–116; for the king's September 6, 1831 proclamation see *Amtsblatt der Königlichen Regierung zu Potsdam...*, September 16, 1831, 219–221.
3. Martens, *Recueil des traités...*, 173.
4. Ibid.
5. Jan Czczyński, *Preussen im Jahre 1831: oder Verfahren der preussischen Militärbehörden gegen...* (Fürth: Korn'sche, 1832), 7.
6. Walerian Kalinka, *Jeneral Dezydery Chłapowski* (Poznan: J. Leitgeber, 1885), 140 and 150; Dezydery Chłapowski, *Pamiętniki: z portretem autora* pt. 2 (Poznan: Nakł. Synów, 1899), 99.
7. "Das Gesetz wegen Bestrafung derjenigen Vergehungen, welche die Übertretung der zur Abwendung der Cholera erlassenen Verordnungen betreffen. Von 15. June 1831," *Amtsblatt...Königsberg*, nr. 26. August 29, 1831, 195.
8. "Bekanntmachungen des Königl OberPräsidiums" nr. 26. June 18, 1831, *Amtsblatt....Königsberg*, June 29, 1831, 200–201.
9. Dankbahr, 1–2.
10. K. Gaszyński, *Notatki oficera polskiego o obchodzeniu się rządu pruskiego z korpusem wojska polskiego weszłego z Litwy do Prus pod dowództwem jenerala Giłguda w czasie 53 dni trwającej kwarantanny* (Paryżu, A. Pinard, 1833), 4–5. The Polish historian Norbert Kasparek makes the point that previous historians have "dismissed in one sentence" the efforts of Generals Rohland and Szymanowski yet "for another 43 hours [they] tried to escape from the [Russian] trap" and were eventually, "forced to follow Chłapowski." Kasparek, 72.
11. Gaszyński, 6; Kalinka, 141.
12. Gaszyński, 8.
13. Dankbahr, 3, 49–50.
14. Ibid., 50.
15. "Kwarantanna pruska," *Gazeta Warszawska*, Nr. 194, VIII 1831, 22, in Kocój, 140; *Amtsblatt der Königlichen Regierung zu Potsdam...*, No. 24, June 24, 1831, 113–117.

Notes. Chapter 12

16. Chad to Palmerston, July 17, 1831, PRO FO 64/173,106; Dankbahr, 13.
17. Dankbahr, 13-14.
18. *Amtsblatt...Königsberg,* August 24, 1831, 306-307.
19. Gaszyński, 11-12 and see also Kasparek, 90.
20. Martens, *Recueil des traités...,* 174.
21. Chad to Palmerston, July 22, 1831, PRO FO 64/173, 132.
22. Kocój, 144.
23. Dankbahr, 49-51.
24. Dankbahr, 4; Kasparek, 91-101.
25. Kasparek, 109.
26. Czczyński, 10; Kasparek, 105.
27. Dankbahr, 6.
28. Gaszyński, 9.
29. Ibid., 10.
30. Ibid.
31. Dankbahr, 8; This fear forced the Prussian government to issue the sanitary report on both camps. See *Amtsblatt...Königsberg,* August 24, 1831, 306-307; in early September the various estates of the districts in Königsberg, still fearful of the infectiousness of the Poles "petitioned the king and asked that the Poles not be placed in Samland to preserve it from the danger of contagion." The king "deigned to ignore their request." Dankbahr, 14.
32. Gaszyński, 10-11.
33. Ibid.
34. *Amtsblatt...Königsberg,* August 29, 1831, 195.
35. Riecke, Bd. 3, 131.
36. Kocój, 142-143.
37. Dankbahr, 13-14; Olkowski, 550.
38. Dankbahr, 6.
39. Kasparek, 106.
40. Ibid., 108.
41. Ibid., 106.
42. Ibid.
43. Dankbahr, 10.
44. Kasparek, 107-108.
45. For example in a report ordered by Rohland concerning clothing needs of the soldiers for units of Rohland's Corps they estimated the need for 1,964 pairs of boots, 1, 491 shirts, 1,414 pants, 798 coats and 445 forage caps. Kasparek, 108.
46. Dankbahr, 6; Gaszyński, 15; Kasparek, 109-110.
47. Dankbahr, 7.
48. Gaszyński, 13.
49. Ibid., 15.
50. Ibid.
51. Ibid.
52. Dankbahr, 9.
53. Dankbahr, 13-14; *Oeffentlicher Anzeiger, Königsberg,* Nr. 24. August 1831, 240; Becker, 48; Olkowski, 550.
54. Wagner, 212-213.
55. Dankbahr, 13-14.
56. Olkowski, 550.
57. Gaszyński, 14.
58. Ibid., 16.
59. Ibid., 17.
60. Dankbahr, 9.
61. Kasparek provides tables for the distribution of the soldiers and officers in the towns and cities that came later after their release from the quarantine camps. Kasparek, 111-115.
62. Dankbahr, 10.
63. Gaszyński, 18.

64. Dankbahr, 10.
65. Kasparek, 105.
66. Kocój, 142.
67. Gaszyński, 18. There was also a mutiny at Schernen on August 22, 1831. See Dankbahr, 9.
68. Kasparek, 105
69. Gaszyński, 18
70. Kasparek, 105.
71. Gaszyński, 18.
72. *Gazeta Warszawska*, 1831, s. 1884; for remarks that this was an exaggerated number see Henryk Golejewski, *Pamiętnik,* ed. Irena Homola et al., t. 1 (Krakow, 1971), s. 365, in Kasperak, 106.
73. Gaszyński, 19.
74. Ibid.
75. Chłapowski, 100; W. Flemig, "Einige Erfahrungen und Ansichten über die Cholera, gesammelt im Jahr 1831, in dem Lager der Polen bei Szernen und unter den dasselbe umgebenden K. Preuss. Truppen," *Cholera-Archiv,* Bd. 3., 267, 276.
76. *Amtsblatt...Königsberg,* August 24, 1831, 309.
77. Ibid., 308.
78. Ibid., 309.
79. Flemig, 267.
80. *Amtsblatt...Königsberg,* August, 24, 1831, 308; Flemig, 268-269, 270.
81. Flemig, 270.
82. Ibid.
83. *Amtsblatt...Königsberg,* August 10, 1831, 265.
84. Flemig, 271.
85. *Allgemeine Medizinisch Zeitung,* 17 August 1831, 1057.
86. Flemig, 287.
87. Kasparek, 106
88. Kalinka, 144-145; and K. Chłapowski, *Wojna na Litwe w Roku 1831* (Krakow, G. Gebethnera i Spółki, 1913), 119.
89. Chłapowski, Pamiętniki, pt. 2, 112 (a letter in defense of his actions going into Prussia is cited here from September 27, 1831. He wrote to Joseph Morawski, a clerk in the resistance in Warsaw, see Kalinka, 145.
90. Chłapowski, *Wojna na Litwe,* 119; J. Tupalski, *General Dezydery Chłapowski...* (Warszawa, 1983), 257 in Kasparek, 106.
91. Ibid.; *Amtsblatt...Königsberg,* 308.
92. *Amtsblatt...Königsberg,* 307.
93. Ibid., 309.
94. *Gaszyński,* 21-22.
95. *Amtsblatt...Königsberg,* 308.
96. For a copy of the oath see Raumer, 516 and for the plan and the imprisonment of those who refused to sign the oath Gaszyński, 19; Raumer, 516-517; Kasparek, 111-112.
97. Gaszyński, 21-22.
98. Ibid., 23.
99. *Amtsblatt...Königsberg,* August 24, 1831, 306; Dankbahr, 9; Kocoj, 142-143.
100. Chłapowski, *Pamiętniki,* 115-116.
101. Martens, *Recueil des traités...,* 173-174.
102. Lorinser Bd. II, 28; There was controversy outside Prussia concerning Dr. Albers, Head of the Prussian delegation to Russia. There was some suspicion that he had been influenced by Rust in his report. See Hawkins, 260.
103. Baltz, 11-12; Lorinser, Bd. II, 26.
104. *Preussische Staats-Zeitung,* September 13, 1831.

105. Raumer, 515.

106. For a comprehensive listing of the complaints against Prussia from the Polish Government during the insurrection and the official answers to them including complaints concerning Prussian cholera policy see Raumer, 501–566. The same complaints were taken up by contemporary émigré publications concerning Prussian policy toward the return of the Poles in Prussia. For example, "The Treatment of the Poles by the Prussian Government and Prussian Officers" *Polonia; or, Monthly reports on Polish affairs*, No. 1 (August, 1832): 175–182.

107. Kasperak, 109; Gaszyński, 13.

108. Kocoj, 143.

109. *Neueste Weltbegebenheiten*, No. 134, August 21, 1831, 560.

110. Brandt, 151–154.

111. Hans Plehn, *Geschichte des Kreises Strasburg Westpreussens in Materialien und forschungen zur wirtschafts- und Verwaltungsgeschichte von Ost und West Preussen* Bd. 2 (Leipzig: Duncker & Humblot, 1900), 310.

112. Brandt, 157.

113. Ibid.

114. Ibid., 158.

115. Ibid.

116. Ibid.; Raumer, 520.

117. General Heinrich von Brandt, *Die Polen in und bei Elbing, Ein Beitrag zur Tagesgeschichte von einem Augenzeugen* (Halle: Kümmel, 1832), 19.

118. Quarantine was reduced to five days. The military was following official regulations. See *Preussische Staats-Zeitung*, September 13, 1831, 1424.

119. *Mémoires officielles sur la Pologne: Précis des négociations entre le Marachel Paskiewitch et Le Commandant En Chef der L'armee Polanaise* (Paris: Michelsen, 1832), 63; see regulations concerning those who transgressed cholera measures in *Amtsblatt der Königlichen Regierung zu Potsdam*, 113–117. These regulations were not repealed until mid–December see *Amtsblatt... Königsberg*, No. 51, December 21, 1831, 557.

120. *Memoires officielles*, 63.

121. Dankbahr, 21–22.

122. Brandt, *Aus dem Leben*, 159 and 165.

123. Ibid., 167.

124. Brandt, *Die Polen in und bei Elbing*, 36.

125. Dankbahr, 31.

126. Brandt, *Die Polen in und bei Elbing*, 37.

127. See Brandt, *Aus dem Leben*, 173; Brandt, *Die Polen in und bei Elbing*, 37–41 for a complete description. Dankbahr 32, notes it is a "truthful representation" of the events at Fischau. See also Raumer, 549–550 for General Rybinski's representation of the events at Fischau and for the King's reply see Raumer, 550–553.

128. *Polonia*, 176.

129. Dankbahr, 36.

130. Ibid., 41.

131. Ibid., 40.

132. Brandt, *Aus dem Leben*, 186–187. Brandt provides an interesting insight into the relationship of the Ministry and the military at the time. Brandt (who was prominently mentioned as the cause of the events at Fischau in the Polonia article on page 180) was asked by General Witzleben, the King's Adjutant General, to write about the Polish refugee story and it be based on documents available in the Foreign Ministry. The King asked that it "be a well written brochure on the subject" and that it be entrusted to Major Brandt. Brandt was told that he would receive the documents he needed as Witzleben had requested them himself. Minister Eichorn refused to supply Brandt with the documents so he asked a friend in the Foreign Ministry for them. He was told that he was "greatly mistaken if a minister to the king will carry out the command immediately of an adjutant general to the king." The king should "ask after the progress of the matter". Brandt asked if he did this what would be the response. The reply was "the matter had already been transferred to a man of great literary reputation." He advised Brandt that matters of diplomacy should be left up to diplomats, not the military." *Brandt*, 187–188. See *Dankbahr*, 32–42 for a discussion of the Polish refugee situation that followed on the publication of Brandt's brochure, *Die Polen in und bei Elbing* (1832).

133. "Dépêche de Ribeaupierre du 1 Septembre 1832," in Martens, *Recueil des traités...*, 184–185.

Conclusion

1. Christian Otto Mylius, *Constitutionum Marchicarum, oder Königl. Preussische.und Churfürstlichen Brandenburgischen* (Berlin, 1755), 328–331; Münch, 57.

2. Münch, 50–53.

3. Pistor, 767.

4. Rex Taylor and Annelie Rieger, "Rudolf Virchow on the Typhus Epidemic in Upper Silesia: an introduction and translation," *Sociology of Health and Illness,* Vol. 6, No. 2 (1984): 205.

5. Taylor, 202.

6. Christina von Hodenberg, "Tapestry of Village Life: Strategies and Status in the Silesian Weaver Revolt of 1844," ed. Jan Kok, *Rebellious Families Household Strategies and Collective Action in the Nineteenth and Twentieth Centuries* (2002), 39.

7. John Post *The Last Great Subsistence Crisis in the Western World* (Baltimore: Johns Hopkins University Press, 1977), 168; Karl-Georg Faber, "Görres, Weitzel und die Revolution (1819)," *Historische Zeitschrift*, 194, Heft 1 (1968): 38–39: and Hans Christoph von Gagern *Mein Antheil an der Politik: Der Bundestag*, Bd. 3 (Stuttgart: Cotta, 1830), 1–2.

8. Nipperdey, 276.

9. For example, see Smitt, 3, 171.

10. Martens, 173.

11. Stefan Hartmann, "Aufsätze und Forschungsberichte Ost- und Westpreussens zur Zeit des polnischen Novemberaufstands in den Berichten der preussischen Verwaltung 1828–1832," Bd. 45, *Zeitschrift für Ostmitteleuropa-Forschung* (1996): 499.

12. As late as 1884 the French Academy received 36 anticontagionist reports as opposed to 109 contagionist reports on the 1884 outbreak of cholera. Anticontagionism still had its adherents. The British government "denied the imported character of the cholera epidemic in Egypt as late as 1885." As a maritime country, Britain was obviously unlikely to accept the need for quarantine. For them it continued to be seen as an impediment to trade. Ackerknecht, 582; and it was not until 1905 that Britain e completely ended its laissez-faire quarantine policy by selecting ports where immigrants could be "inspected and the diseased rejected." See Baldwin, 222.

13. Un Fact Sheet: Combating Cholera in Haiti (February, 2014), http://www.un.org/News/dh/infocus/haiti/Cholera_UN_Factsheet_24%20Feb_2014.pdf.

Bibliography

I. Archival Sources

A. Geheimes Staatsarchive Berlin-Dahlem (GStA PK).

Acta der Königliche Civil Kabinett: Massregln zur Abwehrung zur Cholera in der Haupt-und Residenz Stadt Berlin, GstA PK, Rep. 2.2.1, Nr. 24511, Bl. 143–146.

Rep. 76 VIII C Immediat Commission zur Abwehrung der Cholera.
- Nr. 2 Acta betreffend Conferenz Protocol, May 5, 1831–Feb. 10, 1832.
- Nr. 3 Acta Personalia, May 3, 1831–Feb. 1832.
- Nr. Acta Generalia, May 3, 1831–Feb. 10, 1832.
- Nr. 17 Acta betreffend die auslandischen Aertze, welche mit Beobachtung und die Behandlung der Cholera in den diessietigen Provinzen beschaftigt gewesen sind. May 1831–Feb. 1832.
- Nr. 23 Acta betreffend die Correspondence mit dem Geheimen Cabinet, May 10, 1831–Sept. 10, 1831.
- Nr. 24 Acta betreffend die Correspondence mit den Staatsminister Grafen von Lottum.
- Nr. 25 Acta beteffend die Correspondence mit dem Fursten von Sage Wittgenstein, May 1831–Oct. 1831.
- Nr. 27 Acta betreffend die Correspondence mit dem Ministerio des Innern für Handel und Gewerbe, May 10, 1821–Sept. 10,1831.
- Nr. 28 Acta betreffend die Correspondence mit dem Finanz Ministerio, May 10, 1831–September 1831.
- Nr. 29 Acta betreffend die Correspondence mit dem Ministerio der Geistlichen Unterrichts und Medicinal Angelegenheiten.
- Nr. 43 Acta betreffend die Censur die in den öffentlichen Blatter aufzuanfurhrenden Cholera Artikel, May 1831–Oct. 1831.
- Nr. 51 Acta betreffend den Mess und Markt Verkehr, May 1831–Feb. 1832.
- Nr. 55 Acta betreffend die Correspondence mit der Regierung Franckfurth (Province Brandenburg).
- Nr. 62 Acta betreffend die Sicherstellung den Königlicher Schlosse in Charlottenburg und die Sicherung der hiesigen Palais, August 18, 1831.
- Nr. 83 Acta betreffend den Ausbruch und den Fortgang der Cholera in der Stadt Posen und die Correspondence mit dortigen Regierung, July-Nov. 1831.
- Nr. 115 Acta betreffend die Correspondence mit der Regierung Königsberg Provinz Preussen, May 10, 1831–Nov. 12, 1831.
- Nr. 123 Acta betreffend die westlicher Provinzen..., Sept. 20, 1831–Dec. 1831.

Rep. 76 IXA *Geheime Medizinal Register*
- 3018 Acta betreffend Die Epidemische Krankheit Cholera morbus benannt und die gegen die Verbreitung einschleppung derselben getroffenen Maassregeln, Bd. 1, Jan. 1824–Dec. 12, 1830.
- 3019 Acta betreffend Die Epidemische Krankheit Cholera morbus benannt und die gegen die Verbreitung einschleppung derselben getroffenen Maassregeln, Bd. 2, Dec. 13, 1830–Jan. 17, 1831.
- 3020 Acta betreffend Die Epidemische Krankheit Cholera morbus benannt und die gegen die Verbreitung einschleppung derselben getroffenen Maassregeln, Bd. 3, Jan 18, 1831–Mar. 2, 1831.
- 3021 Acta betreffend Die Epidemische Krankheit Cholera morbus benannt und die gegen die Verbreitung einschleppung derselben getroffenen Maassregeln, Bd. 4, March 1831.

Rep. R77 N.6 Ministerium des Innern und Der Polizei Acta Deutsches Central Archiv: Vol. I. Sec: *Volksaufstaende und Tumult*. Prov. Preussen: Aug. 1, 1831–July 20, 1851.

B. Public Record Office, London (PRO)

Foreign Office: Prussia
- PRO FO 64/174 Chad, July–August 1831.
- PRO FO 64/175 Chad, September–October 1831.

II. Published Primary and Secondary Sources

Abel, Wilhelm. *Agricultural Fluctuations in Europe: From the Thirteenth to the Twelfth Century*. New York: Methuen, 1980.

Abel, Wilhelm. *Massenarmut und Hungerkrisen im Vorindustriellen Deutschland*. Hamburg: Parey, 1974.

Abel, Wilhelm. *Der Pauperismus in Deutschland am Vorabend der Industriellen Revolution*. Dortmund: Gesellschaft für Westfälische Wirtschaftsgeschichte, 1966.

Aberth, John. *Plagues in World History*. New York: Rowman & Littlefield, 2011.

Ackerknecht, Erwin H. "AntiContagionism between 1821 and 1867." *Bulletin of the History of Medicine* 22 (1948): 562–593.

_____. *History and Geography of the Most Important Diseases*. New York: Hafner, 1972.

_____. *A Short History of Medicine*. New York: Ronald Press, 1968.

"Address des magistrats de la Ville de Königsberg au roi de Prusse Frédéric-Guilliame III, en se plaignant au nom de la Prusse Orientale, des vexations, des exigencies des Russe, et du choléra qu'ils ont importé dans le pays." In *Recueil des* Traités, *Conventions et Acts Diplomatiques Concernant la Pologne 1762-1862*, Léonard Chodźko, ed., 833–834. Paris: Brockhaus, 1862.

Albers, Dr. Joh. Christ, et al., eds. *Cholera-Archiv mit Benutzung amtlichen Quellen*, 3 Bd. Berlin: Enslin, 1832.

———. "Pathologische-Therapeutische Wahrnehmungen gesammelt in der Cholera-Heilanstalt des arztlichen Vereines, und mitgetheilt." In Albers, *Cholera-Archiv*, Bd. 2, 85–125.

———. "Report of Dr. Albers, A Prussian Physician at the head of a Commission sent by the Prussian Government to Moscow, to ascertain the nature of the Cholera under date March 9 to 21, 1831." In Hawkins, Bisset. *History of the Epidemic Spasmodic Cholera of Russia; Including A Copious Account of the Disease which Has Prevailed in India, And Which Has Travelled, Under That Name, From Asia Into Europe*, 287–291. London: John Murray, 1831.

Allgemeine Cholera-zeitung: Mittheilungen des Neuesten und Wissenwürdigsten über die Asiatische Cholera. Leipzig, 1831.

Allgemeine Deutsche Biographie. 56 Bd. Leipzig: Duncker & Humblot, 1870–1912.

Allgemeine Medizinische Zeitung (Altenburg).

Allgemeine Zeitung (Augsburg).

Allgemeine Zeitung (München).

"Amtliche Bericht über die Wirkung der Sperr-Massregeln gegen die Cholera enthaltend," in *Verhandlungen der Physikalischen-Medizinische Gesellschaft zu Königsberg über Die Cholera*, 424–441. Königsberg: Bornträer, 1831.

Amtsblatt der Königl. Preuß. Regierung zu Frankfurth a. d. Oder

Amtsblatt der Königl. Preuß. Regierung zu Königsberg

Amtsblatt der Konigl. Preuß. Regierung zu Marienwerde

Amtsblatt der Konigl. Preu. Regierung zu Potsdam und der Stadt Berlin

Archiv für medizinische Erfahrung im Gebiete der praktischen Medizin, Chirugie, Geburtshülfe und Staatsarzneikunde (Berlin)

Artelt, W., and W. Ruegg, eds. *Der Artz und Kranke in der Gesellschaft des 19. Jahrhunderts*. Stuttgart: Enke, 1967.

Artz, Frederick, B. *Reaction and Revolution 1814-1832*. New York: Harper and Row, 1934.

Augustin, Friedrich L. *Die königlich preussische Medicinalverfassung; oder, Vollständige Darstellung aller, das Medicinalwesen und die medicinische Polizei in den königlich preussischen Staaten betreffenden Gesetze, Verordnungen und Einrichtungen*, Bd. 6. Potsdam: Horvath, 1838.

Aubin, Herman, and Wolfgang Zorn, eds. *Handbuch der Deutschen Wirtschafts und Sozialgeschichte*, 2 Bd., Stuttgart: Union Verlag, 1971–1976).

Aus dem Leben des Generals der Infanterie z D. Dr. Heinrich von Brandt. Heinrich von Brandt, ed. 2 Bd. Berlin: Mittler und Sohn, 1868.

Baack, Lawrence, J. *Christian Bernstorff and Prussia*. New Brunswick: Rutgers, 1980.

Baehrel, Rene. "Epidemie et terreur. Histoire et Sociologie." *Archives Historiques de la Revolution Francais* 23 (1951): 113–146.

———. "La Haine De Classe en Temps D'epidemie." *Annales* vii (1952): 351–360.

Baer, Prof. Karl Ernst von. "Bericht über die Veranlassung zum Ausbruche der Cholera in Königsberg." *Cholera Zeitung* (Königsberg, 1831): 26–30.

Baldwn, Peter. *Contagion and the State in Europe, 1830–1930*. Cambridge: Cambridge University Press. 1999.

Baltz, Theodor Friedrich. *Über diesjährige Brechruhr Cholera Epidemie in Berlin*. Berlin: Schultze, 1853.

Barchewitz, Dr. Ernst. *Über die Cholera. Nach eigener Beobachtung in Russland und Preussen*. Danzig: F.S. Gerhard, 1832.

Barnes, Ethne. *Diseases and Human Evolution*. Albuquerque: University of New Mexico Press, 2005.

Becker, F.W. *Letters of the Cholera in Prussia: Letter I to Dr. John Thomson*. London: J. Murray, 1832.

"Bekanntmachung des Allerhöchst genehmigten und bestätigten Regulativs, die sanitätspolizeilichen Vorschriften bei den am häufigsten vorkommenden Krankheiten enthaltend. Vom 28. October 1835." in Friedrich L. Augustin, *Die königlich Preußsche Medicinalverfassung...*," 27–60. Potsdam, Horvath, 1838.

Belke Hans-Jürgen. *Die Preussische Regierung zu Königsberg 1818-1850*. Berlin: Grote, 1976.

"Bericht aus dem Regierungsbezirke Marienwerder für den Monat August 1831." *Preussische Provinzial-Blätter*. Bd. 5, 474–476. Königsberg: Bornträer, 1831.

Berliner Cholera Zeitung (1831).

Bernstorff, Grafin Elise von. *Ein Bild aus der Zeit von 1789 bis 1835. Aus ihren Aufzeichnungen*. ed. Elise von dem Bussche-Kessel, 2 Bd. Berlin: Mittler, 1896.

Blanc, Louis. *The History of Ten Years 1830–1840; or France Under Louis Philippe*, Walter Kelley, trans. 2 vols. Philadelphia: Lea and Blanchard, 1848.

Blasius, Dirk. "Sozialprotest und Sozialkriminalität in Deutschland. Ein Problemstudie zum Vormärz," ed., Heinrich Volkmann und, Jorgen Bergmann. *Sozialer Protest: Studien zu traditioneller Resistenz und kollektiver Gewalt in Deutschland vomVormärz bis zur Reichsgründung*, 212–227. Opladen: Westdeutscher Verlag, 1984:

Bock, Dr. Friedrich, and Dr. Ludwig K Hasenknopf. "Johann Nepomuk Rust," *Veröffentlichungen aus dem Gebiete des Militär-Sanitätswesens. Herausgegeben von der Medizinal—Abtheilung des Königlich Preussischen Kriegsministeriums; Kriegschirurgen und Feldärzte der ersten Hälfte des 19 Jahrhunderts (1795—1848)*." Bd. 2, 301–336. Berlin: A. Hirschwald, 1901

Bohme, Helmut. *An Introduction to the Social and Economic History of Germany*. New York: St. Martins Press, 1978.

Brandt, George. "Die Epidemien in der Provinz Posen in der ersten Hälfte des Jahrhunderts." *Zeitschrift Historische Gesellschaft für Posen* 16 (1901): 103–144.

Brandt, General Heinrich von. *Die Polen in und bei Elbing. Ein Beitrag zur Tagesgeschichte von einem Augenzeugen*. Halle: Kummel, 1832.

Branig, Hans. *Fürst Wittgenstein: Ein preussischer Staatsmann der Restaurationszeit*. Köln: Bohlau, 1981.

Brewster, D. *The Edinburgh Encyclopedia*, 18 vols. Edinburgh: William Blackwood, 1830.

Brierre de Boismont, A. *Relation Historique et Medicale du Cholera Morbus de Pologne*. Paris, Germer-Baillière, 1832.

Briese, Olaf. *Angst in den Zeiten der Cholera I—IV*, Berlin: Akademie Verlag, 2003.

Briggs, Asa. "Cholera and Society in the Nineteenth Century." *Past and Present* 19 (April, 1961): 76–96.

Brockington, C. Fraser. "The Cholera 1831" *Medical Officer*, 96 (1956): 75.

―――. "Public Health at the Privy Council 1831–34." *Journal of the History of Medicine* 16 (1961), 161–185.

Bruford, W.H. *Germany in the Eighteenth Century: The Social Background of the Literary Revival*. Cambridge: Cambridge University Press, 1965.

Burdach, Karl Freidrich. *Rückblick auf mein Leben. Selbstbiographie*, 4 Bd. Leipzig: Voss, 1844.

Burdach, R. "Über den Ursprung der Cholera-Epidemie in Elbing." *Cholera-Zeitung* (Königsberg, 1831): 45–46.

―――. "Verbreitung und Todlickeit der Cholera in Königsberg im Jahr 1831." *Cholera-Zeitung* (Königsberg, 1831): 112–144.

Burnet, MacFarlane. *Natural History of Infectious Disease*, 4th ed. London: Cambridge University Press, 1972.

Chevalier, Louis. *Le choléra, la première épidémie du XIX siècle*. Le Roche-sûr-Yon: Centrale de l'Ouest, 1958.

Chłapowski, Jenerał Dezydery. *Pamiętniki: z portretem autora*. Poznań: Nakładem synów 1899.

Chłapowski, K. *Wojna na Litwe w Roku 1831*. Kraków: G. Gebethnera, 1913.

Chodźko, Léonard, ed. *Recueil des Traités, Conventions et Acts Diplomatiques Concernant la Pologne, 1762–1862*. Paris: Brockhaus, 1862.

Christian, Carl André, ed. *Hesperus: Encyclopädische Zeitschrift für gebildete Leser*. Stuttgart: Cotta,1832.

Ciriacy-Wantrup, Siegfried von. *Agrakrisen und Stockungsspannen zur Frage der langen "Welle" in der Wirtschaftlichen Entwicklung*. Berlin: P. Parey, 1936.

Clark, Christopher M. *Iron Kingdom: The Rise and Downfall of Prussia, 1600–1947*. Cambridge, MA: Belknap Press of Harvard University Press, 2006.

Clausewitz, Paul. *Die Städteordnung von 1808 und die Stadt Berlin*. Berlin: Springer, 1986.

Cockburn, Aiden. *The Evolution and Eradication of Infectious Diseases*. Baltimore: Johns Hopkins University Press, 1963.

Cohnfeld, A. *Ausführliche Lebens-und Regierungs-Geschichte Friedrich Wilhelms III, Königs von Preussen*. 3 Bd. Berlin: Lewent,1840–42.

Conze, Werner. *The Shaping of the German Nation: A Historical Analysis*. New York: St. Martins Press, 1979.

―――. "Vom Pobel zum Proletariat. Sozialgeschichtliche Veraussetzungen für den Sozialismus in Deutschland," *Vierteljahrschrift für Sozial und Wirtschaftsgeschichte* 41 (1954), 333–364.

Craig, Gordon *The Politics of the Prussian Army, 1640–1945*. New York: Clarendon Press, 1956.

Creighton, Charles. *A History of Epidemics in Great Britain*. 2 vols. 2nd ed. London: Cambridge University Press, 1894.

Crosby, Alfred W. *The Columbian Exchange*. Westport: Greenwood Publishing Group, 1972.

Czczyński, Jan. *Preussen im Jahre 1831: oder Verfahren der preußischen Militärbehörden gegen....* Fürth: Korn'sche, 1832.

Curtiss, John Shelton. *The Russian Army Under Czar Nicholas I, 1825–1855*. Durham, NC: Duke University Press, 1965.

Dann, Dr. Edmund. "Bericht über die im Auftrage Eines Hohen Königl. Preuss. Ministerii Behufs der Untersuchung der Cholera nach Russland unternomme Reise." *Archiv fur medizinische Erfahrung* (1832): 118–208, 302–378.

Dankbahr, W. Von. *Der Übertritt der polnischen Corps von Gielgud, Chlapowski und Rybinski auf das Königlich Preußische Gebiet, ihr Aufenthalt daselbst und die angeordnete Entfernung derselben.Unter Benutzung amtlicher Quelle*. Königsberg: Bornträger, 1832.

"Das Gesetz wegen Bestrafung derjenigen Vergehungen, welche die Übertretung der zur Abwendung der Cholera erlassenen Verordnungen betreffen. Von 15. June 1831." *Amtsblatt der Königlichen Regierung zu Potsdam und der Stadt Berlin*, No. 24 (June 24, 1831): 113–117.

De Beaumont-Vassy, Le Vte. *Histoire de mon temps: premier serie: Regne De Louis Philipe-Seconde Republic 1830–1834*. Paris: Perrotin, 1855.

Delaporte, Francois. *Disease and Civilization: The Cholera in Paris, 1832*. Cambridge: MIT, 1986.

"Dem Handel triebenden Publiko der Inn und Ausland ... diesjahrige Martini Messe zu Frankfurt a/O," Abteilung Innern, October, 15, 1831. *Amtsblatt der Regierung zu Marienwerder* No. 43 (October, 28, 1831): 532–33.

"Des Begnadigung derjenigen, welche die zur Abwehrung der Cholera erlassen Verordnungen übertreten haben." *Amtsblatt der Königlichen Preussischen Regierung zu Königsberg* No. 51 (December 21, 1831): 567.

Dettke, Barbara. *Die Asiatische Hydra: Die Cholera von 1831/31 in Berlin und den preussischen Provinzen Posen, Preussen und Schlesien*. Berlin: Walter De Gruyter, 1995.

"Die Quarantaine-Verhältnisse für den Schiffsverkehr zur Abwendung des Einschleppens der Pest und des gelben Fiebers sind geregelt durch das Seitens der Min. der geistl etc. Angel., der auswärtigen Angel., des Innern u. der Finanzen erlassene Reglement vom 30 April 1847." in Dr. Wilhelm Horn. *Das Preussische Medicinalwesen: Aus amtlichen Quellen dargestellt*, 209–212. Berlin: Hirschwald, 1857.

Dieterici Friedrich, W. *Statistische Übersicht der wichtigsten Gegenstände des Verkehrs und Verbrauchs in der Preussischen Staat*. Berlin: E.S. Mittler, 1842.

Dieterici, Friedrich, W. *Der Volkswohlstand im Preussischen Staat. In Vergleichungen aus den Jahren 1816 und von 1828 bis 1832 so wie des neusten Zeit nach statisschen Ermittlungen und dem Gange der Gesetzgebung aus amtlichen Quellen dergestellt*. Berlin: E.S. Mittler, 1846.

Dorwart, Reinhold. *The Prussian Welfare State before 1740*. Bridgewater N.J.: Replica Books, 1971.

Drury, Michael. *The Return of the Plague, British Society and the Cholera 1831–32*. London: Humanities Press, 1979.

Ewald. "Aus den Erlebnissen der Provinz Preussens i. J. 1831 beim ersten Auftreten der Cholera." *Altpreussische Monatsschrift*, 21 (1884): 1–58.

Eck, Dr. W. "Schilderung der hinsichtlich der Erscheinungen, Ursachen und Behandlung der asiatischen Cholera in Berlin gemachten Erfahrungen." In Albers, *Cholera-Archiv*, Bd. 3, 1–102.

"Die Enstehung der Cholera in Pillau und Posen." *Cholera-Zeitung* (Königsberg, 1832): 90–91.

"Epidemic Cholera." *American Journal of the Medical Sciences*, 9 (1831): 441–487.

Evans, Richard J. *Death in Hamburg*. New York: Oxford University Press, 1987.

―――. "Epidemics and Revolutions: Cholera in Nineteenth Century Europe." *Past and Present* 121 (August, 1988): 123–146.

Eversley, David. "Le Choléra en Angleterre." In Chevalier, Louis. *Le Choléra: La Première Épidémie du XIXe Siècle,*

157–188. Le Roche-sûr-Yon: Impr. centrale de l'Ouest, 1948.

"Extract of a Letter from Berlin." Great Britain, Privy Council. *Papers relative to the disease called cholera spasmodica in India, Now Prevailing in the North of Europe*, 59. London: Winchester and Varnham, 1831.

Eylert, R. *Charakter-züge und historische Fragmente aus dem Leben des Königs von Preussen Friedrich Wilhelm III*, 2 Bd. Madegburg: Heinrichshofen, 1844–1847.

Faber, Karl. *Die Haupt- und Residenz-Stadt Königsberg in Preussen*. Königsberg: Grafe und Unzer, 1840.

Fann, Willard R. "The Consolidation of Bureaucratic Absolutism in Prussia, 1815–1827." PhD diss., University of California, 1965.

"Feldmarschall Diebitsch.Vertrauliche Berichte über seinen Feldzug in Polen 1831." *Feldherrn-Stimmen aus und über den Polnischen Krieg vom Jahr 1831*, F. Smitt, ed. 125–244. Leipzig: Winter, 1858.

Felgermann, Major von. *General W.J. von Krauseneck*. Berlin: Reimer, 1851.

Fischer, Alfons. *Geschichte des deutschen Gesundheitswesens*, 2 Bd. Berlin: F. A. Herbig 1933.

Flemig, W. "Einige Erfahrungen und Ansichten über die Cholera, gesammelt im Jahr 1831, in dem Lager der Polen bei Szernen und unter den dasselbe umgebenden K. Preuss. Truppen." In Albers, *Cholera-Archiv*, Bd. 3, 266–297.

Fleischer, Dr. Georg. *Die Cholera Epidemien in Dusseldorf*. Dusseldorf: Triltsch, 1977.

Fodere, F. E. *Recherches historiques et critiques sur la nature, les causes et le traitement du choléra-morbus d'Europe, de l'Inde, de Russie, de Pologne, et autres contrées....* Paris: Levrault 1831.

Forster, Karol. *Powstanie narodu polskiego, w r. 1830–1831*. Berlin: Wydawcy, 1873.

Frejlich, Jozef. "Operacje rosyjskie między Narwią a Dolną Wisłą w lipcu 1831 roku." *Kwartalnik Historyczny* 43 (1929): 187–216.

Frevert, Ute. *Krankheit als politisches Problem 1770–1880*. Göttingen: Vandenhoeck & Ruprecht, 1984.

Gause, Fritze. *Die Geschichte der Stadt Königsberg in Preussen*. 2 Bd. Köln: Ostmitteleuropa in Vergangenheit und Gegenwart, 1968.

Gaszyński, K. *Notatki Officera polskiego o obchodzeniu się rządu pruskiego z korpusem wojska polskiego weszłego z Litwy do Prus pod dowództwem jenerala Giłguda w czasie 53 dni trwającej kwarantanny*. Paryżu: Pinard, 1833.

Gebhart, Bruno. *Wilhelm von Humboldt als Staatsman*. 2 Bd. Stuttgart: Verlag Aalen, 1896, Reprinted, 1965.

Geitl, Franz X. *Die Ergebnisse meiner Beobachtungen über die Cholera vom Jahre 1831–1874*. Munich: C. Kaiser, 1874.

"General Intendant Pogodin, über die Verpflegung des Russiche Armee unter dem Grafen Paskewitz." *Feldherrn-Stimmen*. F. Smitt, ed. 245–260.

Gerecke Anneliese. *Das Deutsch Echo Auf Die Polnische Erhebung von 1830*. Wiesbaden: Isar Verlag, 1964.

Gesetz-Sammlung für die Königlichen Preussischen Staaten, 1831. Berlin: G. Decker, 1832.

Gesetz-Sammlung für die Königlichen Preussischen Staaten, 1832, Berlin: G. Decker, 1833.

Geradin, August et Gaimard Paul. *Du Cholera-Morbus en Russie en Prusse et en Autriche pendant les annees 1831 et 1832*, 3rd ed. Paris: F.G. Levrault, 1831.

Gerlach, Leopold von. *Afzeichnungen aus seinem Leben und Wirken 1795–1877*. 2 Bd. Schwerin: Cotta, 1903.

Giedroyć, Fr. "Lekarze cudzoziemcy w Polsce w roku 1831." *Archiwum Historji I Filozofji Medycyny* 2 (1925):1–24

Goździk, Piotr Władysław. *Cholera w Królestwie polskim w 1831 roku*. Warszawa: Lekarz Wojskowy, 1938.

Granville, A.B. *Travels to St. Petersburgh: A Journey To and From That Capital; Through Flanders, the Rhenish Provinces, Prussia, Poland, Silesia, Saxony, The Federated States of Germany and France*, 2 vols. London: Longman, 1828.

Gray, Marion. "Prussia in Transition: Society and Politics under the Stein Reform Ministry." *Transactions of the American Philosophical Society* 76, Part I (1986): 1–175.

Gregory, George, M.D., "Lectures On the Eruptive Fevers, Delivered At St. Thomas's Hospital in Jan. 1843." *The Medico-Chirurgical Review and Journal of Practical Medicine* 74 (January, 1844): 60–68.

Greville, Charles C.F. *The Greville Memoirs*, 3 vols. London: Spottiswoode, 1874.

Grolman, Carl von. *Leben und Wirken des General der Infanterie und kommandirenden Generals des V. Armeekorps Carl von Grolman*. C. von Conrady, ed., 3 Bd. Berlin: Mittler, 1896.

Haeser, Heinrich. *Lehrbuch der Geschichte der Medicin und der epidemischen Krankheiten*, 3rd ed., 3 Bd. Jena: Mauke, 1875–82.

Hamerow, Theodore, S. *Restoration, Revolution, Reaction: Economics and Politics in Germany 1815–1871*. Princeton: Princeton University Press, 1958.

Hansen, H. V. *Zwei Kriegsjahre Erinnerungen eines alten Soldaten an den Feldzug der Russen gegen die Türken 1828 und den polnischen Aufstand 1831*. Berlin: Miller und Sohn, 1881.

Hamett, John, M.D. "Extracts From Medical Reports, Founded On Actual Observation, And Communicated To The Government, On The Cholera Morbus which Prevailed at Danzig Between the End of May and the First Part Of September, 1831." *The Medico-Chirurgical Review and Journal of Practical Medicine*, New Series, 16 (1832): 305–321.

Hartmann, Stefan, "Aufsätze und Forschungsberichte Ost- und Westpreussen zur Zeit des polnischen November aufstands in den Berichten der preussischen Verwaltung, 1828–1832." Bd. 45, *Zeitschrift für Ostmitteleuropa-Forschung* (1996): 475–505.

Haufsbrand, Dr. "Über die Cholera in Braunsberg," (aus einem K. Regierung zu Königsberg, im December 1831 eingesandten amtlichen Bericht), *Cholera-Archiv*, Bd. 3 (1833): 219–236.

Hawkins, Bisset. *History of the Epidemic Spasmodic Cholera of Russia Including A Copious Account of the Disease which Has Prevailed in India, And Which Has Traveled Under That Name, From Asia Into Europe....* London: J. Murray, 1831.

Helm, Dietrich. *Die Cholera in Lübeck*. Neumunster: Wachholtz, 1979.

Henning, Hans Joachim. "Preussische Sozialpolitik im Vormärz." *Vierteljahrschrift für Sozial und Wirtschaftsgeschichte* 52 (1965): 485–539.

Hille Dr. K. Chr. *Beobachtungen über die asiatische Cholera, gesammelt auf einer nach Warschau im Auftrage der K. Sachs.* Leipzig: Barth, 1831.

Hirsch, August. *Handbook of Geographical and Historical Pathology; Acute Infective Diseases*. Translated by George Creighton M.D., 2 vols. (London: New Sydenham Society, 1883.

Bibliography

Hoffman, Johann Gottfried. "Die Wirkungen der asiatischen Cholera im preussischen Staate wärend des Jahres 1831. Nach den bei dem statistischen Bureau eingegangenen Nachrichten." *Historisch-Philologische Abhandlungen der Koniglichen Akademie der Wissenschaften zur Berlin Aus dem Jahr 1832*, Berlin: F. Dummler, 1834: 33–90.

Holborn, Hajo. *A History of Modern Germany*, 3 vols. NewYork: Knopf, 1964.

Holländer, Eugen. *Die Karikatur und Satire in der Medizin, mediko-kunsthistorische Studie*, 2nd ed. Stuttgart: Ferdinand Enke, 1921.

Holtz, Bärbel. *Das preussische Kultusministerium als Staatsbehörde und gesellschaftlicher Agentur 1817–1934*, 2 Bd. Berlin: Akademie Verlag, 2009.

Homberger, Esther Fischer. *Geschichte der Medizin*. Berlin: Springer-Verlag, 1975.

Hordynski, Joseph, *History of the Late Polish Revolution and the Events of the Campaign*, 4th ed. Boston: Printed for subscribers, 1833.

Horn, Ernst. "Die Contagiosität der Asiatischen Cholera; aus Grunden der Wissenschaft und-Erfahrung nachgeweisen." In Albers, *Cholera-Archiv*, Bd. 2, 1–84.

Horn, Dr. Wilhelm. *Das preussische Medicinalwesen: Aus amtlichen Quellen dargestellt*. Berlin: Hirschwald, 1857.

Huerkamp, Claudia. "Artze und Professionalisierung in Deutschland. Uberlegungen zum Wandel des Arztberufs im 19. Jahrhundert." *Geschichte und Gesellschaft* (1982): 349–382.

Huerkamp, Claudia. "The Making of the Modern Medical Profession, 1800–1914: Prussian Doctors in the Nineteenth Century." Geoffrey Cocks, and Konrad J. Jarausch, eds. *German Professions 1800–1950*, 66–84. New York: Oxford University Press, 1990.

Hufeland, C.W. "Atmosphärische Krankheiten und atmosphärische Ansteckung: Unterschied von Epidemie, Contagion und Infection; ein Beitrag zu den Untersuchungen über die Contagiosität des gelben Fiebers." *Hufeland's Journal* Bd. 57 (July, 1823): 1–54.

———. "Opinion of Hufeland on the Origin and Propagation of Cholera." *The London Medical Gazette* 9 (March 3, 1832): 860.

———. "Verwandtschaft der Cholera mit dem Wechselfieber," *Journal der Practischen Heilkunden* 73 (August, 1831): 126–127.

Ian Inkster, "Marginal Men: Aspects of the Social Role of the Medical Community in Sheffield, 1790–1850." John Woodward, and David Richards, eds. *Health Care and Popular Medicine in the Nineteenth Century England*, 128–163. New York: Holmes & Meier, 1977.

Jameson, James. *Report on the Epidemic Cholera morbus, as it visited the Territories subject to the Presidency of Bengal in the years 1817–1819*. Calcutta: A.G. Balfour, 1820.

Kaczkowski, Karol. *Wspomnienia z papierów pozostałych po ś.p. Karolu Kaczkowskim, General Sztab-Lekarzuwojsk Połiskich, ułożył, Tadeusz Oksza Orzechowski*, 1. Lwów: Gubrynowicza i Schmidta, 1876.

Kalinka, Walerian. *Jeneral Dezydery Chłapowski*. Poznan: J. Leitgeber, 1885.

Kamptz, K. A. von, "Kabinetts Ordre Massregeln gegen die Verbreitung der Cholera 6 September 1831." *Annalen Preußischen Inner Staats-Verwaltung* 15 (1831): 609–612.

Kasparek, Norbert. *Powstańczy epilog Żołnierze listopadowe w dziach klęski i internowania 1831–1832*. Olsztyn: Uniwersytetu Warmińsko-Mazurskiego, 2001.

Kayser, R. *Zur Geschichte der Cholera, speciall der Choleraepidemien in Breslau*. Breslau: Preuss und Jünger, 1884.

Kirchner, Martin. "Die Seuchenbekämpfung unter Berücksichtigung der einschlägigen deutschen und preussischen Gesetzgebung." Dr.von Rapmund, ed. *Das Preussische Medizinal- und Gesundheitswesen in den Jahren 1883–1908*, 196–215. Berlin: Fischer, 1908.

Kitchen, Martin. *The Political Economy of Germany 1815–1914*. London: Croom Helm, 1978.

Klug, Dr. Fr. "Geschichtliche Zusammenstellung derjenigen wissenschaftlichen Erorterungen über die Cholera, welche den von der Verwaltungsbehörde getroffenen früheren Massregeln zum Grunde gelegt worden sind." In Albers, *Cholera-Archiv*, Bd. 1, 1–53.

Kocój, Henryk. *Niemcy a powstanie listopadowe; sprawy powstania listopadowego w niemieckiej opinii publicznej i w polityce pruskiej, 1830–1831; zagadnienia wybrane*. Warszawa: Pax, 1970.

Kocój, Henryk, "Wladze pruskie oraz opinia publiczna Prus i Niemiec wobec powstania Listopadowego." *Roczniki Histororyczne*, 30 (1964): 87–128.

Kollman, Wolfgang. "Die Anfange der Staatlichen Sozialpolitik in Preussen bis 1869." *Vierteljahrschrift für Sozial und Wirtschaftsgeschichte* 53 (1966): 28–52.

Koselleck, Reinhart. *Preussen Zwischen Reform und Revolution*. 3rd. ed. Stuttgart: Klett-Cotta, 1981.

Krehnke, Walter. *Der Gang der Cholera in Deutschland seit ihrem ersten Auftreten bis heute*. Berlin: Schoetz, 1937.

Kunowski, S. "Deutsche Aerzte im Polenaufstand 1831." *Die Medizinische Welt* (December 12, 1931): 1805.

Ladd, Brian. *Urban Planning and Civic Order in Germany, 1860–1914*. Cambridge: Harvard University Press, 1990.

Lammel, Hans-Uwe. "Passer Rusticus Linnaei: Johann Nepomuk Rust (1775–1840) – ein preussischer Medizinalbeamter der Schinkelzeit." *Zeitschrift für ärztliche Fortbildung* 84 (1990): 1066–1070.

Lancet. London, 1844.

Lampe, Richard. *Dieffenbach*. Leipzig: Barth, 1934.

Langer, William, L. *Political and Social Upheaval*. New York: Harper, 1969.

Lanska, D.J. "The Mad Cow Problem in the UK: Risk Perceptions, Risk Management, and Health Policy Development." *Journal of Public Health Policy* 19, no. 2 (1998): 160–183.

Laubert, Manfred. "Beitraege zu Preusssens Stellung Gegenüber dem Warschauer Novemberaufstand V.J. "1830." *Jahrbücher für Kultur und Geschichte der Slaven* 5 (1929): 381–389.

Lempa, Heikki. *Beyond the Gymnasium: Educating the Middle-class Bodies in Classical Germany*. Lanham, MD: Lexington Books, 2007.

Lesky, Erna. "Die österreichische Pestfront an der k.k. Militärgrenze." *Saeculum* 8 (1957): 82–104.

Leslie, R. F. *Polish Politics and the Revolution of November 1830*. London: Athlone Press, 1956.

Lichtenstädt, Jeremias, R. *Die Asiatische Cholera in Russland den Jahren 1829 und 1830*. Berlin: Haude und Spenerschen, 1830.

Longmate, Norman. *King Cholera: Biography of a Disease*. London: Hamish Hamilton, 1966.

Lorinser, Carl, I. *Eine Selbstbiographie Vollendet und herausgegeben von seinem Sohne Franz Lorinser*. 2 Bd. Regensburg: George Joseph Manz, 1864.

Lüdtke, Alf. "The Role of State Violence in the Period of Transition to Industrial Capitalism: The example of

Prussia from 1815–1848." *Social History* 4 (May, 1979): 175–221.

"Manifeste du gouvernement national polonaise, relative à la conduite partiale des Cabinets de Berlin et de Vienne, envers la Russie,Varsovie, le 14 juillet, 1831." In Chodźko, *Recueil des Traités*, 837–839.

Martens, F. de. *Recueil des traités et conventions, conclus par la Russie avec les puissances étrangères: Traités Avec L'Allemagne, 1825–1888*. VIII, St. Petersbourg: Impr. du Ministère des voies de communication, 1888.

McGrew, Roderick E. "The First Cholera Epidemic and Social History." *Bulletin History of Medicine* 25 (1960): 61–73.

———. *Russia and the Cholera 1823–1832*. Madison: University of Wisconsin Press. 1965.

McNeil, William H. *Plagues and People*. New York: Anchor, 1977.

Mémoires officielles sur la Pologne: Précis des négociations entre le Marachel Paskiewitch et Le Commandant En Chef der L'armee Polanaise. Paris: Michelsen, 1832.

"Memorandum der Central-Gesundheits-Behorde in London, die Quarantainen gegen die Cholera betreffend." In Albers, *Cholera-Archiv*, Bd. 1, 118–127.

Morris, R.J. *Cholera 1832 The Social Response to the Epidemic*. New York: Holmes & Meier, 1976.

Müller, J. *Die Polen in der Öffentlicher Meinung Deutschlands 1830–1832*. Marburg: L.G. Elwert, 1923.

Müsebeck, Ernst. *Das Preussische Kultusministerium vor hundert Jahren*. Stuttgart: Cotta 1918.

Mylius, Christian Otto. Corpus Constitutionum Marchicarum, Oder Königl. Preussische. Und Churfürstlichen Brandenburgishen (Berlin, 1755),

Nueste Conversations Lexicon oder Allgemeine deutsche Real Encyclopedie für gebildet Stande, Bd. 12, Wien: Franz Ludwig, 1831.

"Note Officielle du Ministere Des affaires étrangerès du Gouvernment National de Pologne au Cabinet de Berlin, 16 juillet 1831." *La Pologne et La Prusse en 1831*, 3–34. Paris: Pinard, 1832.

Nouvelles de Pologne. Paris: Pinard, Imprimeur du Comité Polonais, 1831.

Olkowski, Zbigniew. "Epidemia Cholery Azjatyckiej W. Prusach Wschodnich W. Latach, 1831–1832." *Komunikaty Mazursko-Warmińskie* 102 (1968): 531–572.

Paret, Peter. "An Anonymous Letter by Clausewitz on the Polish Insurrection of 1830–1831." *Journal of Modern History* 42 (1970): 184–190.

———. *Clausewitz and the State*. New York: Oxford University Press, 1976.

Pertz, G.H., and H. Delbruck. *Das Leben des Feldmarschalls Grafen Neithardt von Gneisenau*, Bd. 5. Berlin: George Reimer, 1864–1880.

Pelling, Margaret. *Cholera, Fever and English Medicine 1825–1865*. New York: Oxford University Press, 1978.

Phoebus, Dr. P. "Cholera-Leichen-Offnungen: Auszug aus einem der Hochlobl. Verwaltungsbehörde des Allerhochstverordneten Gesundheitscomitie für Berlin am 26 Januar d. J. eingerichten Bericht über 69 Cholera-Sectionen." In Albers, *Cholera-Archiv*, Bd. 1, 368–440.

Pirogow, Nicolai I. *Lebensfragen Tagebuch eines Alten Arztes aus dem Russisch en Übertragen von August Fischer*. Stuttgart: Cotta, 1894.

Pistor, M. "Die Medizinalverwaltung auf den einzelnen Gebieten des Oeffentlichen Gesundheitswesens bis zum Schluss des Jahres 1907." *Deutsche Vierteljahrschrift fuer Öffentliche Gesundheits Pflege* 40 (1908): 225–250, 500–554, 749–809.

Pogodin, General, "General Intendant Pogodin, über die Verpflegung des Russiche Armee unter dem Grafen Paskewitz." In *Feldherrn-Stimmen*, F. Smitt, ed., 245–260.

Pollitzer, R. *Cholera*. Geneva: World Health Organization, 1956.

Pologne et La Prusse en 1831. Paris: Pinard 1832.

Post, John, D. "Famine, Mortality and Epidemic Disease in the Process of Modernization." *Economic History Review* 29 (1976): 14–37.

———. *The Last Great Subsistence Crisis in the Western World*. Baltimore: Johns Hopkins University Press, 1977.

Prądzyński, Ignacy. *Pamiętniki generała Prądzyńskiego*. 4 T. Krakowie: Księgarnia Spółki Wydawnczej Polskiej, 1909.

Preussische Provinzial Blätter (Königsberg, 1831–1832).

Preussische Staatszeitung (1831).

Puzyrevskii, Aleksandr Kazemirovich. *Wojna Polska-Ruska 1831*. Warszawa: nakł. Maurycego Orgelbranda, 1899.

Raeff, Marc. *The Well Ordered Police State; Social and Institutional Change through Law in the Germanies and Russia 1600–1800*. New York: Yale University Press, 1983.

Rather, Lleland J., ed. *Disease, Life and Man: Selected Essays, by Rudolph Virchow*. Stanford, CT: Stanford University Press, 1958.

Ramm, Agatha. *Germany 1789–1919*. Oxford: Oxford University Press, 1967.

Raumer, Friedrich von. *Lebenserinnerungen und Briefwechsel*, 2 Bd. Leipzig: Brockhaus, 1861.

———. "Preußens Verhältnisse zu Polen in den Jahren 1831 bis 1832, aus amtlichen Quellen dargestellt." *Vermischte Schriften*, 2 Bd., 501–566. Leipzig: Brockhaus, 1853.

Rehmann, Dr. J. "Die Ankunfts der orientalischen Cholera am Mittelländischen und Kaspischen Meere: Ausbreitung der Cholera in den Russischen Provinzen am Kaspischen Meere bis nach Astrachan." *Hufelands Journal der Practischen Heilkunde*, 59 III Stück. (September, 1824): 3–44.

Reichard, Richard. *Crippled from birth: German social democracy, 1844–1870*, Ames: Iowa State University Press, 1969.

Remer, Carl Julius *Beobachtungen über die epidemische Cholera ges. In Folge in amtlichen Auftr. Gemachten Reise nach Warschau u. mit höhern Orts eingeholter Genehmigung*. Breslau: Joseph Max, 1831.

Richter, O. W. L., Kriminalrichter. "Der Volks-Auflauf in Königsberg am 28. Juli 1831, Mitgetheilt vom Kriminalrichter Richter." *Preussischer Provinzial Blätter* 7 (Königsberg, 1832): 158–170, 263–278.

Riecke, Victor Adolf. *Mittheilungen über die morgenländische Brechruhr*. 3 Bd. Stuttgart: Hoffman,1832).

Rochow, General Theodor von. "Aus den Briefen eines preussischen Militärs zur Zeit Juli Revolution" *Historisch-Politische Blätter für das Catholische Deutschland* 69 (München, 1872): 19–32.

———. *Preussen und Frankreich zur Zeit der Julirevolution, Vertraute Briefe des preussischen General von Rochow an den preussischen Generalpostmeister von Nagler*. Leipzig: Brockhaus, 1871.

Rönne, Ludwig von and Simon, Heinrich. *Das Medicinal Wesen Preussischen Staates*, 2 Bd. Breslau: Aderholtz, 1844.

Rosen, George. "Camaralism and the Concept of Medical Police." *Bulletin of the History of Medicine* 27 (1953): 21–42.

Rosen, George. "The Fate of the Concept of Medical Police, 1780–1890" *Centaurus* 5 (1957): 97–113.

Rosen, George. *From Medical Police to Social Medicine: Essays in the History of Health Care*. New York: Science History Publications, 1974.

Rosenberg, Charles E. "Cholera in Nineteenth Century Europe: A Tool for Social and Economic Analysis." *Comparative Studies in Society and History* 8 (1965–1966): 452–463.

_____. *The Cholera Years: The United States in 1832, 1849, and 1866*, Chicago: University of Chicago Press, 1962.

Rosenberg, Hans. *Bureaucracy, Aristocracy and Autocracy, the Prussian Experience, 1660–1815*. Cambridge, MA: Harvard University Press, 1958.

Rothenberg, Gunther E. "The Austrian Sanitary Cordon and Control of the Bubonic Plague." *The Journal of the History of Medicine and Allied Health* 26 (1973): 15–23.

Ross, Richard S. "The Prussian Administrative Response to the First Cholera Epidemic in Prussia in 1831." PhD diss., Boston College, 1991.

Rowe, Michael, *From Reich to State. The Rhineland in the Revolutionary Age 1780–1830*. New York: Cambridge University Press, 2003).

"Rucksichtlich der dem Min. der G.,U. u. Med. Ang. verbleibenden Angelegenheiten concurrirt das Min. Innern, March 25, 1825." In Ludwig von Rönne, and Heinrich Simon, *Das Medicinal Wesen Preussischen Staats*, 2 Bd. 62–64.

Rudé, George. *The Crowd in History A Study of Popular Disturbances in France and England, 1730–1848*. New York: John Wiley & Sons, 1964.

Rust, Dr. J.N. *Die Medizinalverfassung Preussens, wie sie war und wie sie ist*. Berlin: Enslin, 1838.

Rust, Dr. J.N. "Ein Wort zur Würdigung der Schutzmaaßregeln gegen die Cholera." *Preussische Staatszeitung* (October 12, 1831): 1548

Rust, Dr. J.N. "Sendschreiben des Prasidenten Dr. Rust an Se. Excellenz den königl. preuss. wirklichen Geheimen Rath und Kammerherrn Freyherrn Alexander v. Humboldt." In Albers, *Cholera-Archiv*, Bd.1, 54–85.

Sagarra, Eda. *A Social History of Germany 1648–1914*. New York: Holmes & Meier, 1978.

Sachs, Dr. Albert ed. *Tagebuch über das Verhalten der bösartigen Cholera in Berlin: Eine Sammlung von Aufsätzen pathologisch-therapeutischen gesundheits-polizeilichen und popular-medicinischen Inhalts* (Berlin: Finckh, 1831–32).

Sachs *Repertorisches Jahrbuch für die neuesten und vorzüglichsten Leistungen der....* Dr. L. Posner, ed. 17 (Berlin, 1850).

Samter, Joseph. "Zur Geschichte der Cholera-Epidemien in der Stadt Posen (1831–1873)." *Zeitschrift der Historischen Gesellschaft für die Provinz Posen* 2 (1886): 283–312.

Schiemann, Theodor. *Geschichte Russlands unter Nikolaus I*. 4 Bd. Berlin: G. Reimer 1904–1919.

_____. "Die Sendung des Feldmarschalls Diebitsch nach Berlin September–November 1830." *Zeitschrift für osteuropäische Geschichte*, Bd.1, t.2. (1910–1911): 2–22.

Schlegel, Dr. "Darstellung, der im Regierungs-Bezirk Leignitz vorgekommenen Falle von asiatischer Cholera." In Albers, *Cholera-Archiv*, Bd. 2, 355–392.

Schmedding, A. *Die Gesetze betreffend Bekämpfung ansteckender Krankheiten: und zwar 1. Reichsgesetz betreffend die Bekämpfung gemeingefährlicher Krankheiten vom 30. Juni 1900, 2. Preußisches Gesetz betreffend die Bekämpfung übertragbarer Krankheiten vom 28. August 1905*. Münster: Aschendorf, 1905.

Schnabel, Franz. *Deutsche Geschichte im Neunzehnten Jahrhunderts*, 2ed ed. 4 vols. (Freiberg, 1949).

Schneider, Hans. *Der Preussische Staatsrat 1817–1918: Ein Beitrag zur Verfassungs-und Rechtsgeschichte Preussens*. Berlin: C.H. Beck, 1952.

Schnippel, Emil. "Leichenwasser und Geisterglaube in Ostpreussen." *Zeitschrift der Verein für Volkskunde* 20 (1910): 394–398.

Schnuhr, Dr. J.J.F. "Die Cholera im Johannisburger und Sensburger Kreise des Regierungsbezirk Gumbinnen." In Albers, *Cholera-Archiv*, Bd. 3, 103–164.

Schön, Theodor von. *Weitere Betrage und Nachtrage zu den Papieren des Ministers und Burgrafen von Marienburg Theodor von Schon*, 2 Bd. Berlin: Franz Dunker 1881.

Schwartz, Karl. *Leben des Generals Carl von Clausewitz und der Frau Marie von Clausewitz*, 2 Bd. Berlin: F. Dümmler, 1878.

Scoutetten, H. *Relation historique et médicale de l'épidémie de choléra qui a régné à Berlin en 1831*, 2nd ed. Paris: J. Baillière, 1832.

Sembritzki, Johannes. *Memel im Neunzehnten Jahrhundert: Geschichte der Königlich Preussischen, See—und Handelsstadt, zweiter Theil*. Memel: Siebert, 1900.

Sheehan, James J. *German History 1770–1866*, Oxford: Clarendon Press, 1989.

Shcherbatov, Aleksandr P. *Kampania polska ksiecia Paskiewicza w 1831*. Warsaw, Jana Fiszera, 1899.

_____. *Le feld-maréchal prince Paskévitsch; sa vie politique et militaire d'après des documents inédits*, 7 Tomes. St.-Pétersbourg: Trenké et Fusnot, 1888.

Siegerist, George. "Zur Geschichte Medizin." *Archiv Brandenburgia Gesellschaft fur Heimatkunde der provinz Brandenburg, Berlin* 7 (Berlin, 1901): 1–59.

Sigsworth, E.M. "Gateways to Death? Medicine Hospitals and Mortality 1700–1850." Peter Mathias, ed. *Science and Society, 1600–1900*, 97–110. Cambridge: Cambridge University Press, 1972.

"Sixième circulaire diplomatique du gouvernement national de Pologne, présidé par A. G. Czartoryski, adressée a ses agents à l'étranger, relative à l'envoi, par l'empereur Nicolas I, du médecin russe à Varsovie, et aux motifs qui ont obligé le gouvernement polonais de ne pas le recevoir, Varsovie, le 16 juin 1831." In Chodźko, *Recueil des Traités*, 824–825.

Skrzynecki, General. "Letter Du Généralissme Polonais au Roi de Prusse, 19 Juin 1831." *La Pologne et la Prusse en 1831*, 28–30. Paris: Pinard, 1831.

Smith, F.B. *The Peoples Health 1830–1910*. London: Holmes & Meier, 1979.

Smitt, Fedor, I. ed. *Feldherrn-Stimmen aus und über den Polnischen Krieg vom Jahr 1831*. Leipzig: Winter, 1858.

_____ *Geschichte des polnischen Aufstandes*, 3 Bd. Berlin: Duncker und Humblot, 1848.

Snow, John. *On the mode of Communication of Cholera*, 2nd ed. London: J. Churchill, 1855.

Spazier, Richard Otto. *Ein Geschichte des Aufstandes des Polnischen Volkes in den Jahren 1830 und 1831*, 3 Bd. Altenburg: Fr. Brodhagsche, 1832.

Spielmann, Dr. C. "Regierungspraesident Karl von Ibell

über die preussische Politik in den jahren 1830 und 1831." *Annalen Des Vereins für Naussische Altertumskunde und Geschichtsforschung* 37 (1896): 61–95.

Stagemann, F.A. *Briefe und Aktenstücke zur Geschichte Preussens unter Friedrich Wilhelm III*, Franz Rühl, ed. 3 Bd. Leipzig: Duncker und Humblot, 1902.

Stamm-Kuhlmann, Thomas. "Die Cholera of 1831 Herausforderungen an Wissenschaft und Staatliche Verwaltung." *Sudoffs Acrhiv* 73, no. 2 (1989): 176–189.

_____. *König in Preussens grosser Zeit Friedrich William III. Der Melancholiker auf dem Thron*. Berlin: Siedler, 1992.

Staats und Gelehrte Zeitung des Hamburgischen Unparteiischen (1831)

Stembrowicz, Wiesław. "Pruski Kordon Sanitarny W Okresie Wojny Polska-Rosyjskiej (1830–1831)." *Archiwum Historii Medycyny* 45 (1982): 39–44.

Sticker, George. *Abhandlungen aus der Seuchengeschichte und Seuchenlehre*, 3 Bd. Geissen: Töpelmann, 1912.

Streckfuss, Adolph. *500 Jahren Berliner Geschichte*, 4th ed. 2 Bd. Berlin: Albert Goldschmidt, 1886.

Stromeyer, Dr. Louis. *Skizzen und Bemerkungen von einer Reise nach Danzig und dessen Umgegend*. Hanover: Hahn, 1832.

Stürmer, Theodor. "Der Tod des Russisch Kaiserlichen General-Feldmarschalls Grafen Diebitsch Sabalkansky." Posen: Mittler, 1832.

Sturzbecher, M. *Beitrage zur Berliner Medizingeschichte*. Berlin: Walter de Gruyter, 1966.

Sussman, George, D. "From Yellow Fever to Cholera: A Study of French Government Policy, Medical Professionalism and Popular Movements in the Epidemic." PhD diss.Yale University Press, 1971.

Tilly, Charles, et al. *The Rebellious Century 1830–1930*. Cambridge: Cambridge University Press, 1975.

"The Treatment of the Poles by the Prussian Government and Prussian Officers." *Polonia, or Monthly Reports on Polish Affairs*, No. 1 (August, 1832): 175–182.

Treitschke, Heinrich von. *History of Germany in the Nineteenth Century*, 7 vols. New York: McBride, Nast & Co, 1915–1919.

"Übersicht von dem Dienstleben des am. 18 Nov. 1835 verstorbenen Herrn Polizeipräsident Schmidt." *Vaterlandische Archiv für Wissenschaft, Kunst, Industrie und Agrikultur* 15 (Konigsberg, 1836): 555–566.

Vaterlandische Archiv für Wissenschaft, Kunst, Industrie und Agrikultur (Konigsberg, 1836).

Verhandlungen der Physikalischen-Medicinische Gesellschaft zu Königsberg über Die Cholera. Königsberg, 1831.

Venturini D. Carl. *Chronik des neunzehnten Jahrhunderts, Das Jahr 1831*. Leipzig: Hinrich, 1833.

Volkmann, Heinrich, and Jurgen Bergman, eds. *Sozialer Protest: Studien zu traditioneller Resistenz und kollektiver Gewalt in Deutschland vom Vormarz bis zur Reichsgrundung*. Opladen, 1984.

Wagner, Dr. "Die Verbreitung der Cholera in Preussischen Staate: ein Beweis ihrer Contagiosität." In Albers, *Cholera-Archiv*, Bd. 2, 127–271.

Walker, Mack. *German Home Towns: Community, State and General Estate 1648–1871*. Ithaca, NY: Cornell University Press, 1971.

_____. *Germany and the Emigration, 1816–1885*. Cambridge: Harvard University Press, 1964.

Wasserwerke, Berliner. *Die Wasserversorgung Berlins und die neuen Wasserwerke in ihrer Bedeutung für die Häuserlichkeit und das Familienwohl*. Berlin: Deckerschen, 1857.

Werle, Herman. "Between Public Well-Being and Profit Interests: Experiences of the partial privatization of water supply in Berlin." *Brot für die Welt* (2004): 4. (www.wasser-in buergerhand.de/untersuchungen/berlin_water_privatisation.pdf)

Wildrotter Hans, and Michael Dorrmann, eds. *Das Grosse Sterben Seuchen machen Geschichte*. Berlin: Jovis, 1995.

Winslow, C.A. *The Conquest of Epidemic Disease*. Princeton, NJ: Princeton University Press, 1944.

Winter, Georg, ed. *Die Reorganisation des preussischen Staats unter Stein und Hardenberg. Allgemeine Verwaltungs- und Behördenreform*. Leipzig: S. Hirzel, 1931.

Wasserfuhr, Dr. A. F. "Über die Contagiosität der Cholera." In Albers, *Cholera-Archiv*, Bd. 2, 207–238.

Weese, Dr. "Uber Entstehung, Erkennung, Schultz- und Heilmittel der cholera. Sendschreibung. Des Herren Kreisphysikus Dr. Weese zu Thorn am 17 October 1831 an Hrn. Prof. Cerutti zu Leipzig." *Allgemeine Cholera-Zeitung: Mittheilungen des Neuesten und... von Radius*, Bd. 1, no. 21(November 9, 1831): 161–64; and no. 22 (November 12, 1831): 169–72.

Weinhold C. A. *Von den Übervölkerungen in Mittel-Europa und deren Folgen auf die Staaten und ihr Civilisation*. Halle, Anton, 1827.

Westland, J. *Report of the district of Jessore: its antiquities, its history & its commerce*, 2nd ed. Calcutta, Bengal: Secretariat Office, 1874.

Woodruff, A.W. and Bell, S. A. *Synopsis of Infectious Tropical Diseases*. Bristol: J. Wright, 1968.

Woodward, J. *To do the Sick No Harm*. London: Routledge and Kegan Paul, 1974.

Zacke, Brita. *Koleraepidemien i Stockholm 1834*. Stockholm: Stockholms stadsmuseum, 1971.

Zeitung Für die Elegant Welt (Leipzig, 1831).

Index

Numbers in *bold italics* indicate pages with photographs.

Ackerknecht, E.H. 6, 11, 24, 244
Administrative Authority of Chief, Sanitary Committee 162
Albers, Dr. Johann C. 18–21, 235–236, 238
Allgemeine Zeitung (Augsburg) 170, 174
Alopaeus, Maximilian 41–42, 61, 77, 87–88, 90
Altenstein, Karl Frh. vom Stein zum *10*, 12–13, 16, 18, 20, 30, 33–36, 56, 59, 79, 208–209, 216
Ancillon, Friedrich v. 83, 107–108, 225
Anti-contagion 48, 51, 52, 63, 65, 68, 80, 153, 126, 131, 192, 197–9, 212, 214–215, 220; contagion controversy 196–206, 208–209, 253
Arabia 5, 11
Arnim, Friedrich W.v. 164, 168–170, 187
Asiatic cholera *see* cholera
Astrakhan 5, 12, 16, 20
Aszecken 233, 235–238
Austria 5, 7, *10*, 12–13, 15–16, 20, 38, 41, 90, 203, *205*, 207, 218, 244
Austrian-Turkish Border *10*, 15–16, 203, 207–208, 244

Baer, Dr. Karl Ernst v. 124–125, 133, 198
Baldwin, Peter 3, 244
Baltic Sea 75
Barchewitz, Dr. Ernst 18–22, 69, 79
Bärensprung, Friedrich 164
Bassewitz, Friedrich M.v. 170
Becker, Dr. F.W. 5–6, 175–177, 185, 189–90, 194, 199
Belgium *10*, 39–40, 107; Belgian question 39
Below, Gustav A.v. 70, 156

Bengal 5, 16
Berlin *10*, 19, 21–22, 26–27, 29, 31, 37–38, 40, 43, 56, 60, 69, 79, 88–90, 93–94, 102, 108, 146, 148, 152, 155, 157, 158, 160–165, 167–171, 173, 177, 179, 183, 185–187, 189–197, 201, *205*, 206, 209–211, 213, 221, 225, 248–249; demonstration 180; employment 179–180
Berliner Cholera Zeitung (Berlin) *178*–179, 191*–93*, 196, 210
Bernstorff, Graf Albrecht 18, 38–41, 54, 90, 108, 206
Bombay 5, 16
Boston 232
Brahe River 101
Brandt, Gen. Heinrich v. 89–90, 96–97, 99, 103, 239
Brenn, Gustuv v. 12–14, 16, 18, 36, 79, 150, 216
Bresen (Danzig) 80, 81, 84
Breslau 44, 107, 177, 213
Brierre de Boismont, Dr. A. 45–49
Bromberg 99, 100–102, 177
Brussels 39
Burdach, Dr. Karl F. 22, 69, 121–122, 131, 133, 147, 156

Cabinet Order of February 2, 1832 214–15
Cabinet Order of June 15, 1831 115, 212, 225, 228
Cabinet Order of November 22, 1831 212
Cabinet Order of October 9, 1831 210, 212
Cabinet Order of September 6, 1831 214
Calcutta 5
cameralism 24, 246
Canitz, Karl Ernst v. 89, 95, 97, 100
Carlsbad Decrees 7

Central Cholera Commission (St. Petersburg) 19, 20
Central Health Committee, Poland 43–44, 46–53, 57
Chad, George 74, 82–83, 107–108, 149, 160, 167, 174, 179–180, 197, 225–226
Chapłowski, Gen. D. 222–224, 226, 233, 235, 237–238
charitable organizations 189
Charlottenburg 167, 170, 171
Chernyshev, Alexander 93, 100
Chief Sanitary Committee for Berlin 158, 160–161, 163–164, 168–169, 171, 186–*188*, 190, 192
Cholera Archiv (Berlin) 21, 125
Cholera Commission 14, 16–18, 56
cholera, etiology 5
cholera hospitals: death rates in Berlin hospitals 191; Poland *47*, 49, *50*, 55; prejudice against hospitals 179, 187–*188*; Prussia 58, 66, 119, 130, 132, 155, 163, 179, *188*–191; therapies 66, 192
cholera, Poland: in army 7, 10; border, 7, 20; contagion policy, 46; controversy between military and civilian authorities, 45–48; foreign doctors, 52–53; outbreak; 7, 10–11, 40–41, 43–48, 50–51
cholera, Prussia: Berlin 165–171, 183–185, 213; Breslau 177; Bromberg and surrounding areas, 101–102; Danzig, 62–63, 65–72; East Prussia; 115–117; Königsberg; 118–124; Memel, 127, 234; Posen, 103–106; Thorn and surrounding areas, 100–1
cholera *vibrio* 5, 253
Cholera Zeitung (Königsberg) 120, 123–124, 127, 147, 153, 198–199
Civil Protection Committees (Berlin) 158, 161, 163, 186–187, 189–92, 194, 218

Index

Civilian and Military Commission (Prussia) 241
Clausewitz, Claus v. 39, 84, 91, 95–96, 103–104, 106–107
Congress of Vienna 40, 247
Constantine Pavlovich, Grand Duke 41
contagion 3, 6, 7, 43, 48, 53, 57, 60–61, 67–69, 78–82, 84, 86, 103, 149, 153, 108, 111, 120, 123, 126, 131, 156, 186, 191–199, 207, 214–215, 218–220, 228, 246, 253
contagion controversy 5, 69, 195, 196–206, 208–209; Poland 48–52, 253; *see also* anti-contagion
Contagious Diseases Law of 1835 215–220, 246
Contagious Diseases Law of 1905 (Germany) 220
Cöslin 176–177
Cracow 17
Czartoryski, Adam 41, 46

Dankbahr, W.v. 225, 227–229, 231
Dann, Dr. Edmund 18–21
Danzig 18, 21, 53, 59, 61–62, 64–78, 80–81, 83–85, 87–88, 90–93, 95, 102–104, 113–14, 146, 153, 155–157, 160, 170, 174, 177, 201, 210, 213, 215, 215, 240–42, 244, 248
Danzig Sanitary Commission 62, 64–72; recommendations 64, 66–67, 69, 71, 72, 121
Dębe Wielkie, battle of 86
Diebitsch, Field Marshal I.I. Graf 38–40, 42–43
Dirschau 63–64, 76, 81, 113, 241
Doctors Commission to Russia 16–22, 244
Dwernicki, Gen. J. 225

East Prussia 18, 22, 32, 40, 64, 75, 110, 156, 170, 176, 212, 222, 227, 231, 236–238, 240, 251
Eichorn, Karl F. 57
Elbe River 170, 203, 210
Elbing 64, 70, 153, 241
England 3, 6, 20, 38–40, 43, 221, 252
Europe 3, 6, 9–*10*, 15, 24, 38, 53, 61, 225, 253
Evans, Richard 3, 4
Ewald, Johann F. 78–79, 114, 128–129, 133–134, 139–140, 155–156

Fischau riot, 241–242
Fischhausen 237
Flahaut, Charles de 109
Flemig, Dr. W. 233–234, 236
Flottwell, Eduard, H.v. 41, 57, 61, 104–105, 115, 170
Foy, Dr. François 49, 51, 53, 57
France 4, 6, *10*, 38–41, 43, 45, 53, 57, 90, 107, 109, 115, 144, 175, 182, 192, 207, 221, 232, 241, 250
Frankfurt an der Oder 176–177, 212
Frederick William, Crown Prince of Prussia 70, *159*
Frederick William, elector 26
Frederick William II, King 27, 54
Frederick William III, King 7, 20, 38, 39, 42, 59, 77, 83–84, 91, 237, 251
French Revolution (1830) 9, 38–39, 41, 144, 207, 247, 250–251
Frische Nehrung 7–8, 80

Ganges Delta 9, 16
Gaszyński, Konstanty 229–230, 232–233, 236–237, 239
General Medical Council, Poland 44–49
germ theory 5, 253
Germany 3, 5, 43, *205*–206, 253
Gielgud, Gen. Antoni 221–226, 228, 240–241, 251
Gneisenau, Field Marshal August Graf Neidhardt v. 40, 56–57, 61, 90, 94–96, 99–100, 103–104, 106–107
Graefe, Dr. Charles F.v. 14–16, 57
Grochów, battle of 42, 86
Grodno 93
Gumbinnen 18

Haiti 253
Hake, Karl G.A.E.v. 79
Hamburg 3–5, 253
Hamburger Magazin (Hamburg) 208
Hamett, Dr. John 84
Hansen, H. 98–99
Hardenburg, Karl A. Fürst v. 29–34
Hartungsche Zeitung (Königsberg) 133
Hela (Danzig) 80–81
Hindenburg, Gen. Beckendorff v. 90, 93, 96, 99
Hindustan 5
Holland 39
Holm (Danzig) 66
Horn, Dr. Ernst 4–5, 14–16, 60, 169, 208–209
Horodyski, Andreas 96
Hufeland, Dr. C.W. 199, 201–202, 204, 206, 210–212, 214, 220
Humboldt, Alexander v. 16, 209, 214
Humboldt, William v. 28–29, 31
Hungary 5, 203, 235

Iganie, battle of 7, 20, 43–44, *50*, 60, 87, 204
Immediate Commission to Prevent Cholera 7, 11, 17, 20, 22, 36, 56, 57, 59, 61, 64, 67–71, 74, 76, 78–85, 94–96, 103–104, 114, 120–122, 125, 127, 129–130, 147, 151–153, 154–155, 157–158, 160–165, 170–173, 175–177, 181–182, 196, 201–202, 207, 210–219, 221–222, 228–229, 231, 238, 244–245, 248–249, 251
India 5, 9, 12, 16, 203
Inowrazlaw 101–102

Jahrbücher für Wissenschaftliche Kritik 202–203
Justi, Johann H.G.v. 24

Kaczkowski, Dr. Karol 44–*47*, 49–52
Kaluszyn 44
Kiev 18, 20
Kleszczewo 88
Klewitz, Wilhelm A.v. 3366
Koch, Robert 5, 253
Königsberg 18, 22, 40, 64, 68–69, 71, 73, 75–76, 78–83, 87, 90, 95, 97, 103–104, 110, 113–114, 117–121, 123–128, 130–131, 135, 145–148, 151–155, 158, 160, 173, 177, 180, 201, 210, 213, 221–223, 227, 231, 236–237, 247–249
Königsberg Physical and Medical Society 122–123
Krafft, Gen. Karl August A.v. 56, 82, 135, 139–140, 143, 152, 156, 224, 226–227, 232, 235, 237
Krehnke, Walter 102
Kronstadt 21, 77
Krukowiecki, Gen. Jan 48–*50*, 228
Krümmungen 240
Kulivecha, battle of 89
Kursk 40

Lautenburg 240
lazaret 18–19, 52, 66, 67, 102–104, 106, *116*, 119–120, 138–140, 146–148, 151, 161–162, 184, 202, 229, 234–235, 240, 247; ineffective 113–14; living conditions 112–113; regulations for travelers and goods 111–112
Le Brun, Dr. M 45
Le Gallois, Dr. N. 45–46
Leo, Dr. Leopold 44, 49, 51, 66
Lithuania 13, 20, 22, 61, 73, 75, 86, 93, 110, 115, 124, 223, 235 soldiers in quarantine camps 235, 239
London 39, 57, 192
Lorinser, Dr. Carl 21, 202–203, 206–210, 212, 214, 238
Louis Philippe King of France 9, 38–37

Madgeburg 176–177
Madras 5
malaria 204
Malcz, Dr. Wilhelm 45–48, 51–52